*Facial Pain*

# Facial Pain

**Parker E. Mahan,** D.D.S., Ph.D., F.A.C.D.
Distinguished Service Professor and Director of
Dental Occlusion and Facial Pain Center
University of Florida
College of Dentistry
Gainesville, FL


**Charles C. Alling, III,** D.D.S., M.S., D.Sc. (Hon), F.A.C.D.
Private Practice
Oral and Maxillofacial Surgery
Birmingham, Alabama

*Third Edition*

Lea & Febiger · *Philadelphia* · *London* · *1991*

Lea & Febiger
200 Chester Field Parkway
Malvern, Pennsylvania   19355-9725
U.S.A.
(215) 251-2230
1-800-444-1785

**Library of Congress Cataloging-in-Publication Data**

Mahan, Parker E.
    Facial pain / Parker E. Mahan and Charles C. Alling III—3rd ed.
        p.      cm.
    Rev. ed. of: Facial pain / edited by Charles C. Alling III, Parker
E. Mahan, 2nd ed. 1977.
    Includes bibliographical reference.
    Includes index.
    ISBN 0-8121-1252-0
    1. Facial pain.  I. Alling, Charles C. 1923–        II. Title.
    [DNLM: 1. Facial Pain.   WE 705 M214f]
RC936.M28   1991
617.5′2—dc20
DNLM/DLC                                              90-13278
for Library of Congress                                    CIP

Reprints of chapters may be purchased from Lea & Febiger in quantities of 100 or more.

PRINTED IN THE UNITED STATES OF AMERICA

Print number:  5  4  3  2  1

*This book is dedicated, with love,*
*to Lorraine N. Mahan and Laura F. Alling*
*who kept two families functioning*
*during the five years we devoted, with pleasure,*
*to the writing of this edition.*

# Preface

The human face is the most complex and expressive portion of the body. All the primary senses channel through the face, life's triumphs and tribulations are reflected in the face, and the world first knows the human creature by the face. For most people, there is an element of truth in the milk maid's line from the nursery rhyme, "'My face is my fortune, Sir,' she said." Happily for the human race, behavior and intellect become more important than facial features in the course of selected acquaintanceships that extend over one's lifetime. Sensitive to pain—real, imagined, and recalled—the face is the central area of interest, study, and treatment by several of the healing sciences.

This third edition represents the work of two authors rather than the 20 contributors who wrote the second edition. The text has been completely reorganized into 18 chapters that, the authors believe, best describe their combined experience of 75 years of treating patients with craniofacial pain and dysfunction. It is organized to be of efficient use by busy clinicians who are treating patients, by students in lecture rooms and study halls, and by laboratory and clinical scientists.

This text features the clinical application of basic sciences to the diagnosis and treatment of facial pain and dysfunction; it reflects the excitement of this time in history when the understanding of basic science foundations is being renewed, along with new applications in clinical procedures. The management of pain in the maxillofacial region requires a multidiscipline approach because of the different anatomic, physiologic, and psychosomatic factors that interact in the face. The authors have worked together to apply concepts to the diagnosis and management of facial pain from neuroscience, physiology, anatomy, oral and maxillofacial surgery, general dentistry, pathology, neurosurgery, internal medicine, neurology, clinical psychology, psychiatry, otorhinolaryngology, oral pathology, orthopaedic surgery, physical therapy, pharmacology, and anesthesiology. Thus the text will be of interest to the clincial diagnostic disciplines, laboratory scientists, health science students, interns, residents, and, especially, clinicians who treat patients with facial pain.

*Gainesville, Florida*
*Birmingham, Alabama*

Parker E. Mahan
Charles C. Alling, III

# Acknowledgments

We could not begin to express adequate appreciation to the many persons who have stimulated and broadened our interest in facial pain and who have, with great patience, helped us understand some of its pathophysiology and methods of management. We wish to recognize in a special way a host of colleagues and associates who have made this third edition possible.

We are especially grateful to the 18 contributors to the second edition of this book upon whose writings we have built this edition.

The University of Florida College of Dentistry Deans Don Allen and Donald Legler have been most supportive. Our colleagues at the University of Florida Facial Pain Center have been resources of understanding and knowledge and include Drs. Robert Bates, Barry Loughner, Michael Henry, Brian Fuselier, Peter Benoit, and Henry Gremillion.

Our gratitude goes to the following doctors who generously gave us textual and illustrative materials, insights, and review: oral and maxillofacial surgeons Rocklin Alling, Eugene Messer, Robert Ord, Hugh Brindley, Michael Koslin, Simon Weinberg, and Michael Nealis; psychologists Vernon Pegram and Daniel Doleys; neurologists Gordon Kirschberg and John Schottland; otorhinolaryngologists Edwyn Boyd, Keith Kreutizger and Donald Wittich; and rheumatologist David McLain.

Dr. Charles Porter assured that the vast educational resources of the AMI Brookwood Medical Center of Birmingham, Alabama, were available to us. At the Center, Miss Lucille Moor, Medical Librarian, and Mr. William Davis, Supervisor of Instructional Resources, willingly provided definitive library research and incomparable photographic illustrations. Appreciation is extended to Mr. Samuel Collins for his amplification of concepts with his medical illustrations.

We are especially appreciative of the continuing support of Mr. Christian "Kit" Spahr and the other officers and the staff of Lea & Febiger. Our sincere thanks to Mr. Raymond Kersey, Executive Editor, for his leadership and occasional gentle inspirational spurring! Epitomizing the attention to detail that leads to excellence were Ms. Susan Hunsberger, Project Editor of the Manuscript Editing Department; Mr. Samuel Rondinelli, Production Manager; and Ms. Elizabeth Frazier, Assistant Production Manager. Their dedication to the publication of this third edition made our tasks even more pleasant.

*Gainesville, Florida*
*Birmingham, Alabama*

Parker E. Mahan
Charles C. Alling, III

ix

# Contents

## VI.   *ORAL AND NASAL CAVITIES AND SALIVARY GLANDS*

# Part I

# The Patient in Pain

# Understanding the Patient in Pain

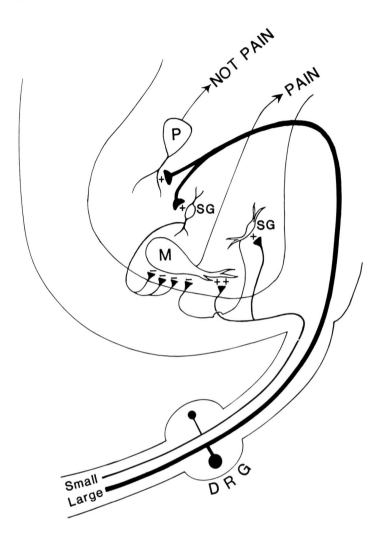

*Fig. 1–3.* Basic anatomy of the central inhibitory balance theory. DRG, dorsal root ganglion; M, large marginal neuron subserving pain; SG, substantia gelatinosa (gating) cells; P, pyramidal cell not believed to subserve pain. This theory states that the small fibers not only massively activate the marginal neuron, but also activate an impotent inhibition of the M neuron via the SG neuron. The large fibers massively inhibit the M neuron (pain) via the SG and activate the supposedly non-noxious pyramidal cell.

In recent years, investigators identified a series of polypeptides called endorphins and enkephalins that serve as endogenous opiates and obtund pain as do the opiate drugs.[9] Their discovery sparked new hope that a new class of analgesics could be produced that would not have the addicting, respiratory depression and other side effects of the narcotic analgesics now on the market.[10,11] Findings of studies so far indicate that amino peptidases in body fluids hydrolyze the polypeptides so rapidly that lasting analgesia cannot be produced by these compounds. Continuing research with these compounds may overcome these problems and provide a new approach to pain control.

## Classification of Pain Patients

The International Association for the Study of Pain has defined chronic pain as pain that has lasted longer than 6 months. The 6-months criteria is rather arbitrary in that some patients can take on the characteristics of chronic pain in a few months. Pain can be grossly divided into two groups: (1) acute pain, which has lasted less than 6 months; and (2) chronic pain, which has lasted longer than 6 months. Most patients with acute pain do not suffer more than a few weeks before their pain is resolved.

The authors have found it helpful to classify pain into six classes, taking into account the acute and chronic categories just mentioned. This classification is based on temporal aspects of pain as proposed by Crue.[12]

1. *Acute pain* is typically sharp pain that lasts a maximum of a few days, such as acute periapical abscess. It responds to antibiotics, nonsteroidal anti-inflammatory or narcotic medication, and defin-

itive treatment of the lesion. The development of drug dependence or tolerance in a nonaddicted patient is not a problem.

2. *Subacute pain* lasts a few weeks, such as cellulitis. It is typically controlled by procedures that resolve the inflammation, such as incision and drainage with supportive medication, analgesics and/or narcotics. Again, drug dependence or tolerance in a nonaddicted patient is not a problem.

3. *Recurrent acute pain* is ongoing acute pain brought on by continuous excitation of inflammation, such as that seen in association with rheumatoid and hypertrophic osteoarthritis and disk disease. In patients with these conditions, daily function continuously activates pain mechanisms. Pain of this type is difficult to control and patients often pressure the clinician to write repeated narcotic prescriptions. These patients usually do not respond to tricyclic antidepressant medication used as analgesics or to the combination of tricyclic and phenothiazine medication. If the painful condition is not remedied in a short time, some patients develop drug dependence and tolerance. Most of these individuals, however, have little problem discontinuing the narcotic medication when the pain has resolved.[13]

4. *Ongoing acute pain of neoplasia* is continuing pain resulting from the growth of a tumor. The pain occurs in response to tissue and nerve damage at the periphery of the tumor as it expands. The pain can actually be used as an indicator of growth of the tumor. When the tumor shrinks in response to irradiation or antimetabolite therapy, the pain subsides. This pain can usually be controlled with adequate doses of narcotics and, unfortunately, drug dependence and tolerance are not an important consideration because the life expectancy is often short.

5. *Chronic pain with coping* is pain that has lasted longer than 6 months but the patient is able to cope with the continuous noxious perception. Such pain usually begins with acute trauma or a peripheral pathologic process, but some unknown, potentiating central nervous system mechanisms take over and the pain continues. This pain appears to be centralized in that central mechanisms in the pain system remain active. This pain can often be controlled with tricyclic antidepressants or the combination of tricyclics and phenothiazine medication, which alter norepinephrine and serotonin metabolism at central synapses and dopamine metabolism in subcortical nuclei.

6. *Chronic pain with inadequate coping* is pain that has lasted longer than 6 months and that renders the patient unable to function and thus completely disabled. These patients beg the clinician for strong medication and any mutilating operation that might relieve their suffering. These patients may commit suicide or undergo a psychotic break, the mental equivalent of suicide, when their clinicians refuse to perform any further nerve block or surgical procedure or to prescribe more medication. Such patients can often benefit from the care of psychiatrists, who are skilled in suicide prevention methods.

The major emphasis in this book is on the diagnosis and treatment of patients with pain that is classified in groups 2, 3, and 5. If these patients can be diagnosed and treated in time, individuals with the subacute and recurrent acute pain can often avoid becoming chronic pain patients, and those in the chronic pain group can often improve their coping skills to the point that pain no longer destroys their quality of life. All six classes of pain are discussed in the various chapters.

## References

1. Lewis C.S.: The Problem of Pain. New York, The Macmillan Co., 1959.
2. Coggeshall R.E.: Afferent fibers in the ventral root. Neurosurgery, 4:443, 1979.
3. Chung J.M., Lee K.H., Kim J., and Coggeshall R.E.: Activation of dorsal horn cells by ventral root stimulation in the cat. J Neurophysiol, 54:261, 1985.
4. Light A.R. and Metz C.B.: The morphology of the spinal cord efferent and afferent neurons contribut-

ing to the ventral roots of the cat. J Comp Neurol, 179:501, 1978.

5. Melzack R. and Wall P.D.: Pain mechanisms: A new theory. Science, 150:971, 1965.

6. Hongo T., Jankowska E., and Lundberg A.: Postsynaptic excitation and inhibition from primary afferents in neurons of the spinocervical tract. J Physiol (Lond), 199:569, 1968.

7. Melzack R. and Wall P.D.: The Challenge of Pain. New York, Basic Books, 1982.

8. Kerr F.W.L.: Pain, a central inhibitory balance theory. Mayo Clin Proc, 50:685, 1975.

9. Hughes J., et al.: Identification of two related pen-tapeptides from the brain with potent opiate agonist activity. Nature, 258:577, 1975.

10. Dickenson A.H.: A new approach to pain relief? Nature, 320:681, 1986.

11. Morley J.S.: Structure-activity relationships of enkephalin-like peptides. Annu Rev Pharmacol Toxicol, 20:81, 1980.

12. Crue B.L.: The neurophysiology and taxonomy of pain. In Management of Patients with Chronic Pain. Edited by S.F. Brena and S.L. Chapman. New York, S.P. Medical and Scientific Books, 1983.

13. Porter J. and Jick H.: Addiction rare in patients treated with narcotics. N Engl J Med, 302:123, 1980.

# Part II

# *Diagnostic Basics*

# 2

# *History and Physical Examination*

Making the correct diagnosis is the most important, and often the most difficult, part of patient management. When dealing with chronic pain, the final diagnosis may be obscured by the patient's perception of the cause as well as by the doctor's biases based on his or her education and experience.

As an example, the patient often determines that because a pain is located in the facial areas or in the teeth that the problem is of dental origin; the patient either may not understand or want to understand that a systemic or psychopathologic element may underlie the chief complaint, especially if the pain was first noted coincident with the onset of a dental malady or after a dental procedure. Likewise, the doctor may be so oriented to either occlusal therapy, surgery, or another method that multiple adjustments of the occlusion or even multiple surgical procedures may be performed in what may be vain hopes of adjusting the pain away or of excising the pain from the body.

Thus, we may have a situation of both parties, the patient and the doctor, using the same words and talking about different things but with a mutual desire for a rapid initiation of a treatment plan. The best insurance against establishing the wrong treatment plan is to obtain a medical and dental history and to perform a physical evaluation.

The identification of a facial pain patient may be through knowledge acquired from a referring source, by the patient's response to a request for a statement of the chief complaint, or by findings discovered in the normal course of medical or dental treatment.

## Chronic Pain Patient Questionnaire

For the chronic pain patient, the acquisition of the medical history and physical evaluation may be assisted through the use of a standardized questionnaire. Use of a Patient Response Form (Fig. 2–1) assures the inclusion of elements that could be overlooked in a dialogue directed specifically to the chief complaint and findings. An effective step, when time and circumstances permit, is to send the form to the patient for completion before the initial examination. The patient and the patient's support group of family and friends

then have an opportunity to reflect on the scope of the facial pain, as included in the questions. At the initial consultation, the doctor acknowledges, with appreciation, the completion of the form. In some instances, the doctor may use the form as a guide, completing it during an initial consultation with the patient.

After receiving the completed chronic pain patient questionnaire from the patient, attention is directed to acquiring a standard medical and dental history that includes the regional facial pain problems in the context of the overall health status of the patient. The chronic pain patient form is evaluated by the doctor between, not during, consultations with the patient.

## Routine History and Physical Examination

The acquisition of the routine baseline history and physical examination are best accomplished by having the patient in a suitable and comfortable, perhaps nonclinical, area. The doctor should have a close physical relation to the patient, with care not to invade the patient's personal space. The posturing of the patient and doctor should convey the professional attitude of true concern for the patient as an individual. We recommend making entries in the patient's chart as the initial step during acquisition of the history, the chief complaint, and the present illness.

### Chief Complaint

The response to a request for the chief complaint may evoke a variety of statements as ambiguous as: "I'm here because I have TMJ;" "You are supposed to tell me what my problem is;" "My (sister, mother, father, dentist, physician, doctor, friend) told me I have a problem;" "I was (in a fight, in an automobile accident, under general anesthesia) (1 year, years) ago, and I was advised by a lawyer to see you about my clicking jaw joint." Or, the patient may respond with identification of having a specific somatic pain or problem related, as examples, to meniscus subluxation or dislocation, myospasm, or headache.

We emphasize careful attention to the

words used by the patient to describe the chief complaint, because the words may have deep diagnostic significance. The exact wording of the chief complaint should be recorded to assist in directing the treatment.

When recording the chief complaint, we ask the patient to use one finger and point to the location of the complaint. The patient often responds by placing the hand on the side of the face. If this occurs, our response is, "No, we need to be more specific. Just take one finger and outline the location of the pain on the face." If the patient cannot localize the pain in this manner, the pain perhaps is diffuse, involves a systemic malady, or is chronic pain that has become centralized. Combining the verbal complaint and the patient's location of the pain through pointing allows an early assessment of the system that likely is involved: musculoskeletal, vascular, neurologic, psychophysiologic, or the sinal and dental areas. The clinician, however, should resist the temptation to jump forward to a diagnosis before a full history, physical examinations, and associated studies and consultations have been completed.

### Present Illness

The patient's ability and interest in identifying the onset, the course, and the previous treatments of the chief complaint must be noted with specifics as to when, what, where, why, and how. The antecedent history is helpful in planning the ongoing treatment and should be taken with care and in detail to provide a rational treatment plan that avoids problems that were encountered in earlier treatments.

### Past Medical History

Forms are often used (Fig. 2–2) for the past medical history and review of systems. The doctor acquires and then records the family, social, and occupational histories in the progress notes of the chart.

The patient may be informed that questions regarding the past medical history will include areas not directly related to the facial pain problems. To hear and understand the patient's responses to the past medical history

is instructive. Coupled with the direct interview techniques of acquiring the chief complaint, onset, course, and previous treatments of the present illness, the past medical history helps to make the diagnosis and treatment plan clear in the doctor's mind. The diagnostician should maintain an investigative attitude and avoid the pitfall of permitting associations and relationships of complaints and historical information to sway the formulation of a diagnosis and treatment plan, bearing in mind, however, that these associations and relationships may fit a syndrome. The doctor should invest the time to acquire all the information available by completing the entire analysis.

### Review of Systems

The review of systems further focuses the patient's and the doctor's attention on the total individual as well to produce positive findings that bear on or alter the final diagnosis and treatment plan.

Countless examples are well known of the effect of various systemic influences on the oral cavity. The secondary or augmented response of the cardiovascular system to pharmacotherapeutic agents, the history of lesions or conditions of the gastrointestinal tract indicative of impaired abilities to assimilate nutrients or of being bellwethers of psychopathologic maladies, the history of diabetes in the patient or in the patient's family that would compromise repair, the ingestion of psychotropic agents, and the presence of other joint and muscle problems are examples of significant findings in a review of systems. The common denominator point is that the stomotognathic system is an integral part within the complex of systems.

### Family History

The family history, usually recorded in the progress notes, is important in cases involving patients suspected or known to have diabetes, one of the anemias, allergies, and diseases of the cardiovascular, respiratory, nervous, vascular, digestive, and musculoskeletal systems. The patient coming from a pain-ridden family burdened by diseases

# PATIENT'S QUESTIONNAIRE

Patient Name      Date      Time

What is your problem, your **chief complaint**, in your own words?

We will discuss these forms when we have our appointment. Meanwhile, please answer as much as possible and return in the enclosed envelope.

Check **all** areas where you now have pain or problems.

**HEADACHE**    Right Left
Forehead
Side of head
Back of head
Sinus
Migraine

**SHOULDERS**

**EARS**
Decreased hearing
Dizziness
Ringing, hissing or crickets
Aches
Sensitivity to sounds
Sensation of fluid

**EYES**
Pain behind eyes
Tearing
Sensitivity to light
Narrowing of visual fields
Abnormal eyeball pressure

**FACE**    Right Left
Above mouth & mid-ear
Below mouth & mid-ear
In area of ear & TMJ
Below ear & TMJ
Behind ear & TMJ
In front ear & TMJ
Inside ear & TMJ

**NASAL SINUS AREAS**    YES
Blood or pus from nostrils
Post-nasal drip
Runny or stuffy nose
Allergic rhinitis
Persistant sore throat
Tight throat

**TOOTHACHES**

**GINGIVAL OR GUM INFLAMMATIONS**

**DIZZINESS**

**NECK**
Do you hear grinding and clicking noises when you turn your head & neck?

1

**JAW MOVEMENT PROBLEMS**    YES
Limited opening
Limited side movement
Locks open
Locks closed
Does not move smoothly
Clicking or popping sensation in jaw joint (TMJ)
Grinding sensation in (TMJ)
Clenching
Gnashing or grinding of teeth at night or during the day
Awaken with teeth or jaw muscles tired

**UNUSUAL SENSATIONS IN MOUTH SOFT TISSUES**    YES
Numb feeling
Pain
Burning
Tingling
Gritty
Salty taste
Metallic taste

Which of **all** of the preceding is the **greatest** pain or problem? When did it first occur?

What previous treatments have you received? What has been the result of the treatments? (Continue on back of sheet, if necessary).

2

*Fig. 2–1.* Chronic pain patient questionaire.

PLEASE FILL IN SOLIDLY, WITH PENCIL, THE AREA OF YOUR GREATEST PAIN OR PROBLEM. CROSSHATCH, WITH PENCIL, OTHER PROBLEM AREAS.

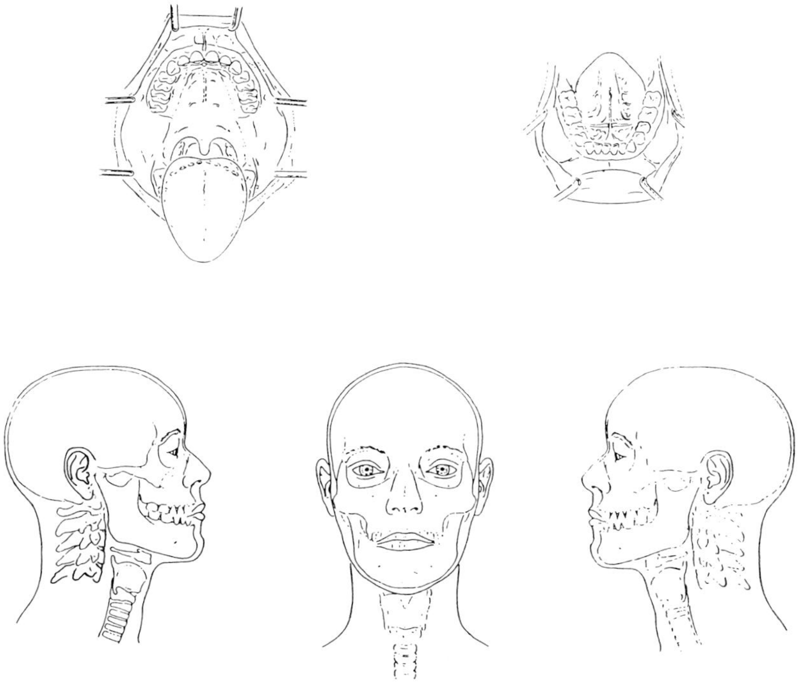

PLEASE INDICATE YES IF APPROPRIATE

YES ☐☐☐☐☐

Do you sleep on your back,
side,
stomach,
random?

Have you been in an accident involving your head?

Do you use a foam pillow,
feather pillow,
no pillow?

Do your teeth fit together comfortably?

Is your face straight or is your upper or lower jaws too long or too short?

Have you ever had orthodontic treatments?

For the pain you **now** have,
have you worn a bite plane; night guard or other appliances?

have your teeth been ground or equilibrated?

have your teeth received crowns, bridges, periodontal or gum treatments, root canals, extractions?

have you had TMJ injections or operations?

**HAVE YOU EVER HAD:**

YES ☐☐☐☐☐☐☐☐☐☐☐☐☐☐☐☐☐

backaches difficult to treat
migraine headaches
whiplash injury
thyroid gland operation
appendectomy
hysterectomy
tonsillectomy
mastoid operations
ear operations
spastic colon
mouth ulcers
stomach ulcers
high blood pressure
heart trouble
thoracic outlet syndrome
prescriptions for thyroid,
mood elevators
tranquilizers
high blood pressure

**DO YOU:**

YES ☐☐☐☐☐☐

bite your cheeks or nails
chew gum daily
smoke a pipe, cigar or cigarettes
chew food on one side
open hairpins with teeth
chew tobacco or dip snuff
have frequent sour stomach taste

PLEASE LIST DOCTORS CONSULTED AND MEDICINES PRESCRIBED; continue on back of sheet, if necessary.

4

3

Left Side

Right Side

*Fig. 2-1.* Chronic pain patient questionaire (continued).

PLEASE INDICATE THE PRESENCE AND INTENSITY OF THE FOLLOWING PERTAINING TO YOUR AREA OF **GREATEST** PAIN OR PROBLEM.

| | Never | Sometimes | Frequently | Always |
|---|---|---|---|---|
| Touching or tapping causes pain | | | | |
| Worse in morning | | | | |
| Worse in afternoon and evening | | | | |
| Awakens you at night | | | | |
| Worse when moving jaws | | | | |
| Lasts less than 5 minutes | | | | |
| Like worms burrowing | | | | |
| Like nails being driven | | | | |
| Interferes with work | | | | |
| Interferes with hobbies | | | | |
| Has caused swelling | | | | |
| Has caused redness or blushing | | | | |
| Has caused blanching or whitening | | | | |
| Causes you to cry easily | | | | |
| Is uncomfortable, not painful | | | | |
| Hurts to yawn | | | | |
| Hurts when eating | | | | |
| Hurts on top of skull | | | | |
| Hair roots seem to hurt | | | | |
| Produces a numb feeling | | | | |
| Produces paralysis of face | | | | |
| Occurs when closing mouth | | | | |
| Occurs when opening mouth | | | | |
| Is in bone | | | | |
| Is in soft tissues | | | | |
| Is in jaw-joint (TMJ) | | | | |
| Is in ear | | | | |
| Is in cheeks | | | | |
| Is in nose | | | | |
| Is in maxillary sinuses | | | | |
| Is in frontal sinuses____ | | | | |
| Is in teeth | | | | |
| Is in soft tissues of mouth | | | | |
| Is in eyes | | | | |
| Is behind eyes | | | | |
| Have problem moving eyes | | | | |
| Have problem seeing | | | | |
| Has produced pus | | | | |

5

PLEASE CIRCLE WORDS AND PHRASES THAT DESCRIBE YOUR PAIN.

| | | | | |
|---|---|---|---|---|
| Steady | Occurs at end of day | Cold | Non-localized | Deep |
| Localized | Contracting | Severe | Moving | Dull |
| Heavy | Hot | Disabling | Light | General |
| Constant | Throbbing | Pinching | Blunt | Squeezing |
| Pulsating | Spreading | Hard | Not bothersome | Numb |
| Morning | Expanding | Numb | Fleeting | Growing |
| Expanding | Exploding | Burning | Twisting | Pressing |
| Varying | | Tingling | Hurts when standing | Hurts when eating |
| Hurts more when reclining | | Short duration | Bothersome | |
| Constant | | Unbearable | Bearable | |
| Long duration | | Intermittant | Hurts on weekdays | |
| Specific | | Intense | Hurts on weekends | |
| Often | | Sharp | Hurts when awakening | |
| | | Stretching | Hurts when going to bed | |
| Aching | | Lancinating | Punishing | |
| | | Electric-like | | |
| | | Knife-like | | |
| | | Awakens you at night | | |

6

*Fig. 2-1.* Chronic pain patient questionaire (continued).

PATIENT'S NAME: _____ AGE: _____ SEX: _____ RACE: _____

INFORMANT: _____ DATE: _____ CLINIC NO.: _____

CLOSEST RELATIVE: _____ PHONE: _____

## PAST MEDICAL HISTORY

NO            YES            COMMENTS

☐ Care of physician? (who, why) ☐

☐ Serious illnesses? ☐

☐ Serious injuries? ☐

☐ Hospital admissions? ☐

☐ Operations? (what, when, where) ☐

☐ Transfusions? (why, when) ☐

☐ Pregnancies? (past, present) ☐

☐ Allergies? (food, drugs, other) ☐

☐ Present medications (kinds, dosage) ☐

☐ Illicit drugs (quality, quantity) ☐

☐ Alcohol (quality, quantity) ☐

☐ Tobacco (quality, quantity) ☐

LAST PHYSICAL EXAMINATION: _____ DATE: _____ WHY: _____

## REVIEW OF SYSTEMS

| NEG | | POS | COMMENTS | NEG | | POS | COMMENTS |
|---|---|---|---|---|---|---|---|
| **CARDIOVASCULAR:** | | | | **ENDOCRINE:** | | | |
| ☐ | Angina pectoris | ☐ | | ☐ | Diabetes | ☐ | |
| ☐ | Myocardial infarction | | | ☐ | Adrenal disorders | | |
| ☐ | Congenital heart defect | | | ☐ | Thyroid disorders | | |
| ☐ | Rheumatic fever | | | ☐ | Parathyroid disorders | | |
| ☐ | Rheumatic heart disease | | | ☐ | Steroids | | |
| ☐ | Murmurs | | | ☐ | Other: | ☐ | |
| ☐ | Hypertension | | | | | | |
| ☐ | Stroke | | | **GENITOURINARY:** | | | |
| ☐ | Other: | ☐ | | ☐ | Kidney Infections | ☐ | |
| | | | | ☐ | Veneral disease | | |
| **RESPIRATORY** | | | | ☐ | Other: | ☐ | |
| ☐ | Tuberculosis | ☐ | | | | | |
| ☐ | Emphysema | | | **HEMATOPOIETIC** | | | |
| ☐ | Asthma | | | ☐ | Anemia | ☐ | |
| ☐ | Shortness of breath | | | ☐ | Bleeding disorders | | |
| ☐ | Dyspnea on exertion | | | ☐ | Anticoagulants | | |
| ☐ | Orthopnea | | | ☐ | Leukemia | | |
| ☐ | Edema | | | ☐ | Other: | ☐ | |
| ☐ | Other: | ☐ | | | | | |
| | | | | **NEUROLOGIC:** | | | |
| **GASTROINTESTINAL/LIVER** | | | | ☐ | Epilepsy | ☐ | |
| ☐ | Ulcers | ☐ | | ☐ | Convulsions | | |
| ☐ | Bleeding | | | ☐ | Psychiatric treatment | | |
| ☐ | Hepatitis | | | ☐ | Faints/Spells | | |
| ☐ | Jaundice | | | ☐ | Tranquilizers | | |
| ☐ | Cirrhosis | | | ☐ | Other: | ☐ | |
| ☐ | Other: | ☐ | | | | | |
| | | | | **MUSCULOSKELETAL** | | | |
| | | | | ☐ | Bones | ☐ | |
| | | | | ☐ | Muscles | | |
| | | | | ☐ | Joints | | |
| | | | | ☐ | TMJ | | |
| | | | | ☐ | Other: | ☐ | |

*Fig. 2–2.* Past medical history and review of systems.

should be identified. Family members may "sell" their sphere of problems to the patient; a parent may recount personal pain problems and firmly identify the similarity of the recalled pains with the child's chief complaint of facial pain or dysfunction.

## Social History

All oral and maxillofacial maladies are reflected, to a greater or lesser degree, in the patient's psyche; the patient usually strongly identifies the mouth and face with their own image perception. Although the patient may seek a rapid and easy solution for somatic complaints, the patient may make statements and inferences during the acquisition of the history indicative of whether or not psychic depressions are significant factors contributing to the chief complaint (see Chapter 5).

Certain physiologic symptoms may help to identify psychic depression: sleep disturbance, appetite disturbance, severe and recurring constipation or diarrhea, spastic colon, low back pain, fatigue, lack of interest in sex, fibromyalgia, decreased pleasure, and oral mucosal inflammations and ulcerations.

If, as the history and physical examination proceed, the patient shows signs of sadness, a feeling of worthlessness, a negative outlook on life, or a loss of interest in a normal life, the identification of depression is more certain.

On the other hand, a patient may display either no or minimal evidence of depression, may have a "can-do" attitude, and may do most things well. The patient may regard the chief complaint in a balanced and rational context, and somatic treatment will more likely be associated with a high success rate.

Somatic therapy for a magnified complaint in a psychophysiologically disabled patient probably is doomed to failure. Consultation with the family physician, a psychiatrist, or a psychologist is usually indicated when the patient is psychologically troubled.

## Occupational History

The history of the patient's occupation is an extension of the social history. Responses of the patient to the physical environment en-countered for most of the waking hours has a direct bearing on his or her physical and mental health. Interactions with family, peers, subordinates, and superiors; the level of satisfaction with the occupation; and an indication that the work is considered meaningful and useful by the patient may be ascertained in the occupational history.

## Physical Examination

The examination of any portion of the body consists of four components: inspection, palpation, percussion, and auscultation. These four words and the procedures that they represent have stood the test of time. Clinicians around the world use these words for communicating with clarity. They describe every type of examination. Even as a hammer is an extension of an arm, an automobile is an extension of the legs, and computers are extensions of the brain, so medical imaging, dental and medical laboratory studies and tests, and consultations are extensions of these four basic components of a physical examination.

The initial aspect of the physical examination of a facial pain patient is taking and recording the vital signs. As the doctor takes the pulse, often while an assistant takes the blood pressure, the physical contact with the patient is indicative both of concern for the total patient and of competence by the doctor. A useful technique is to count the pulse rate for 15 to 30 seconds and, still holding the pulse, count the respirations for 15 to 30 seconds. When the patient knows that the respirations are being recorded, the patient may voluntarily or involuntarily alter the breathing rate.

The regional physical examination of the oral and maxillofacial tissues and contiguous regions may be recorded on any of several different formats. For simplicity, as well as completeness, many clinicians use standardized forms (Fig. 2–3). After the usual identifying data are gathered and the initial signs are recorded, a routine of inspection, palpation, percussion, and auscultation of the various regions and structures of the stomatognathic system follow.

## PHYSICAL EXAMINATION

PATIENT'S NAME:_____ REG. NO._____

INFORMANT (if other than patient)_____

A. General appearance and findings _____

B. Prostheses, health aids or appliances_____

C. Vital signs: BP_____ , P_____ , R_____ , Wgt_____ , Hgt_____ , Age_____

| | NORMAL | | ABNORMAL | COMMENT | | | NORMAL | | ABNORMAL | COMMENT |
|---|---|---|---|---|---|---|---|---|---|---|
| | | D. Craniofacial skeleton | | | | | | F. Intraoral tissues | | |
| 1. | ☐ | Cephalic index | ☐ | | | 1. | ☐ | Breath | ☐ | |
| 2. | ☐ | Orthognathic relations | ☐ | | | 2. | ☐ | Saliva | ☐ | |
| 3. | ☐ | TMJ | ☐ | | | 3. | ☐ | Lips | ☐ | |
| 4. | ☐ | Other | ☐ | | | 4. | ☐ | Commissures | ☐ | |
| | | | | | | 5. | ☐ | Buccal mucosa | ☐ | |
| | | | | | | 6. | ☐ | Retromolar areas | ☐ | |
| | NORMAL | | ABNORMAL | COMMENT | | 7. | ☐ | Pharynx | ☐ | |
| | | E. Extraoral tissues | | | | 8. | ☐ | Soft palate | ☐ | |
| 1. | ☐ | Cutaneous tissues | ☐ | | | 9. | ☐ | Hard palate | ☐ | |
| 2. | ☐ | Auricular structures | ☐ | | | 10. | ☐ | Tongue | ☐ | |
| 3. | ☐ | Ocular structures | ☐ | | | 11. | ☐ | Floor of mouth | ☐ | |
| 4. | ☐ | Nasal structures | ☐ | | | 12. | ☐ | Gingiva | ☐ | |
| 5. | ☐ | Sinal structures | ☐ | | | 13. | ☐ | Occlusal relations | ☐ | |
| 6. | ☐ | Thyroid cartilage | ☐ | | | 14. | ☐ | Other | ☐ | |
| 7. | ☐ | Thyroid gland | ☐ | | | | | | | |
| 8. | ☐ | Trachea | ☐ | | | | | | | |
| 9. | ☐ | Cervical chains | ☐ | | | | | | | |
| 10. | ☐ | Parotid space | ☐ | | | | | | | |
| 11. | ☐ | Submandibular spaces | ☐ | | | | | | | |
| 12. | ☐ | Submental triangle | ☐ | | | | | | | |
| 13. | ☐ | Salivary glands | ☐ | | | | | | | |
| 14. | ☐ | Myofascial tissues | ☐ | | | | | | | |
| 15. | ☐ | Neurological | ☐ | | | | | | | |
| 16. | ☐ | Other | ☐ | | | | | | | |

G. Preventive dentistry

1. Oral hygiene
   ___ Poor ___ Average ___ Excellent
2. Dental health motivation
   ___ Poor ___ Average ___ Excellent
3. Previous dental care
   ___ Poor ___ Average ___ Excellent
4. Nutrition
   ___ Poor ___ Average ___ Excellent

*Fig. 2–3.* Physical evaluation.

## Facial Pain Analysis

The mobilization of objective information about the chronic pain the patient is enduring is assisted by following a routine that keeps subjective views at a minimum. A preliminary diagnosis should be possible by combining information gleaned from the routine baseline histories and physical examinations, the patient-generated history form, and the following examinations and analyses. In view of the admonition to resist shortcuts on the route to establishing a diagnosis, a routine sequence should be developed for the examination. For convenience, we often use a facial pain analysis form (Fig. 2–4) to record neurologic system, vascular system, musculoskeletal system, dentition, occlusal function, temporomandibular, psychopathologic, and other head and neck maladies.

### Neurologic Pains

The patient may locate the pain in one of the distributions of a cranial nerve (CN) or a branch of the nerve. The pain is often described as being of short duration but of great intensity. An abbreviated cranial nerve examination is often indicated by the chief complaint (Fig. 2–5).

### Cranial Nerves

The abbreviated cranial nerve examination includes assessment of the following.

**CN I, Olfactory Nerve.** Have the patient smell, using one nostril at a time, to identify common odiferous substances such as vanilla flavoring, banana oil, and vinegar.

**CN II, Optic Nerve.** Examine each eye for general function and acuity by an eye chart, or by having the patient read from a printed page. Check the visual fields by having the patient gaze at a point directly ahead while the examiner moves wiggling fingers or some other target into the visual fields from the superior, inferior, medial, and posterior-lateral directions, asking the patient to indicate when the fingers or the target is first observed. If the pupil or pupils are cloudy, if the patient experiences pain in the orbital region, or if a test for glaucoma has not been performed recently, the patient should be re-ferred to an ophthalmologist for a pressure test.

**CN III, Oculomotor Nerve; CN IV, Trochlear Nerve; and CN VI, Abducens Nerve.** Covering each eye in turn, have the patient gaze at a small target, such as the tip of a pen or pencil, and follow it carefully. Move the target vertically and then horizontally to assess the ability of the eye to track the target without nystagmus. The patient who cannot track the target or who perceives a double target should be referred to an ophthalmologist. The levator palpebrae superioris is innervated by CN III, and drooping of the upper eyelid may be indicative of an injury to CN III.

**CN V, Trigeminal Nerve.** To evaluate the sensory components of CN V, ask the patient if numbness or tingling of the face has been noticed. Using a pledget of cotton formed into a point, like a pointed instrument, ask the patient to close the eyes and report "right" or "left" when they feel the light touch of cotton. Touch the chin, cheek, or forehead to check for sensitivity to light touch in the three divisions of the trigeminal nerve. If the response to light touch is not normal, a blunt and sharp test is initiated. Place the blunt handle and then the sharp end of a sterile dental explorer or other device against the face, and ask the patient to report which stimulation is blunt and which is sharp. The sharp test is best for testing the mucosa inside the mouth.

To estimate the activity of the motor components of CN V, palpate the areas of the temporalis and masseter muscles as the patient first opens the mandible against resistance and then clenches the teeth. Hold the patient's mandible in a firm closed position and ask the patient to open. An appreciation of bilateral and equal pressure from the depressor muscles is a normal finding. The temporalis and masseter areas should feel soft to palpation during this phase of the test. Then, ask the patient to clench the teeth. Palpation of the masseter and temporalis areas should reflect bilateral and equal muscle contractions.

**CN VII, Facial Nerve.** Ask the patient to close the lips and blow against the cheeks. Air will leak out the corner of the mouth on the side of a paresis (Bell's palsy). Then put an index finger in the infraorbital region and pull downward on the skin, asking the patient to close the eyelids tightly. The eyelid will remain open on the affected side. Then ask the patient to raise the forehead in "wonder and amazement," but the forehead will not wrinkle or elevate the eye brow on the affected side. A noteworthy fact is that a small percentage of patients with Bell's palsy have pain around the lobe of the ear from involvement of the nerve intermedius of CN VII. This pain continues for a few weeks and should be treated with analgesics or synthetic narcotics, as indicated.

**CN VIII, Stato-Acoustic Nerve.** Move to the right and left lateral of the patient and speak a sentence softly, asking the patient to repeat the sentence. Ask the patient if dizziness occurs when they stand up from sitting or if it occurs spontaneously to test for vestibular function. Nystagmus when the head is still is evidence of a pathologic process, if the condition is not congenital.

**CN IX, Glossopharyngeal Nerve.** The patient typically reports difficulty in swallowing if a pathologic process involves CN IX. The best test is to apply a cotton-tipped applicator, dipped into a flavored solution, to the dorsum of the tongue or the affected side. Solutions of salt, lidocaine, sugar, and vinegar can be used to test for sensations of salty, bitter, sweet, or sour. Touch only the tongue posterior to the sulcus terminalis and circumvallat papillae. Ask the patient to identify the taste sensation. Apply the same test to the anterior two thirds of the tongue to test for chorda (CN VII) tympani nerve function. Taste may be affected in a patient with Bell's palsy.

Parenthetically, a patient will experience intractable coughing if a hair falls into the external auditory meatus and lodges against the tympanic membrane when the patient is being prepared for surgery. The surgeon should place cotton in the ear before shaving the area, if required.

**CV X, Vagus Nerve.** The patient with injury to the vagus nerve may develop hoarseness of the voice. Remember that the vagus nerve innervates a small zone in the pinna of the ear and under the lobe of the ear in some patients. The patient will also have difficulty swallowing when the vagus nerve is affected because it richly innervates the pharyngeal plexus.

**CN XI, Accessory Nerve.** The patient with CN XI injury typically shows atrophy of the trapezius and sternocleidomastoid (SCM) muscles. To test for CN XI function, place the palm of the hand on the patient's forehead and ask the patient to bend the head forward. In patients with CN XI injury, the SCM muscles are asymmetric as they bulge out in the neck. Then, place the hands on top of the shoulders and press downward while asking the patient to raise or shrug the shoulders. Weakness is evident on the affected side.

**CV XII, Hypoglossal Nerve.** The patient with a hypoglossal nerve injury has atrophy of the tongue on the affected side. Dysarthria and difficulty in swallowing also are noted. To test for injury, such as a fracture of the occipital bone across the hypoglossal canal, ask the patient to "stick out the tongue." The tongue is flaccid to palpation and deflects toward the affected side. The patient typically is not able to push out the cheek with the tongue on the affected side.

When cranial nerve dysfunction is identified, the patient should be referred immediately to a neurologist or neurosurgeon for diagnosis and treatment.

### Cervical Nerves

Remember that the second and third cervical nerves, rather than CN V-3 (mandibular division of the trigeminal nerve), innervate the angle of the mandible, and that osseous, myofascial, and neurologic maladies of the posterior cervical muscles, spine, and nerves may be sensed in the mandibular area.

The pain of cardiac muscle ischemia can be referred to both angles of the mandible, but more frequently, it is referred to the left angle. The possibility exists that the only complaint of an ischemic heart attack will be sensed in the mandible. A 63-year-old man had pain in the symphyseal area of the mandible that moved up both sides of the mandible, down the neck, and into the upper chest. The patient was referred for evaluation of temporomandibular joint (TMJ) dysfunction, because he had a loud crepitus and clicking in both TM joints. He had no TM joint pain with

**FACIAL PAIN ANALYSIS**

PATIENT'S NAME _____

DATE _____

**1**

**NEUROLOGIC SYSTEM**

| | Yes | No |
|---|---|---|
| Taste aberration | | |

**Light touch sensibility**

| | Right Normal | Right Abnormal | Left Normal | Left Abnormal |
|---|---|---|---|---|
| V-1 distribution | | | | |
| V-2 distribution | | | | |
| V-3 distribution | | | | |

| | Yes | No | | Yes | No |
|---|---|---|---|---|---|
| Facial paresthesia | | | | | |

**Vision**

| | Right Yes | Right No | Left Yes | Left No | |
|---|---|---|---|---|---|
| Does eyelid droop? | | | | | (CN III) |
| Does eyeball track vertically? | | | | | (CN III & IV) |
| Does eyeball track laterally? | | | | | (CN IV) |

COMMENTS ON NEUROLOGIC EXAMINATIONS
_____
_____
_____
_____
_____
_____
_____
_____
_____
_____
_____

**Facial paralysis**

| | Right Normal | Right Abnormal | Left Normal | Left Abnormal |
|---|---|---|---|---|
| Lip blowing test | | | | |
| Lower eyelid closure | | | | |
| Lift eyebrows | | | | |

| | Yes | No | | Yes | No |
|---|---|---|---|---|---|
| Pain below ear | | | | | |

**Tongue**

| | Right Yes | Right No | Left Yes | Left No |
|---|---|---|---|---|
| Geographic | | | | |
| Fungiform papilla present | | | | |
| Bald (beefy, red) tongue | | | | |

**Trigger points**

| | Yes | No |
|---|---|---|
| Are there facial or oral trigger points producing pain? | | |
| Does swallowing trigger pain in the ear or throat? | | |

**VASCULAR SYSTEM**

HEADACHES, history of

| | Yes | No |
|---|---|---|
| Migraine | | |
| Cluster | | |
| Tension | | |
| Sinus | | |

Tenderness of

| | Right Yes | Right No | Left Yes | Left No |
|---|---|---|---|---|
| Facial artery | | | | |
| Superficial temporal a | | | | |
| Carotid sinus | | | | |

COMMENTS ON HEADACHES AND VASCULAR SYSTEM
_____
_____
_____
_____
_____
_____
_____
_____
_____
_____
_____

**SALIVARY GLANDS**

| | Parotid right | | Parotid left | | Submandibular right | | Submandibular left | | Sublingual right | | Sublingual left | | Minor | |
|---|---|---|---|---|---|---|---|---|---|---|---|---|---|---|
| | N | Ab | N | Ab | N | Ab | N | Ab | N | Ab | N | Ab | N | Ab |
| Morphology on palpation | | | | | | | | | | | | | | |
| Tenderness | | | | | | | | | | | | | | |
| Masses | | | | | | | | | | | | | | |
| Secretions | | | | | | | | | | | | | | |

COMMENTS ON SALIVARY GLAND EXAMINATIONS
_____
_____
_____
_____
_____
_____
_____
_____

**LYMPHATICS**

| | Right N | Right Ab | Left N | Left Ab |
|---|---|---|---|---|
| Submental | | | | |
| Submandibular (Diagastric) | | | | |
| Deep (anterior) cervical chain | | | | |
| Superficial (posterior) cervical chain | | | | |

COMMENTS ON LYMPHATICS EXAMINATIONS (size, texture and tenderness)
_____
_____
_____
_____

**2**

**MYOSPASMS**

Palpations

| | Right Yes | Right No | Left Yes | Left No |
|---|---|---|---|---|
| Masseter muscle | | | | |
| anterior-superior quadrant | | | | |
| posterior-superior quadrant | | | | |
| middle zone | | | | |
| inferior zone | | | | |
| Temporalis muscle | | | | |
| anterior zone | | | | |
| posterior zone | | | | |
| Sternocleidomastoid muscle | | | | |
| superior zone | | | | |
| middle zone | | | | |
| inferior zone | | | | |
| Diagastric muscle | | | | |
| anterior belly | | | | |
| posterior belly | | | | |
| Splenius capitis muscle | | | | |
| Trapezius muscle | | | | |
| superior zone | | | | |
| middle zone | | | | |
| inferior zone | | | | |
| Medial pterygoid muscle | | | | |
| inferior zone | | | | |
| middle zone | | | | |
| Lateral pterygoid muscle | | | | |

**ORTHOGNATHIC RELATIONS**

Major facial skeletal deformity

| | Yes | No |
|---|---|---|
| Maxillary retrognathism | | |
| Maxillary prognathism | | |
| Mandibular retrognathism | | |
| Mandibular prognathism | | |
| Apertognathism | | |
| Long face | | |
| Short face | | |
| Other | | |

COMMENTS ON FACIAL SKELETAL RELATIONSHIPS
_____
_____
_____

**3**

*Fig. 2–4.* Facial pain analysis form.

## Panel 4

**OCCLUSION AND DENTITION**

Mobility (0-3)
Vitalo-meter Reading

1  2  3  4  5  6  7  8  9  10  11  12  13  14  15  16

X = Missing or unerupted teeth
P = Pain on percussion
C = Pain to cold
H = Pain to heat

R                                                                 L

32  31  30  29  28  27  26  25  24  23  22  21  20  19  18  17

Vitalo-meter Reading
Mobility (0-3)

**COMMENTS:**                    Tooth #

Open or recurrent decay _____
Crowns or larger restorations _____
Fracture or craze lines _____
Presence of implants _____
State of oral hygiene _____

Angle's occlusal classification _____

I    II₁    II₂    III

4

## Panel 5

**OCCLUSAL FUNCTION**

|            | Group Function | Cuspid rise | Balanced |
|------------|----------------|-------------|----------|
| Right side |                |             |          |
| Left side  |                |             |          |

|                                          | Right |    | Left |    |
|------------------------------------------|-------|----|------|----|
|                                          | Yes   | No | Yes  | No |
| Centric prematurity                      |       |    |      |    |
| Lateral deviation in slide from RC to IP |       |    |      |    |
| Lateral guidance by posterior teeth      |       |    |      |    |
| Lateral retrusive guidance               |       |    |      |    |
| Balancing interference                   |       |    |      |    |
| Protrusive guidance on posterior teeth   |       |    |      |    |
| Teeth in crossbite (#)                   |       |    |      |    |

|                       | Excessive | Inadequate |
|-----------------------|-----------|------------|
| Interocclusal distance |           |            |

**OCCLUSION AND DENTITION**

1. Dental arch formation (alignment of the teeth)

2. Compensating curvatures of the dental arches (curved occlusal planes)

3. Compensating curvatures of the individual teeth (curved axes)

4. Angulation of individual teeth in relation to various planes (including root form)

5. Functional form of the teeth at their incisal and occlusal thirds

6. Facial relations of each tooth in one arch to its antagonist or antagonists in the opposing arch in centric occlusion

7. Occlusal contact and intercusp relations of all the teeth of one arch with those in the opposing arch in centric occlusion

8. Occlusal contact and intercusp relations of all the teeth during the various functional mandibular movements

9. Summary

COMMENTS ON OCCLUSAL FUNCTIONS

_____
_____
_____
_____

5

## Panel 6

**TEMPOROMANDIBULAR JOINT**

Palpation
**Static**

|                                                      | Right |      |    | Left |      |    |
|------------------------------------------------------|-------|------|----|------|------|----|
|                                                      | Yes   | Slgt | No | Yes  | Slgt | No |
| Lateral pole, closed                                 |       |      |    |      |      |    |
| Lateral pole, open                                   |       |      |    |      |      |    |
| Anterior lateral superior condylar head, impact loading |   |      |    |      |      |    |

Auscultation (crepitus)

|       |              | Coarse |    | Fine |    |
|-------|--------------|--------|----|------|----|
|       |              | Yes    | No | Yes  | No |
| Right | Vertical     |        |    |      |    |
|       | Right lateral |       |    |      |    |
|       | Left lateral |        |    |      |    |
| Left  | Vertical     |        |    |      |    |
|       | Right lateral |       |    |      |    |
|       | Left lateral |        |    |      |    |

(Picture of dynamic points, early, late, crest, end point)

**Dynamic**

|       |                  | Early | Late | Crest | End pt |
|-------|------------------|-------|------|-------|--------|
| Right | Opening movement |       |      |       |        |
|       | Closing movement |       |      |       |        |
| Left  | Opening movement |       |      |       |        |
|       | Closing movement |       |      |       |        |

Range of motion in millimeters

|                | mm | Deviation |   |
|----------------|----|-----------|---|
|                |    | L         | R |
| Maximum vertical |  |           |   |
| Protrusive     |    |           |   |
| Right lateral  |    |           |   |
| Left lateral   |    |           |   |

Auscultation (click)

|       |                 | Early | Late | Crest | End pt |
|-------|-----------------|-------|------|-------|--------|
| Right | Opening vertical |      |      |       |        |
|       | Closing vertical |      |      |       |        |
|       | Right Lateral   |       |      |       |        |
|       | Left Lateral    |       |      |       |        |
| Left  | Opening vertical |      |      |       |        |
|       | Closing vertical |      |      |       |        |
|       | Right Lateral   |       |      |       |        |
|       | Left Lateral    |       |      |       |        |

COMMENTS ON MUSCLE AND TMJ EXAMINATIONS (Including meniscus subluxation and dislocation)

_____
_____
_____

6

## Panel 7

**IMAGERY FINDINGS**

Temporomandibular joint

|                |                     | Right |    | Left |    |
|----------------|---------------------|-------|----|------|----|
|                |                     | Yes   | No | Yes  | No |
| Glenoid Fossae | Normal contours     |       |    |      |    |
|                | Irregular surface   |       |    |      |    |
|                | Sclerotic           |       |    |      |    |
|                | Enlarged            |       |    |      |    |
|                | Other               |       |    |      |    |
| Articular Eminences | Normal contours |       |    |      |    |
|                | Flattened           |       |    |      |    |
|                | Steep               |       |    |      |    |
|                | Osteophyte          |       |    |      |    |
|                | Central radioluceny |       |    |      |    |
|                | Sclerotic           |       |    |      |    |
|                | Other               |       |    |      |    |

| Frontal view | | Ovoid | Flat | Angular | Round | Concave |
|---|---|---|---|---|---|---|
|  | right |  |  |  |  |  |
|  | left |  |  |  |  |  |

|                |                  | Right |    | Left |    |
|----------------|------------------|-------|----|------|----|
|                |                  | Yes   | No | Yes  | No |
| Condyles       | Lateral view, normal contours | |  |      |    |
|                | Ely's cysts      |       |    |      |    |
|                | Sclerosis        |       |    |      |    |
|                | Erosion – Medial / Lateral / Central | | |  |    |
|                | Atrophy          |       |    |      |    |
|                | Osteophytes Spike – Posterior / Middle / Anterior | | | | |
|                | Shelf – Anterior / Posterior |  |  |   |    |
|                | Plateau – Middle / Lateral |  |  |     |    |
|                | Displacement     |       |    |      |    |
|                | Other            |       |    |      |    |

| Bilateral symmetry of intracapsular spaces | No | Yes |
|---|---|---|
| Angle of condylar long axes to sagittal plane (SMV) | No | Yes |

Arthrograms

|                               | Right |    | Left |    |
|-------------------------------|-------|----|------|----|
|                               | Yes   | No | Yes  | No |
| Normal superior cavity outline |      |    |      |    |
| Normal inferior cavity outline |      |    |      |    |
| Anterior subluxation of disc   |      |    |      |    |
| Anterior dislocation of disc   |      |    |      |    |
| Disc perforation               |      |    |      |    |
| Disc adhesions – superior cavity |    |    |      |    |
| – inferior cavity              |      |    |      |    |

and other medical imagery

|                        | Yes | No | Month/year |
|------------------------|-----|----|------------|
| Panoramic, routine     |     |    |            |
| Transpharyngeal, TMJ   |     |    |            |
| Transcranial, TMJ      |     |    |            |
| Panoramic, TMJ         |     |    |            |
| Transorbital, TMJ      |     |    |            |
| Submental vertex       |     |    |            |
| Laminographic, TMJ     |     |    |            |
| Arthrograms            |     |    |            |
| Paranasal sinus views  |     |    |            |
| Cephalometric views    |     |    |            |
| Periapical views       |     |    |            |
| Occlusal views         |     |    |            |
| Bite wing views        |     |    |            |
| CT scan                |     |    |            |
| Bone scan              |     |    |            |
| N.M.R.                 |     |    |            |
| Thermograms            |     |    |            |

COMMENTS ON IMAGERY FINDINGS

_____
_____
_____
_____
_____
_____
_____
_____

7

*Fig. 2–4.* Facial pain analysis form (continued).

**NEUROLOGIC SYSTEM**

|  | Yes | No |
|---|---|---|
| Taste aberration |  |  |

Light touch sensibility

|  | Right | | Left | |
|---|---|---|---|---|
|  | Normal | Abnormal | Normal | Abnormal |
| V-1 distribution |  |  |  |  |
| V-2 distribution |  |  |  |  |
| V-3 distribution |  |  |  |  |

|  | Yes | No |  | Yes | No |
|---|---|---|---|---|---|
| Facial paresthesia |  |  |  |  |  |

Vision

|  | Right | | Left | |  |
|---|---|---|---|---|---|
|  | Yes | No | Yes | No |  |
| Does eyelid droop? |  |  |  |  | (CN III) |
| Does eyeball track vertically? |  |  |  |  | (CN III & IV) |
| Does eyeball track laterally? |  |  |  |  | (CN IV) |

Facial paralysis

|  | Right | | Left | |
|---|---|---|---|---|
|  | Normal | Abnormal | Normal | Abnormal |
| Lip blowing test |  |  |  |  |
| Lower eyelid closure |  |  |  |  |
| Lift eyebrows |  |  |  |  |

|  | Yes | No |  | Yes | No |
|---|---|---|---|---|---|
| Pain below ear |  |  |  |  |  |

Tongue

|  | Right | | Left | |  |
|---|---|---|---|---|---|
|  | Yes | No | Yes | No |  |
| Geographic |  |  |  |  |  |
| Fungiform papilla present |  |  |  |  |  |
| Bald (beefy, red) tongue |  |  |  |  |  |

Trigger points

|  | Yes | No |
|---|---|---|
| Are there facial or oral trigger points producing pain? |  |  |
| Does swallowing trigger pain in the ear or throat? |  |  |

COMMENTS ON NEUROLOGIC EXAMINATIONS

_____

_____

_____

_____

_____

_____

_____

_____

_____

*Fig. 2–5.* Neurologic system evaluation.

eating and the mandible had a normal range of motion. The patient could relieve the chest, neck, and facial pain by resting. Consulation with a cardiologist revealed significant coronary artery blockages. The patient underwent a cardiac and lifestyle rehabilitation program with successful results.

Occipital headaches may occur in individuals with C2 and C3 pathologic involvement, such as nerve entrapment in the posterior cervical muscles. This pain can be differentially diagnosed by greater auricular nerve and posterior nerve anesthetic blocks.

### Vascular Pains

Vascular pains in the head and neck are usually of one of two types: the migrainous or vasodilating type or the arteritis type. The major migrainous types observed by the authors are classic migraine, common migraine, and cluster headache. The common arteritis types are giant cell arteritis (temporal arteritis) and carotid system arteritis with carotidynia.

The patient with cluster variant of migraine usually indicates the pain is in, around, or behind the eye and no evidence of a pathologic process of the eye, such as acute glaucoma, is noted. The pain is often described as throbbing and is accompanied or followed by headaches. Classification of headache is often a differential diagnosis in patients with chronic facial pain.

### Migrainous Type and Migraine Headaches

The patient with classic and common migraine often describes the pain as throbbing;

it often involves one half of the cranium and sometimes extends into the face (Fig. 2–6).

If the headache is of the cluster type, the headache may last 1, 2, 3, or 8 days and then begins to taper off. The patient may be free of headaches for weeks or months before it recurs. To test for cluster headache, place an oxygen mask over the patient's nose and mouth, and ask the patient to breathe normally while administering 7 liters per minute of 100% oxygen for 3 minutes. About 80% of patients with cluster headache gain relief with this test.

Classic and common migraine do not respond to breathing 100% oxygen. The relief obtained in the cluster patient may be short-lived or it may continue for days and even weeks. These patients are often supported by such preparations as ergotamines, beta-blockers, calcium channel blockers, or compounds such as Midrin (isometheptene mucate).

Migrainous headaches may need to be differentiated from sinal and muscle contraction headaches. The patient with sinus headache typically points to the region of the maxillary antrum or, in the event of a frontal sinus headache, to the lower frontal bone. These patients often describe symptoms of nasal drainage with evidence of infection occurring coincident with these headaches.

Tension headache, which is now called *muscle contraction headache*, can often be diagnosed by combining the history of the headache with an examination of muscles by palpation.

### Temporal Arteritis

In patients 55 years of age and older, palpation of the arteries of the face is particularly important. The facial artery is palpated easily by running the index finger along the inferior border of the mandible in the region of the antigonal notching at the anterior margin of the masseter muscle.

The superficial temporal artery is palpated by placing the index finger just above the base of the pinna of the ear above the roof of the glenoid fossa. The tissue is relatively soft in this region, and if excessive pressure is applied with the index finger, no pulse from the superficial temporal artery is perceived. A good technique is to palpate the two sides simultaneously, pressing inward and then easing off gradually until the pressure allows the pulsating to occur. In patients 55 years of age and older, a painful flat mass or a firm matchstick-like artery with no pulse on one side and normal pulsations on the opposite side is suggestive of giant cell or temporal arteritis. This condition is discussed in Chapter 13.

### Carotidynia

The carotid pulse is palpated just anterior to the SCM muscle at the level of the hyoid bone. The painless side is palpated first. As soon as the pulsation is perceived, apply pressure and ask the patient to note the amount of discomfort. Then, palpate the painful side, and ask the patient to compare the painful

HEADACHES, history of

|  | Yes | No |
|---|---|---|
| Migraine |  |  |
| Cluster |  |  |
| Tension |  |  |
| Sinus |  |  |

Tenderness of

|  | Right | | Left | |
|---|---|---|---|---|
|  | Yes | No | Yes | No |
| Facial artery |  |  |  |  |
| Superficial temporal a. |  |  |  |  |
| Carotid sinus |  |  |  |  |

COMMENTS ON HEADACHES AND VASCULAR SYSTEM

_____

_____

_____

_____

_____

_____

_____

*Fig. 2–6.* Vascular system evaluation.

side to the control side. Painful carotidynia may be of the vasodilating or migrainous type or it may be an arteritis type of carotidynia. If the sedimentation rate is elevated, the carotidynia is more likely of the arteritis type than of the vasodilating type.

### Salivary Gland Maladies

In healthy subjects, the submandibular glands, often the sublingual glands, but seldom the parotid glands, are palpable. In patients with pathologic changes of salivary gland, palpation reveals firmness and swelling in the parotid region, in the submandibular gland region, or in the floor of the mouth, the sublingual gland region (Fig. 2–7). If the findings of inspection or palpation disclose masses in the major salivary glands, further studies could include sialograms, computed tomographic (CT) scans, and nuclear medicine imaging.

If the patient complains of xerostomia, the major glands can be inspected for function as follows. For the parotid gland, take two 5 × 5 cm cotton gauzes and place one in each

| | Parotid, right | | Parotid, left | | Submandibular, right | | Submandibular, left | | Sublingual, right | | Sublingual, left | | Minor | |
|---|---|---|---|---|---|---|---|---|---|---|---|---|---|---|
| | N | Ab | N | Ab | N | Ab | N | Ab | N | Ab | N | Ab | N | Ab |
| Morphology on palpation | | | | | | | | | | | | | | |
| Tenderness | | | | | | | | | | | | | | |
| Masses | | | | | | | | | | | | | | |
| Secretions | | | | | | | | | | | | | | |

COMMENTS ON SALIVARY GLAND
EXAMINATIONS

_____

_____

_____

_____

_____

_____

_____

*Fig. 2–7.* Salivary glands evaluation.

hand. With one hand, grasp the corner of the mouth on the affected side; evert the cheek and pull the corner of the mouth outward. With the other hand, blot the everted cheek mucosa. While lifting the gauze off the mucosa, firmly caress the parotid gland and the duct by moving fingers from below the ear posterior to the angle of the mandible, then superiorly to the TM joint area, and then forward just inferior to the zygomatic arch. Observe the parotid papilla and note the quantity or the absence of secretions. Crystal clear serous fluid is the normal finding. Cloudy milky fluid is abnormal and should be collected for microbiologic culture and sensitivity studies and other medical laboratory examinations.

To examine the function of the submandibular and sublingual glands, ask the patient to open wide and to elevate the tongue to the roof of the mouth. Press a 5 × 5 cm cotton gauze into the floor of the mouth in the midline while pressing the tongue downward, thus drying the floor of the mouth. When the 2 × 2 gauze is removed, and the patient's tongue is released from the pressure, press extraorally on the submandibular region and push up into the floor of the mouth, watching for normal clear mucous saliva to occur and flush out of the submandibular gland duct (Wharton's duct) orifice lateral to the lingual frenum in the anterior floor of the mouth. Occasionally, the saliva spurts over the lower teeth during this test. The submandibular and sublingual glands may drain through the same duct or separate ducts, and multiple small openings for the sublingual gland along the plica sublingualis may be noted.

To examine the function of the minor salivary glands, give the patient a small amount of concentrated commercial, astringent mouthwash. Astringent mouthwashes stimulate the simple tubular alveolar minor salivary glands. Ask the patient to open wide and to tilt the head up so the light is reflected across the palate. Blot the palate immediately with a 5 × 5 cm gauze, remove the gauze, and observe the palate. Little crystal-clear dots or mounds of saliva, which is a mucous type saliva, are noted if the minor salivary glands are functioning normally.

## Lymphatic Maladies

With localized areas of inflammation in the oral and maxillofacial tissues, the lymph nodes draining the region may become swollen and painful (Fig. 2–8). Palpation begins beneath the chin for submental lymphadenopathy and lymphadenitis, moving posteriorly medial to the inferior border of the mandible into the digastric (submandibular) triangle; the palpation of the submental and submandibular spaces is most accurately performed bidigitally, with a stabilizing finger intraorally and the palpating fingers extraorally. Next, the palpation is directed inferiorly along the anterior margin of the SCM muscle; the posterior side of the SCM muscle is supported by the fingers of the nonpalpating hand. The anterior border of the SCM is then supported and the posterior border of the SCM muscle is palpated. These palpations of the borders of the SCM should disclose tender or swollen deep cervical chain or superficial cervical chain nodes.

Usually, lymph nodes responding to infection are tender to palpation and, although enlarged, are soft in consistency; this presentation is termed lymphadenitis. Lymphadenopathy—firm in consistency, fixed to surrounding tissues, and nonpainful to palpation—may indicate nodes bearing metastatic neoplasms or chronic, fibrotic nodes from past infection.

## Musculoskeletal System Disorders

Musculoskeletal system disorders are characterized by the patient indicating pain in the area overlying the TMJ, masseter, and/or the temporalis muscle mass. The pain is often of long duration and feels like an overwhelming ache. Muscle tenderness to palpation does not provide a diagnosis; it merely aids in making the diagnosis. The pain may be related to mandibular movements, noxious bruxing or clenching, painful clicking of the TM joint (indicating a painful subluxation of the disk); or blocked movement of the mandible (indicating a dislocation of the disk).

### Myospasms

Muscle pain and dysfunction can be diagnosed by using the history of painful or limited contraction and a systematic palpation of the head and neck muscles (Fig. 2–9). The palpation of head and neck muscle is described in Chapter 7. All of the major muscles of mastication, except the lateral pterygoid, may be palpated. The lateral pterygoid muscle is provoked by placing the thumb on the chin and asking the patient to protrude forward against the thumb. The painful lateral pterygoid muscle produces pain beneath and deep to the zygomatic arch on the affected side during this test.

A number of factors may cause the lateral pterygoid muscle to respond as painful in the provocation test. These factors include painful TM joint degenerative arthritis on the same side as the tender pterygoid. Also, a patient receiving phenothiazines, such as Compazine, may develop painful pterygoids. A pterygomandibular space infection produces both limitation of mandibular movements and painful medial and/or lateral pterygoid muscles, and occlusal factors such as a lateral deviation in the slide from retruded contact to intercuspal position or balancing

**LYMPHATICS**

| | Right | | Left | |
|---|---|---|---|---|
| | N | Ab | N | Ab |
| Submental | | | | |
| Submandibular (Diagastric) | | | | |
| Deep (anterior) cervical chain | | | | |
| Superficial (posterior) cervical chain | | | | |

COMMENTS ON LYMPHATICS EXAMINATIONS (size, texture and tenderness)

_____

_____

_____

_____

_____

_____

_____

*Fig. 2–8.* Lymphatic system evaluation.

**MYOSPASMS**

Palpations

| | Right | | Left | |
|---|---|---|---|---|
| | Yes | No | Yes | No |
| Masseter muscle | | | | |
| anterior-superior quadrant | | | | |
| posterior-superior quadrant | | | | |
| middle zone | | | | |
| inferior zone | | | | |
| Temporalis muscle | | | | |
| anterior zone | | | | |
| posterior zone | | | | |
| Sternocleidomastoid muscle | | | | |
| superior zone | | | | |
| middle zone | | | | |
| inferior zone | | | | |
| Diagastric muscle | | | | |
| anterior belly | | | | |
| posterior belly | | | | |
| Splenius capitis muscle | | | | |
| Trapezius muscle | | | | |
| superior zone | | | | |
| middle zone | | | | |
| inferior zone | | | | |
| Medial pterygoid muscle | | | | |
| inferior zone | | | | |
| middle zone | | | | |
| Lateral pterygoid muscle | | | | |

*Fig. 2–9.* Myospasm evaluation.

interferences may be involved in pterygoid tenderness to palpation.

*Facial Skeletal Deformities*

Some facial skeletal deformities result in head and neck pain and dysfunction (Fig. 2–10). In patients, for example, who have developed a skeletal anterior open bite, an apertognathism, by age 20 or 30 years often experience temporal and/or occipital headaches, temporal and facial pain, and sometimes TMJ pain bilaterally. To determine whether or not the anterior open bite is causing the pain, the patient is fitted with a full arch occlusal splint, providing support and guidance for the anterior teeth or at least support as far forward as the canines with lateral guidance. If these patients, who have been functioning only on second molars, get 100% relief of their temple and occipital headache, tightness across the face, and TMJ pain, the anterior open bite function is likely causing the headaches and the face aches.

With the great attention to detail that is necessary to manage the intricacies of occlusal relations, it is possible to overlook facial skeletal deformities that carry the alveolar processes and teeth to abnormal relationships. Clinical clues to the presence of facial skeletal deformities are seen when the patient must strain the lips and soft tissues over the chin to close the rima oris, when a smile reveals excessive mucoperiosteum apically from the anterior dentition, and when inspection of the profile discloses prognathism or retrognathisms of either or both the mandible and maxilla. Rapid and reliable assessment of the facial skeleton is possible by using Jacobson's templates over lateral cephalometric films, as described in Chapter 8.

*Occlusion and Occlusal Pathofunction-Related Pain*

When the pain is localized in and about the upper and lower dental arches, the teeth are inspected as follows (Fig. 2–11). Probe the gingival sulcus around the teeth for depth and evidence of infection or inflammation. Evaluate any tender teeth by thermal tests, electrovitalometer tests, and by percussion.

**ORTHOGNATHIC RELATIONS**

Major facial skeletal deformity

| | Yes | No |
|---|---|---|
| Maxillary retrognathism | | |
| Maxillary prognathism | | |
| Mandibular retrognathism | | |
| Mandibular prognathism | | |
| Apertognathism | | |
| Long face | | |
| Short face | | |
| Other | | |

COMMENTS ON FACIAL SKELETAL RELATIONSHIPS

_____

_____

_____

_____

_____

_____

_____

_____

*Fig. 2–10.* Orthognathic relationships.

In these tests, the patient is asked to respond. Watch the pupil of the eyes for dilations indicative of painful stimulus responses. The tests are directed at the area of possible pathologic involvement, and contiguous teeth and comparable teeth in the opposite side are stimulated to verify the validity of the patient's responses. During the percussion tests, beside seeking painful and nonpainful responses, be aware of the sound evoked by the percussing instrument, usually the handle of a mouth mirror, as it strikes the teeth; a crisp, musical quality ring indicates the tooth is normal, healthy bone; a dull sound is produced by a tooth not supported in a periodontally sound area.

**Occlusal Pathofunction.** The details of examination of occlusal function are presented in Chapter 9. If the examination of occlusal function demonstrates, for example, posterior interference in protrusion, the patient often complains that they had no pain or discomfort until a crown was seated, and examination of the crown may show that it has been adjusted several times. Another possibility is an excessively high lingual cusp on a lower molar crown that interferes with protrusive movement. This location is checked by using articulating ribbon and having the

patient make a protrusive movement. A triangular ridge that extends up to the cusp tip on lower lingual cusps that interferes with protrusive movements is easy to overlook. The patient experiences complete relief of pain and discomfort when the triangular ridge is adjusted clear of the protrusive excursion.

A plunger cusp may be noted in the area of a deep infrabony pocket, for example, on the mesial of the last mandibular molar. This region is examined by elevating the posterior mandible as described in Chapter 9, with marking ribbon between the teeth to determine the presence of a mesial incline on the lower molar and a distal incline on an upper lingual cusp of the opposing molar that would drive the lower molar distally when biting down. If the incline has been built into a crown on the lower second molar, the lower last molar will be deflected distally when the patient bites, opening up the mesial embrasure between it and the next molar. The food being masticated is then driven into this space between the teeth, and when the mouth opens in the chewing stroke, the last molar moves forward, pumping the food down into the mesial embrasure. If these interfering inclines on the mesial of the lower cusps are

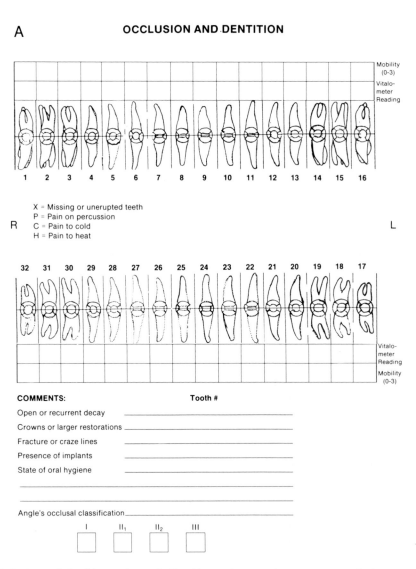

*Fig. 2–11.*   Occlusion and dentition analyses. A, Dentition and supporting structures analysis.

**B**

**OCCLUSAL FUNCTION**

|  | Group Function | Cuspid rise | Balanced |
|---|---|---|---|
| Right side |  |  |  |
| Left side |  |  |  |

|  | Right | | Left | |
|---|---|---|---|---|
|  | Yes | No | Yes | No |
| Centric prematurity |  |  |  |  |
| Lateral deviation in slide from RC to IP |  |  |  |  |
| Lateral guidance by posterior teeth |  |  |  |  |
| Lateral retrusive guidance |  |  |  |  |
| Balancing interference |  |  |  |  |
| Protrusive guidance on posterior teeth |  |  |  |  |
| Teeth in crossbite (#) |  |  |  |  |
|  | Excessive | | Inadequate | |
| Interocclusal distance |  |  |  |  |

## OCCLUSION AND DENTITION

1. Dental arch formation (alignment of the teeth)

2. Compensating curvatures of the dental arches (curved occlusal planes)

3. Compensating curvatures of the individual teeth (curved axes)

4. Angulation of individual teeth in relation to various planes (including root form)

5. Functional form of the teeth at their incisal and occlusal thirds

6. Facial relations of each tooth in one arch to its antagonist or antagonists in the opposing arch in centric occlusion

7. Occlusal contact and intercusp relations of all the teeth of one arch with those in the opposing arch in centric occlusion

8. Occlusal contact and intercusp relations of all the teeth during the various functional mandibular movements

9. Summary

COMMENTS ON OCCLUSAL FUNCTIONS

_____

_____

_____

_____

_____

_____

*Fig. 2–11.* Continued. B, Analyses of occlusal functions.

adjusted, the infrabony pockets reossify and the teeth become firm.

**Arch Form.** The arch form of the patient can be significant in that the patient with a square arch form typically has short heavy muscles. These patients do considerable damage to their teeth when they are bruxists. They hypertrophy their masseter muscles and likely develop a parotid-masseteric hypertrophy traumatic occlusion syndrome, as discussed in Chapter 17.

The patient with a tapering arch form may demonstrate lateral bulging in the preauricular area when the mouth opens wide and the condyles pass anterior to the articular eminence onto the anterior incline. The noncreptis joint sound that results is discussed in Chapter 10.

**Curved Occlusal Planes.** In examining the curve of Spee, the dentist may take note of an excessive occlusal curve on one side and a reversed curve on the opposite side. These patients often have a history of experiencing chronic myofascial pain dysfunction syndromes. When these patients are to have restorative dentistry, or when treatment is required because they are no longer able to cope with their troublesome complaints, the dentist must correct the reversed curve of Spee, which typically requires full upper and lower restoration of the dentition.

**Angulation of Teeth Positions.** In the occlusal examination of a pain patient, teeth in distoversion or mesioversion deserve special attention. These teeth often interfere in the centric relation closure arc, and the interference may produce the pumping action of a plunger cusp as described previously. Adult patient's teeth in linguoversion and buccoversion often can be adjusted to function in those positions without orthodontic alignment. The procedure for occlusal adjustment of a tooth in crossbite does not follow the usual rules for equilibration, because the cuspal relationships are different in a crossbite function. Rotated teeth typically produce interferences in at least one functional excursion, because the transverse ridges interfere with an opposing cuspal guide path.

**Occlusal Contacts in Centric Relationships.** When posterior teeth do not occlude in intercuspal position, the TMJ are examined

with the purpose of determining whether or not a joint space is increased. The growth of a tumor and hemarthrosis or edema in the joint space can lower a condyle and open the occlusion between the posterior teeth.

When an anterior bite is opened, the clinician should examine for any factor that will shorten the height of the ramus. This situation arises after fracture of the condylar neck as well as in patients with advanced rheumatoid arthritis when the condyle has eroded, decreasing its vertical dimension. The patient with rheumatoid arthritis may give a history of rapid development of an anterior open bite.

**Occlusal Contacts During Mandibular Movements.** Crossover abrasive facets are typically seen in the incisal edges of the twelve anterior teeth. In the patient with crossover bruxism, obvious notching of the teeth, with shiny abraded surfaces, is evidence of the diagnosis of crossover bruxing. Two apparent signs of bruxism are elevator muscle tenderness and more pronounced abrasive facets on the teeth than could be produced by diet or is appropriate given the age of the patient. Therefore, advanced abrasive facets are an indication that the patient has been or is a bruxist.

**Isometric Mandibular Posturing.** Isometric mandibular posturing is an unusual type of noxious habit. Patients do not brux or clench the teeth together but, at a small amount of opening, they antagonistically contract elevator muscles against depressor muscles. The muscles may become hypertrophic and TM joint intracapsular painful dysfunctions may occur similar to that affecting the patient who clenches or bruxes. This condition can also be treated with the repeat timer method of biofeedback (see Chapter 9).

*Temporomandibular Joint Pain*

**Static Palpation.** Static palpation is used to determine whether or not equal palpating pressure bilaterally on the lateral poles, the lateral posterior of the condyles, and then with superior loading of the condyles produce unilateral or bilateral pain or tenderness (Fig. 2–12). Only 48% of patients with TM joint degenerative arthritis have tenderness at one lateral pole of the condyle, and almost all of

**TEMPOROMANDIBULAR JOINT**

Palpation

**Static**

|  | Right | | | Left | | |
|---|---|---|---|---|---|---|
|  | Yes | Slgt. | No | Yes | Slgt. | No |
| Lateral pole, closed |  |  |  |  |  |  |
| Lateral pole, open |  |  |  |  |  |  |
| Anterior lateral superior condylar head, impact loading |  |  |  |  |  |  |

(Picture of dynamic points: early, late, crest, end point)

Auscultation (crepitus)

|  |  | Coarse | | Fine | |
|---|---|---|---|---|---|
|  |  | Yes | No | Yes | No |
| Right | Vertical |  |  |  |  |
|  | Right lateral |  |  |  |  |
|  | Left lateral |  |  |  |  |
| Left | Vertical |  |  |  |  |
|  | Right lateral |  |  |  |  |
|  | Left lateral |  |  |  |  |

**Dynamic**

|  |  | Early | Late | Crest | End pt. |
|---|---|---|---|---|---|
| Right | Opening movement |  |  |  |  |
|  | Closing movement |  |  |  |  |
| Left | Opening movement |  |  |  |  |
|  | Closing movement |  |  |  |  |

Range of motion in millimeters

|  | mm | Deviation | |
|---|---|---|---|
|  |  | L | R |
| Maximum vertical |  |  |  |
| Protrusive |  |  |  |
| Right lateral |  |  |  |
| Left lateral |  |  |  |

Auscultation (click)

|  |  | Early | Late | Crest | End pt. |
|---|---|---|---|---|---|
| Right | Opening vertical |  |  |  |  |
|  | Closing vertical |  |  |  |  |
|  | Right Lateral |  |  |  |  |
|  | Left Lateral |  |  |  |  |
| Left | Opening vertical |  |  |  |  |
|  | Closing vertical |  |  |  |  |
|  | Right Lateral |  |  |  |  |
|  | Left Lateral |  |  |  |  |

COMMENTS ON MUSCLE AND TMJ EXAMINATIONS (Including meniscus subluxation and dislocation)

_____

_____

_____

_____

*Fig. 2–12.* Temporomandibular joint analyses.

rheumatoid arthritis patients have bilateral condylar pole tenderness. The degenerative arthritic tenderness typically is unilateral or one side is more tender than the other. The patient with tenderness to palpation behind the condyle in the wide open position, i.e., the lateral posterior of the condyle, often has an anteriorly displaced disk with retrodiskal inflammation.

The patient with tenderness on bilateral superior loading of the condyles into the fossa likely has an anterior displaced disk with retrodiskal tissue that is innervated and inflamed, along with hyperplasia of endothelium in the blood vessels within the joint space. No pain whatsoever on superior loading of the condyle does not necessarily mean that the disk is in a normal position in that joint. Such a patient may have a loud reciprocal click with opening and closing. We have classified this click as the eighth type of noncrepitus joint sound in Chapter 10.

**Dynamic Palpation.** When the static palpation is completed, the dynamic palpation is performed as follows. With the index fingers placed just anterior to the tragus, ask the patient to open and close slowly. Note where in the open and/or closing that a deflection of tissue occurs and identify which direction of deflection the tissue takes. The patient repeats the opening and closing movements of the mandible until the approximate location of the opening click is localized, in the first fourth, one half, two thirds, or three fourths of opening or at full opening; the closing click is localized in the same manner. The location of opening and closing clicks are recorded. Noting the direction of deflection of tissue at the time of the click is important in differentiating the first and second types of noncrepitus joint sounds (see Chapter 10).

**Auscultation Devices.** Many auscultation devices can be used to evaluate TM joint function, including Doppler units, the digital stethoscope, electronic stethoscope, and standard stethoscopes. The authors have noted that a Doppler unit amplifies crepitus beyond what one can detect with the standard stethoscope. The click type sound with meniscus-condyle discoordination is obviously audible, yet it is not amplified to the extent that crepitus is amplified when using

Doppler techniques. When using Doppler instruments the transducer head must be held lightly against the skin in the lubricating medium and any extraneous movement of the transducer head produces a loud crackling sound that obscures crepitus. Courses in instruction in its use are needed before a Doppler unit can be used reliably. Doppler auscultation may have a high correlation to anatomic and pathologic findings during subsequent surgery. It is a cost effective method for analyzing, as an outpatient modality, the progress of patients.[1]

**Stethoscopic Auscultation.** When the TM joint is auscultated with a standard stethoscope, the contralateral TMJ should be palpated simultaneously. If a sound is audible at the instant that a deflection of tissue is perceived under the palpating finger, the meniscus-condyle discoordination is probably located on the palpated side rather than on the auscultated side.

The TM joint is auscultated both vertically and horizontally. The patient opens and closes the mouth slowly. Then, with the teeth slightly separated, the mandible is moved slowly to the right and left maximally. If auscultation does not include both vertical and horizontal function, some crepitus may be missed in the degenerative arthritic patient. Degenerative arthritis may be silent with opening and closing, but loud crepitus may be heard at one lateral extreme. From 33 to 50% of patients with normal joints have a sound at the approach of maximum opening and when just leaving maximum opening.[2,3] The normal joint may be silent only within the usual functional range. A deflection of the skin beneath the stethoscope at maximum opening owing to condylar movement often initiates a sound that is mistaken for a joint sound.

Crepitus is typically equated with degenerative changes in the joint. Fine crepitus is typically associated with fibrillation or roughening of the bony articular surfaces or the surface of the disk, whereas coarse crepitus is associated with perforation of the disk. Popping, clicking, or snapping sounds are typically associated with a displacement of the disk during function.

**Range of Mandibular Motion.** The range

of motion is measured and recorded. The maximum amount of vertical opening is measured as described in Chapter 10, and the maximum opening vertically should be 45 or more millimeters. This distance is typically equal to placing three fingers sideways between the incisal edges of the anterior teeth. Protrusive movements of the mandible should be approximately 10 mm, with a range of 6 to 14 mm, and right and left lateral movements should be approximately 8 mm, with a range of 6 to 11 mm in the adult. Asymmetry in maximum lateral movement is an indication of pathology of dysfunction. If the patient moves 8 mm to the right but only 2 or 3 mm to the left, the right condyle is not translating as it should. Lack of translation may be the result of intra-articular fibrosis, blocking by a displaced disk, or spasm or contracture in the elevator muscles.

**Meniscus Dysfunction Test.** The tests for meniscus dysfunction summarized in this chapter are described in Chapter 10. The *cotton roll test* is used in the patient with degenerative arthritis to determine whether or not a splint would be beneficial. The patient bites down into the cotton rolls placed between the posterior teeth. After the patient bites maximally the second or third time, the cotton rolls are removed and the patient bites maximally without cotton rolls in place. The patient is then asked which hurts more, biting on the cotton rolls or biting on the teeth. The patient that gets relief from the arthralgia when biting on the cotton rolls will benefit from the use of a bite splint. If pain increases with biting on the cotton rolls, a splint would not be of benefit.

The *protrusive-retrusive test* not only identifies or helps to identify an anterior displaced disk, but also helps to identify the registration for the mounting of an anterior repositioning splint. The patient's casts are mounted just anterior to the retrusive click when performing this test. The patient protrudes until a click occurs keeping the anterior teeth together. Then, the mandible is retruded to the point that the patient feels the disk is just ready to click. The patient with an anterior displaced disk can identify this point precisely. The patient then opens the mouth and taps the teeth right at that position, typically

reproducing the position with accuracy. This area is the location of the registration for the construction of an anterior repositioning splint.

The *repositioned trapped disk test*, as described in Chapter 10, is often called the romancing test. The patient opens the mandible until the opening click occurs. The clinician grasps the mandible with a bimandibular manipulation, torquing superiorly as the condyle disk assembly is gently manipulated (romanced) up into the fossa while slowly closing the mouth. Pressure is maintained at all times superiorly at the angle of the mandible; if the condyle disk assembly can be seated all the way into the roof of the fossa, then the disk is considered recapturable, i.e., it is not foreshortened, it still has a concavity, and it has a sufficiently thick posterior band to position itself behind the condyle if repositioning splint therapy is attempted.

The *temporary malocclusion test*, sometimes called the instant malocclusion test, demonstrates that a small shim, the anterior displaced disk, can be manipulated into and out of position, lowering or raising the condyle that opens or closes the occlusion of the posterior teeth beneath that condyle. The clinician can also use this demonstration to teach the patient that the problem is in the joint, not in the teeth.

The details of these four tests for determining whether or not an anterior displaced disk can be recaptured are described in Chapter 10.

## Imaging

Different types of TM joint radiographs may be used when screening a pain patient for a suspected intra-articular origin of pain (Fig. 2–13).

### Screening Radiographs

Screening images often are the lateral transcranial radiograph or a panoramic TM joint view. With these images, the lateral lip of the glenoid fossa is examined for the contour, whether a steep or flat eminence is present, whether the surface of the fossa lateral margin is smooth or irregular, whether the surface is sclerotic, whether the articular eminence is

**IMAGERY FINDINGS**

Temporomandibular joint

| | | | Right | | Left | |
|---|---|---|---|---|---|---|
| | | | Yes | No | Yes | No |
| Glenoid Fossae | Normal contours | | | | | |
| | Irregular surface | | | | | |
| | Sclerotic | | | | | |
| | Enlarged | | | | | |
| | Other | | | | | |
| Articular Eminences | Normal contours | | | | | |
| | Flattened | | | | | |
| | Steep | | | | | |
| | Osteophyte | | | | | |
| | Central radioluncency | | | | | |
| | Sclerotic | | | | | |
| | Other | | | | | |

| | | | Ovoid | Flat | Angular | Round | Concave |
|---|---|---|---|---|---|---|---|
| Condyles | Frontal view | right | | | | | |
| | | left | | | | | |

| | | | Right | | Left | |
|---|---|---|---|---|---|---|
| | | | Yes | No | Yes | No |
| | Lateral view, normal contours | | | | | |
| | Ely's cysts | | | | | |
| | Sclerosis | | | | | |
| | Erosion | Medial | | | | |
| | | Lateral | | | | |
| | | Central | | | | |
| | Atrophy | | | | | |
| | Osteophytes | Spike | Posterior | | | | |
| | | | Middle | | | | |
| | | Shelf | Anterior | | | | |
| | | | Lateral | | | | |
| | | | Posterior | | | | |
| | | Plateau | Middle | | | | |
| | | | Lateral | | | | |
| | Displacement | | | | | |
| | Other | | | | | |

| | No | Yes |
|---|---|---|
| Bilateral symmetry of intracapsular spaces | | |
| Angle of condylar long axes to sagittal plane (SMV) | o | o |

Arthrograms

| | Right | | Left | |
|---|---|---|---|---|
| | Yes | No | Yes | No |
| Normal superior cavity outline | | | | |
| Normal inferior cavity outline | | | | |
| Anterior subluxation of disc | | | | |
| Anterior dislocation of disc | | | | |
| Disc perforation | | | | |
| Disc adhesions — superior cavity | | | | |
| Disc adhesions — inferior cavity | | | | |

and other medical imagery

| | Yes | No | Month/year |
|---|---|---|---|
| Panoramic, routine | | | |
| Transpharyngeal, TMJ | | | |
| Transcranial, TMJ | | | |
| Panoramic, TMJ | | | |
| Transorbital, TMJ | | | |
| Submental vertex | | | |
| Laminographic, TMJ | | | |
| Arthrograms | | | |
| Paranasal sinus views | | | |
| Cephalometric views | | | |
| Periapical views | | | |
| Occlusal views | | | |
| Bite wing views | | | |
| CT scan | | | |
| Bone scan | | | |
| N.M.R. | | | |
| Thermograms | | | |

COMMENTS ON IMAGERY FINDINGS

_____

_____

_____

_____

_____

_____

_____

_____

_____

_____

_____

_____

*Fig. 2–13.*  Imagery findings.

pneumatized, and whether the fossa is enlarged. The articular eminence is examined for contour, the presence or absence of an anterior incline; the character of an inclined plane, possible erosions and flattening; and the presence of osteophytes spurs. A pneumatized eminence could have significance if surgical contouring of the eminence is planned. These air cells often are easily identified in lateral transcranial and panoramic TM joint radiographs. We have noted a common presence of mastoid air cells in the eminence of patients who have the number 3 and 4 type of joint sounds. These patients have a short, bulbous articular eminence with an anterior incline. The condyle is positioned, not only anterior to the crest of the eminence in the open view, but also superior to the lateral lip of the articular eminence.

From the frontal view the condyles are often asymmetric, but a rounded or bulbous condyle noted unilaterally typically indicates the involvement of a pathologic process.[4,5]

## Degenerative Arthritis

Ely cysts, as described in Chapter 11, are marrow spaces filled with collagen beneath eroded articular surfaces in joints with degenerative arthritis. When degenerative arthritis goes into its fourth stage or in the reparative stage, the articular surface often appears sclerotic. When the articular surface of the condyle displays irregular erosions, degenerative arthritis is included as the primary differential diagnosis. An atrophied condyle is typically associated with the erosion that occurs in rheumatoid arthritis.

## Displaced TM Joint Disks

A posterior inferior placement of the condyle in a lateral, transcranial radiograph is not pathognomonic of an anteriorly displaced disk. It often coincides, however, with the other examination data and is confirmatory of an internal derangement or anterior displaced disk in a patient. Because normal joints show condyles that are posteriorly displaced, superiorly displaced, and anteriorly displaced, this condylar position is not pathognomonic of a specific problem.

## Arthographic Examinations

The use of TM joint arthrography is described in Chapter 3. The authors use five indications for performing arthrography. First, to identify an internal derangement, we use a fluoroscopic inferior cavity arthrogram. The fluid can be observed to deflect back and forth on the bottom of the disk with opening and closing while viewing the fluoroscope. Second, arthrography reveals perforations of the disk. An inferior cavity arthrogram is performed, but 3 ml rather than 1 or 1.5 ml of dye are injected into the cavity; the radiograph displays dye filling both cavities. Third, arthrographic laminograms identify defects in form of both the superior and the inferior cavity. The laminographic arthrogram visualizes the fluid as it deflects into concavities in either the condyle or the glenoid fossa-articular eminence. Fourth, fibrous adhesions prevent the flow of the dye into the region that is adhered by fibrosis. In the inferior cavity, if the lateral pole of the condyle is adherent to the disk, the dye does not flow into that region during opening and closing in the views on the fluoroscope. The fifth indication for arthrography is if it is required for records to verify clinical findings. The use of other medical imaging techniques are discussed in Chapter 3.

## Other Medical Imaging Modalities

Magnetic resonance imaging (MRI), an application of nuclear magnetic resonance spectroscopy, is not hazardous to the patient, aside from the effect of the magnetic field on metallic objects. The resulting images may display the soft tissues in exquisite detail. As MRI technology evolves, it will be even more useful in analyses of the TM joint.

Computer tomography (CT) is produced by a combination of x-ray scanning and digital computer technology. The resultant images are optically clear slices of the antomy being examined. The TM joint, for example may be observed without superimposition of overlying and underlying structures. The CT program may be instructed to provide images that emphasize either hard or soft tissue structures. Three dimensional reconstructions are possible to show stunning details as viewed from all the different planes. Color coding of the images of structures may be produced with special equipment and programs.

### Sinal Pain

The acute problems of the sinus usually are simple to identify, but the chronic, unusual problems of inflammations and neoplasia are made difficult by neurologic factors of referred pain and radiated pain, as described in Chapter 16. The pains originating from the sinal areas may mimic those of musculoskeletal, vascular, neurologic, and psychopathologic origin.

### Psychopathology

When asked to indicate precisely the location of the pain, the patient may have a problem in indicating a single location, and often describing or indicating the pain as bilateral. The patient uses words that have emotional connotation, such as "punishing pain." The patient's behavior may seem inappropriate to the chief complaint pain. The history reveals signs of psychopathology such as a description of unrealistic signs and symptoms and body language of extreme stress, as described in Chapter 5. A preliminary indication of psychopathology can be determined by using the Impath program. In this analysis, the patient is placed before a computer terminal and is asked to just answer Y or N, yes or no, to the questions displayed on the screen monitor of the computer. The IMPATH:TMJ[6] microcomputer assessment of behavioral and psychosocial factors in cranial and mandibular disorders provides an immediate analysis as soon as the patient has completed answering the questions. The patient must answer each question, because the computer does not go to the next question until the patient enters either a Yes or No (Fig. 2–14). A patient can leave no blanks in questions they do not wish to answer. Significant insight into behavior and psychosocial factors in the life of the patient are provided by this program. A relative disadvantage of this technique is that a patient may take 1 or 2 hours to complete the examination, so the computer terminal is occupied for extended periods for each patient.

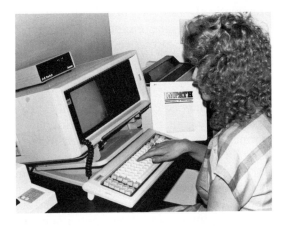

*Fig. 2–14.* IMPATH:TMJ microcomputer assessment. Typical scene of patient responding to questions asked by the computer program.

An advantage is that the program provides a detailed printout for the clinician as well as a shorter version that may be given to the patient.

Another excellent program for diagnosing psychologic factors is provided by the TMJ Scale.[7,8] The TMJ Scale provides a comprehensive assessment of individuals and of groups of patients with TMJ-related disorders. As a clinical investigative assessment, it affirms the " . . . basic premise that TMJ disorders cannot be defined by using a . . . single symptom approach for evaluation and management."[9] As a practical tool for individual patient evaluation, the TMJ Scale gives the doctor a patient-generated device to provide a multidimensional assessment of signs and symptoms of somatic and psychologic maladies related to the TM joint as compared to odontogenic disorders.

## References

1. Davidson S.L.: Doppler auscultation: an aid in temporomandibular joint diagnosis. J Craniomand Disord Facial Oral Pain, 2:128, 1988.
2. Muhl Z.F., et al.: Occurrence of TMJ sounds with jaw movement. J Dent Res, 65:335, 1986.
3. Gay T., et al.: The acoustical characteristics of the normal and abnormal temporomandibular joint. J Oral Maxillofac Surg, 45:397, 1987.
4. Yale S.H., et al.: An epidemiological assessment of mandibular condyle morphology. Oral Surg, 21:169, 1966.
5. Emmering T.E.: A new approach to the analysis of the functional surfaces of the temporomandibular joint. Oral Surg, 21:603, 1967.

6. Fricton J., Nelson A., and Monsein M.: Impath: Microcomputer assessment of behavioral and psychosocial factors in cranial mandibular disorders. J Craniomandib Pract, 5:372, 1987.

7. Lundeen T.F., Levitt S.R., and McKinney M.W.: Evaluation of TMJ disorders by clinician ratings. J Prosthet Dent, 59:202, 1988.

8. Levitt S.R., McKinney M.W., and Lundeen T.F.: The TMJ Scale: Cross-validation and reliability studies. J Craniomandib Pract, 6:18, 1988.

9. Levitt S.R., Lundeen T.F., and McKinney M.W.: Initial studies of a new assessment method for temporomandibular joint disorders. J Prosthet Dent, 59:490, 1988.

# 3

# *Imaging*

In 1895, Wilhelm Konrad Roentgen, a German physicist, obtained an x-ray image of his wife's hand and thus opened the door for the development of noninvasive information about the interior of the body. Conventional radiographic equipment and techniques improved during the next 50 years, mostly for studies of lung and bone, and in the 1950s, ultrasonography and nuclear medicine studies became available. As computers developed and were married to radiographic imaging capabilities, an explosion in new techniques occurred, including computed tomography (CT), magnetic resonance imaging (MRI), and single photon emission computed tomography (SPECT).

Images are now an adjunct to clinical diagnoses. As a permanent technical record of the patient's condition at the time the image was obtained, imaging can be repeated later and the images utilized for comparison studies. Therefore, medical imaging allows assessment of both form and function and registers the response to therapy or the rate of progression of a disease process.

Techniques especially applicable to head and neck imaging, and that are discussed in this chapter, are film radiography using outpatient dental equipment; xeroradiography; linear tomography; both linear and corrected polycycloidal arthrography; CT; nuclear medicine and SPECT studies; Doppler information; thermograms; and ultrasonography.

Traditional radiography remains a standard for outpatient and many inpatient examinations for the foreseeable future because of the high resolution of images, many indications and applications, and world-wide availability and understanding of the interpretations. Improvements of standard techniques applicable to dentistry have been made, however, including polycycloidal corrected tomography, temporomandibular joint (TMJ) arthrography, image subtraction, and xeroradiography.

Polycycloidal corrected tomographs of the TMJ provide clear laminographic planes every 1 or 2 mm of the condyle and glenoid fossa as viewed from both the anterior aspect perpendicular to the long axis of the condyle and from the lateral aspect in line with the axis of the condyle. Arthrograms of the TM joint

have been used to validate the clinical impressions of subluxation versus dislocation of the meniscus, perforations in the menisci, defects in form of articular surfaces, and fibrous adhesions. Xeroradiography, a diagnostic imaging technique, involves a photocopying process to record radiographic images; when compared to conventional film views, these images have a wider exposure latitude and greater detail and density differences. Arthroscopic examinations can capture detailed views of the superior joint space. CT can display static views of the details of bone and soft tissues. MRI provides graphic details of soft tissue.

The repertory of diagnostic methods includes evolving techniques that are changing "radiologic examinations" to "medical imaging." Signals generated by radioactive labeling isotopes, by tomography, by magnetic nuclear scanning, and by ultrasonography have been married to computer techniques to be converted into images. The images, in many instances, are available either color coded or in the usual black, white, and shades of grey. Medical imaging techniques of special interest are CT, nuclear imaging, SPECT, ultrasonography, and MRI. The latter two methods and thermography, a topical registration of minute temperature changes, do not involve exposure to radiation and, hence, may be attractive from a biologic health standpoint.

## Outpatient Radiography of the TM Joint

For decades, outpatient, extraoral radiography of the TM joint using dental and panoramic equipment has been a fundamental tool in assessing the TM joint. The most common techniques are the transcranial, the transpharyngeal, the transorbital, and the panoramic views. Techniques recommended for achieving these views are designed to meet these objectives: to produce minimal distortion of the images; to meet radiologic standards of safety; to keep the patient in a standardized, comfortable position; to have the alignment of the patient, machine, and film easily visualized; and, in one variation of the transcranial view, to keep the number of accessories to a minimum by using only a lead apron for the patient and a ruler for estimating the direction of the central ray. The radiologic safety factors are met by having the target-to-skin distance no less than 20 cm, keeping the x-ray beam diameter confined to the size of the film, and, when using cassettes, using high speed intensifying screens and film.

The variation in the normal anatomy of the condyle and condylar neck need to be appreciated (Fig. 3–1). The condyle has several variations in form as visualized from an anterior aspect. The anterior neck of the condyle has a variety of configurations for insertion of the lateral pterygoid muscle. The fossa for insertion of the lateral pterygoid muscle may be so deep that it may resemble a central lesion of the condylar neck when viewed on a radiographic film. Anecdotal histories recount surgical explorations, and in at least one case, excision of the head and neck of the condyle based, in part, on the radiographic representation of the pterygoid muscle insertion fossa that resembled a central radiolucent lesion of the condylar neck. These two variations of normal, the variety of condylar heads and the variations of contours of the anterior aspect of the condylar process, must be appreciated when studying images of the area.

## Transcranial Radiographs

The transcranial radiograph displays the lateral one half to one third of the condyle (Fig. 3–2). The appearance of the condyle varies depending on the position of the central ray and its intersection with the cortical margins of the condyle. The need for the head to be oriented to permit passage of the central ray without being obscured by the petrous portion of the temporal bone produces an oblique view of the condyle and its articulating surface. The angulation to the sagittal plane of the long axis of the condyle varies among individuals, and this angulation must be considered when interpreting a radiographic image of the condyle. The superior-inferior angle of the central ray, however, may produce an image in which the joint space appears reduced if the central ray is either too low[1] or, as the authors have found, too high.

A variety of angle boards and head holders have been devised to orient the patient's head (Fig. 3–3). These devices endeavor to produce the best angle for the central ray to enter the contralateral side of the patient's head with the objective of passing in planes that compensate for the angle of the long axis of the condyle to the sagittal plane and for the angle

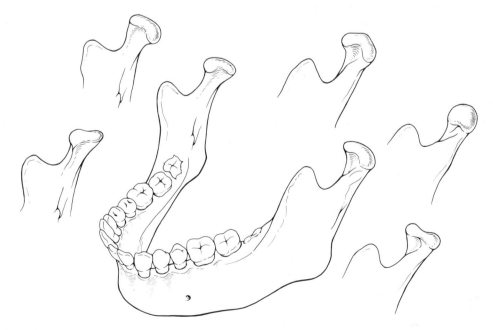

*Fig. 3–1.*   Variations in osseous anatomy of mandibular condyles.

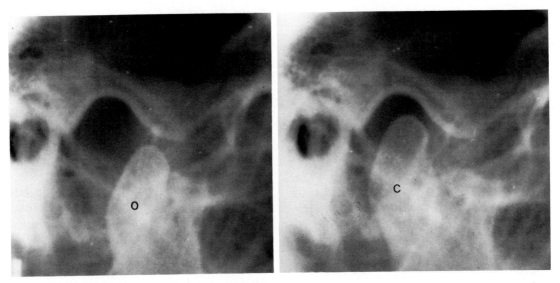

*Fig. 3–2.*   Transcranial lateral radiograph of the mandibular condyle in open and closed positions. The bony outlines of the glenoid fossa, articular eminence, and external auditory canal are clearly seen. The mandibular condyle is identified seated within the glenoid fossa in the closed views (c). With the mouth open (o), the mandibular condyle can be seen anteriorly translocated to the level of the articular eminence; there is no objective means of determining whether the limit of condyle excursion has been reached during filming. Note that the condylar lateral pole is always superior, regardless of the configuration of the condyle, and the medial pole is inferior in the transcranial lateral projection film. In this film, the normal texture of the cancellous bone in the condyle can be seen, and there are no scleroses, osteophytes, or irregularities apparent on the articulating surface of the condyle.

that avoids the petrous portion of the temporal bone. The objectives that Lindblom described in 1936 are fundamental: first, to project the condyle "onto the plate (film) in pure profile . . . ," and second, to direct the beam through as few bony areas as possible.[2] The pure profile objective is not possible with transcranial views, but variations of the technique have been used by many practitioners to the benefit of their patients. Aquilino and associates, however, found that even with a dry skull, condyle and fossa relationships cannot be classified reliably by evaluation of TM joint views produced by using lateral oblique transcranial techniques.[3]

### Mongini-Preti Craniostat

Because it is adjustable and it is used by the authors, the Mongini-Preti Craniostat is described. The patient is positioned in the Craniostat with ear plugs in each ear, the nose tip is aligned with a plastic marker, a resting plate is then fixed against the occiput, and a plastic support is adjusted against the nasion.

When the patient is comfortably positioned, the angle of the Craniostat arm is set at 25° to the horizontal plane and 17° to the coronal plane of the patient's head. The indicator light is turned on and the Craniostat arm is adjusted so that the light on the patient's face is located over the lateral pole of the condyle just anterior to the tragus. The light is then turned off and the cassette holder is moved against the patient's face. The x-ray tube is positioned against the collimator housing. The film in the cassette is positioned to the first marker, the patient closes into the intercuspal position, and the film is exposed. The cassette is moved to the second marker, the patient is instructed to position the mandible at rest or at maximum opening, as desired, and the film is exposed. Often a radiograph of the TM joint is needed to show a condylar change of position when a splint or dental restoration is in place so additional exposures are made with the appliance in position.

After imaging one side, the Craniostat arm is removed, turned 180°, and replaced in its holder. The procedure, as just described, is repeated for the opposite side.

Because of the long target-to-film distance with the Craniostat, the image of the TMJ

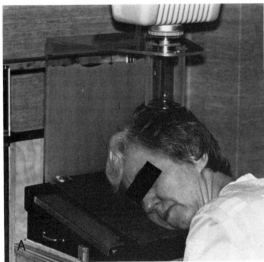

*Fig. 3–3.* Transcranial radiographic techniques for the TM joint. A. Updegrave angle board. B. AXA (Anatomical x-ray aligner) head and film holder. C. Mongini-Preti Craniostat. D. Position of machine and patient without using accessories.

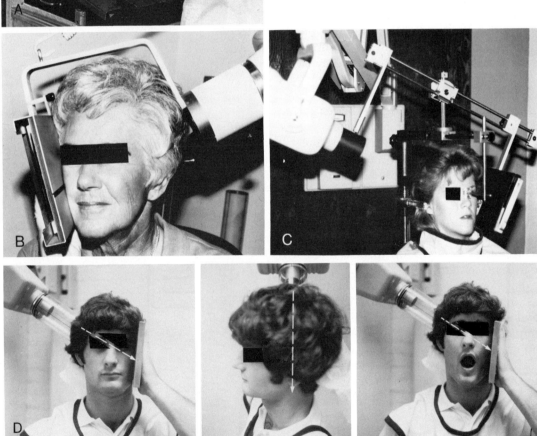

structures is not enlarged appreciably, which provides an image of the joint without the slight artifact of enlargement from diverging beams of x-rays.

For examination of an adult, the technical settings of the x-ray unit are: 75 kVp, 10 mA, and 48 impulses.

### Transcranial Technique without Accessories

A reasonable view may be obtained without the use of an angle board or a modified x-ray machine. The vertical angulation of the x-ray beam is set at 25° inferiorly. To pass the central ray tangentially to the condyle, a point of entry of the central ray is established by measuring 6 cm vertically above the superior edge of the condyle and 3 cm posteriorly. The horizontal angulation of the x-ray beam is chosen so that the central ray emerges at the articulation to be examined; a ruler or rod is useful to position the head of the x-ray machine to deliver the central ray on the course described. The central ray is centered by sighting first over the patient's head and then sighting from in front of the patient. Exact centering of the point of exit of the central ray is most important in this technique.

The film holder is placed against the zygomatic arch, angle of the mandible, and the ear. The holder is supported by the palm of the hand of the patient. To show a second view of the articulation on the same film, the film holder is shifted to bring a new area of film adjacent to the TMJ, and a different position of the condyle (open, rest, or closed) may be recorded.

For examination of an adult, the technical settings of the x-ray unit are 70 kVp, 15 mA, and 10 impulses when using a short cone, 20 impulses when using a long cone. A lead diaphragm containing a 1-cm circular aperture must be inserted within the cone to decrease the scattered radiation and to concentrate the x-ray beam to the size of the film to be exposed.

### Transpharyngeal Radiographs

A transpharyngeal radiograph provides a tangential view of the medial pole of the condyle, which is not seen in a lateral transcranial radiograph. This view is helpful when path-

ologic involvement of the medial pole is suspected. In children, the condyle is not well ossified and does not register on a lateral transcranial radiograph, because the x-ray beam passes through the parietal bone, the brain posterior to sella turcica, and the roof of the glenoid fossa before striking the surfaces of the joint. With the transpharyngeal radiographs, the target-to-film distance is short and only a thin plate of bone of the mandibular ramus below the sigmoid notch, the pterygoid muscles, palatine tonsils and the air of the oral pharynx affect the beam of x-rays before reaching the TM joint structures (Fig. 3–4).

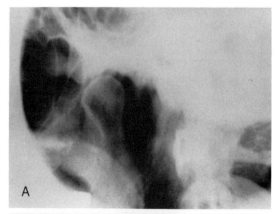

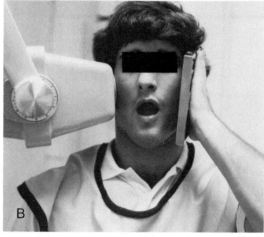

*Fig. 3–4.* Transpharyngeal radiographic technique for the TM joint. A. Normal, asymptomatic condylar process of the patient viewed with the transpharyngeal technique. Note that the condylar lateral pole is always anterior, regardless of the configuration of the condyle, and the medial pole is posterior in the transpharyngeal film. B. Transpharyngeal radiographic technique. A pillow may be added to support the cassette.

To produce a transpharyngeal radiograph, the target-to-skin distance must be no less than 8 inches (20 cm) to meet radiologic standards. This standard distance may be achieved by using a recessed head x-ray machine with the cone removed; the collimation and filtration units are left in place with the x-ray head lightly touching the face. With a nonrecessed head machine, the 20-cm measurement is made with a cone of an appropriate length, or if the cone is removed, from the x-ray port of the machine to skin. The patient is upright in the chair with the head supported. The x-ray housing is positioned against the preauricular region of the face and angled superiorly 10°. The patient opens the mouth widely and moves the mandible toward the x-ray head as far as possible. The translating condylar lateral pole is palpated during this movement, and the assistant places a finger on the lateral pole and holds it as the patient maintains the mandible in the lateral position. The palpation and holding of the lateral pole may be accomplished, in some instances, by the patient. The clinician or radiologic technologist stands in front of the patient and adjusts the x-ray head vertically so the central ray passes through the palpating finger tip. The clinician or technologist moves behind the x-ray head and rotates it horizontally to direct the central beam through the condyle as indicted by the palpating finger tip. The palpating finger is removed, and the patient maintains the mandibular position. The cassette is positioned perpendicularly to the central ray on a pillow on the patient's shoulder, and the patient holds the cassette against the face.

The film is exposed at 75 kVp, 10 mA, and 6 impulses (1 per 10 second). The process is then repeated for the opposite side.

### Transorbital Radiographs*

The transorbital radiograph provides a frontal view of the mandibular condyle (Fig. 3–5). The frontal view assists the clinician in

*We extend our appreciation to Dr. Jaru R. Patel, the University of Alabama School of Dentistry, and Mr. Albert Richards, University of Michigan School of Dentistry, for their instruction and assistance with many of the outpatient radiographic techniques.

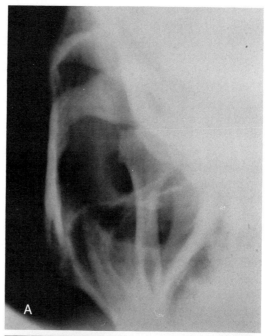

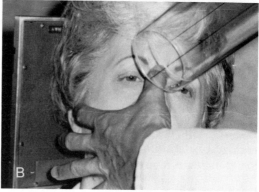

*Fig. 3–5.* Transorbital view of the TM joint condyle. A. Note osteophytes on the lateral margin of the condyle; these were not visible on transcranial, transpharyngeal, tomographic, and panoramic x-ray views. B. Position of the patient and equipment to produce a transorbital frontal view of the condyle.

interpreting images produced from the lateral aspect. Normally shaped condyles may be misinterpreted as involving pathologic changes on the basis of their appearance on a lateral view. For example, an excessive amount of cortical plate may be perceived from a lateral view (this has been called marbleized bone) when the patient actually has a flat condyle, the x-ray beam simply having passed down the long axis of the cortex. Similarly, an interpretation of a decreased or irregular cortical covering of the condyle may result from an image in which the x-ray beam passed through a condyle that is domed or triangular or is flat but steeply angulated in reference to the sagittal plane. On a few occasions, osteophytes and arthritic changes that could not be detected with other radiologic views, including lateral perspective linear tomograms, have been disclosed with a transorbital view.

The transorbital view is produced with the patient positioned comfortably seated or reclining; the positioning is not critical if the alignment between the central ray, the patient's head, and the x-ray film plate is correct. The film is positioned behind the patient's head at right angles to the central ray. The central ray is directed through the inner canthus area of the eye on the same side as the TMJ being examined. The patient's mouth is open, bringing the condyle anterior and slightly inferior on the articular eminence of the temporal bone, and the exposure is made. On some individuals, because of anatomical variations, it is not possible to produce this x-ray view.

## Panoramic Radiographs

Panoramic x-ray equipment can produce excellent lateral views of the TM joint. The radiographs are similar to those produced by the transpharyngeal views with the advantage that a closed mouth position, with the condyle seated in the glenoid fossa, is possible. This image is obtained because the panoramic view is a modified laminographic technique and the spinal column does not completely obstruct the passage of the x-ray beam.

The lateral views of the TM joint may be produced by two different techniques (Fig. 3–6). One technique produces two or three images per side, four to six images on the same film. The patient's head is lowered by adjusting the guides that govern the vertical position of the patient's head. This positioning moves images of the TM joint to the horizontal central part of the film. A series of exposures are made of the TM joint, as indicated, with the patient closing firmly in centric, opening to the rest position, and then wide opening. Before each exposure, with

machines that can be reversed, the x-ray tube and the film holder are returned to the beginning position for the side being examined.

Alternatively, with similar patient positioning, standard rotation of the tube and film is performed with the production of an image of the entire mandible in the selected condyle to fossa position.

For examination of an adult, the technical settings of the x-ray unit are 90 kVp, 12 mA, and exposure at 2 seconds to produce six images (three per side) and 3 seconds to produce four images (two per side). Standard exposure is used for production of an image of the total mandible. The plane of focus is adjusted according to the machine being used; e.g., when using the GE Panelipse machine, the usual plane of focus is at 9 cm.

A logical modification for the panoramic view of the condyle was described by Chilvarquer and associates.[4] They positioned the patient to permit the central ray to pass along the assumed long axis of the condyle. The result was greater anatomic clarity than that achieved with the conventional position in which the central ray passes from anterior to posterior at an acute angle to the long axis of the condyle.

## Digital Image Enhancement

The process of digital subtraction consists of scanning radiographic images and digitizing with a pixel by pixel format. Intensity values of the digitized second image are subtracted from the original radiograph to produce a third, subtracted image. The third image has enhanced contrast and crisp margins and is useful for analysis of the mandibular condyle.[5] Digital imaging processing is applied to periapical and panoramic radiographs.[6,7]

## Xeroradiography

Xeroradiography (XR) differs from conventional radiography in that the radiograph is replaced by the technology used in the Xerox office copier. This system is a photoelectrostatic rather than the conventional photochemical process, and it is based on the properties of materials known as photocon-

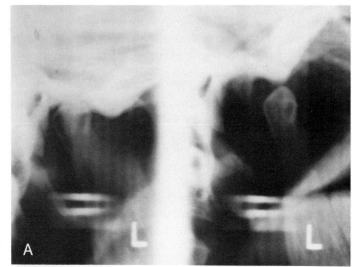

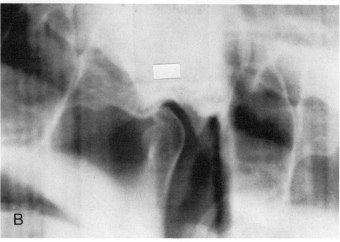

*Fig. 3–6.* A. Panoramic images in the lateral projection, with the mouth open and closed show the bony structures of the TM joint. In this tomographic image, the bony structures of the mandibular condylar process are relatively well seen. It is noted that the tomographic artifact effectively obscures the corresponding structures in the glenoid fossa. The nature of the tomographic blurring in panoramic units does not allow fine-section discrimination of bony structures as would be obtained with conventional radiographic tomography. The main value of these images is that some confusing overlying shadows are obscured, allowing a relatively clear view of the condylar process. B. Double-headed condyle as viewed with a panoramic radiograph. This was an incidental finding without history, signs or symptoms of a malformed condyle.

ductors. These materials do not conduct electric current in the dark, but become conductive when they interact with electromagnetic radiation, such as light or x-rays. In XR, a plate of aluminum coated with photoconductive selenium is the image receptor. A uniform charge is placed on the surface of the selenium to sensitize it for exposure. The charged plate is placed in a light-tight cassette, which is then used like an x-ray film. When a remnant x-ray beam from an object being examined reaches the plate, it is discharged at any particular area in an amount proportional to the intensity of beam falling on the area. The initial uniform charge on the selenium surface partly and variably dissipates, forming an electrostatic charge pattern that corresponds to the various radiodensities in the examined part. The electrostatic latent image is developed by passing oppositely charged particles over the plate. These particles are attracted to the variably charged areas of the surface in proportion to the intensity of the remaining charge. The powder image on the plate is either fused to paper or laminated between a transparent and a translucent sheet of plastic. In the former case, the image is viewed by reflected light, whereas the latter image is visible by either reflected or transmitted light. The charging and processing of the plates is done automatically in a light-tight processor that requires only a source of electric current, and the plates are reusable for about 1000 times. The process is fast and convenient, and produces dry, permanent images.[8]

Although differences in the image characteristics can be described, the XR is superior to the conventional radiographic image in certain important respects. It has a broader recording latitude, providing visible images of air, fat, water, cartilage, and bone with excellent detail on the same film (Fig. 3–7).[9] The second feature that contributes to the excellent image produced by the XR process is the so-called *edge enhancement effect*. This phenomenon is unique to the photoelectrostatic process, and it results in an exaggeration of the boundaries between areas of different densities, whether the differences are large or small. This intensification of the boundaries is the result of more toner particles being deposited at the higher charged side of the boundary and less toner at the lower charged side, enhancing the boundary and producing high local contrast.[10,11] Also, the xeroradiograph has better resolution and less granularity.

The XR is a low-radiation imaging system. The Xerox systems require only about one third to one half the radiation exposure used for conventional radiography.[9]

## Tomography

A variety of other terms are used to describe tomography: planigraphy, stratigraphy, and laminagraphy. Tomography minimizes or eliminates the unwanted shadows of superimposed structures so that, for the most part, only a picture of the structure to be examined remains. This is accomplished by synchronously moving the film in one direction and the x-ray source in the opposite direction (Fig. 3–8).

### Linear Tomography

The linear motions of the film and x-ray source cast the images of the structure at a particular level of interest (which is the focal plane or the pivot point of movement) on the same area of the moving film and generate relatively sharp images. The images of structures above and below this level of interest are projected progressively over the film, resulting in some blurring (caused by a widening of their individual edges and a reduction of their densities). This technical procedure effectively enhances the visuali-

zation of the images that are of interest by increasing their radiographic contrast.

### Multidirectional Tomography

When the long axes of linear structures are oriented more or less parallel with the film and point more or less in the same direction of film and tube movement, their images are not blurred on the linear tomogram, even though they lie outside (above or below) the focal plane. Sharp thin-section tomographs, however, can be obtained if the tube and film are moved synchronously in a pattern of nonlinear directions. Various movements have been engineered into x-ray machines: circular, elliptical, hypocycloidal, and trispiral. The circular tomographic movement results in the poorest and the hypocycloidal and trispiral movements produce the sharpest images.[12]

### Polycycloid Corrected TM Joint Radiographs

Dunn et al. wrote that, " . . . it is seen that the medial pole of the condyle is more posterior than the lateral pole. If tomograms were made by passing a ray at right angles, then the central ray would make a lateral cut on one portion but an oblique cut on another. In fact, most of the cuts would be oblique rather than lateral. Therefore, it is necessary to position the patient's head so that the medial and lateral poles of the condyle are in a direct line, so that the central ray passes along the entire width of its long axis. This is called corrected tomography. To accomplish this, a submental vertex radiograph of the condyles is taken first. On this radiograph, a horizontal line is then drawn posterior to the condyles, either through an area at both external auditory meatuses (transmeatal line) or perpendicular to the midline of the palate."[13] Lines are then drawn from the lateral poles of the condyles to the medial poles until they contact the original horizontal line. The angles thus created are measured. The patient's head is positioned so that the tomogram cuts pass through the long axes of the condyles (Fig. 3–9).

With the usual 2-mm cuts, 15 to 20 lateral images of the condyles are available. Additional detailed imaging information is avail-

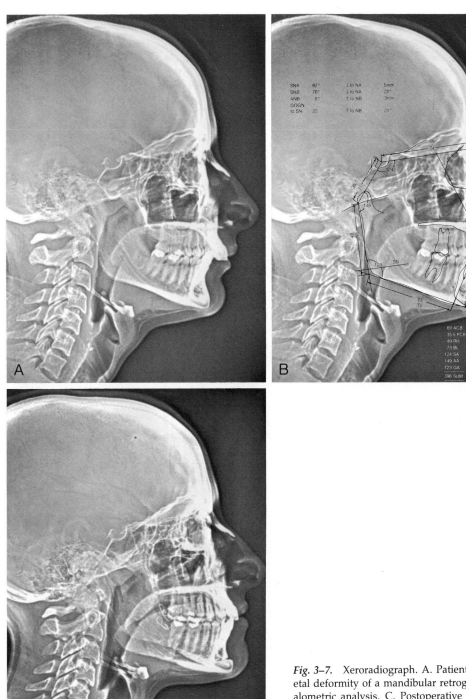

*Fig. 3–7.* Xeroradiograph. A. Patient with a facial skeletal deformity of a mandibular retrognathism. B. Cephalometric analysis. C. Postoperative view following bilateral sagittal rami advancing osteotomies and horizontal advancement of the anterior base of the mandible. (Courtesy of Dr. Eugene J. Messer, Carpinteria, California)

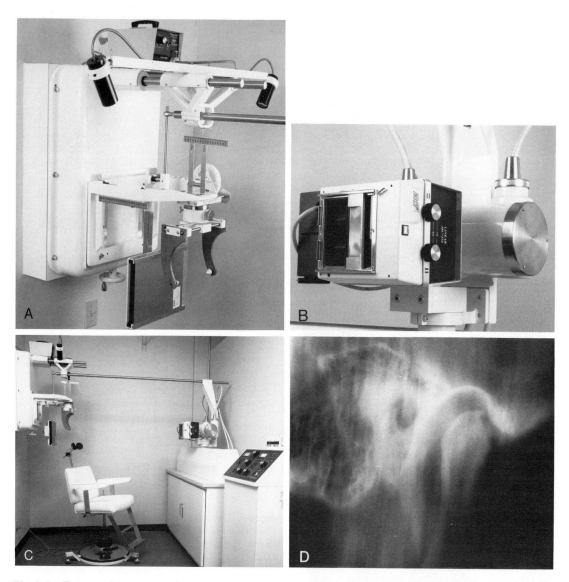

*Fig. 3–8.* Tomographic imaging of the TM joint. A–C. Outpatient radiographic equipment, the Quint-Sectograph, that will produce extraoral single plane and tomographic views of the craniofacial skeleton, including the TM joint. D. Linear tomographic view of the TM joint: a painful TM joint caused by the condylar exostosis which protruded through the disk. The patient was managed by removal of the exostosis and repair of the perforated disk.

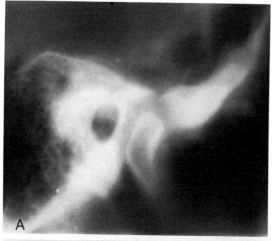

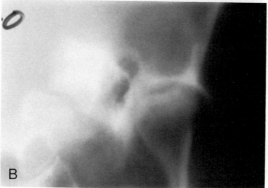

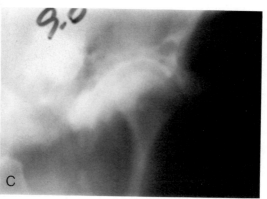

*Fig. 3–9.* Polycycloidal corrected (for the long axis of each condyle) tomographic images. The views, with 2 mm slices, are obtained in both lateral and frontal projections of the condyles, corrected in all cases for the long axis of each condyle as measured from submental vertex views. Examples from different patients disclosed: A. Lateral projection with an incidental finding of the absence of the osseous roof to the glenoid fossa in an asymptomatic joint. B. Frontal projection displays sclerotic bone on the condyle in a patient with an anterior dislocation (chronic closed lock) of the disk. C. Frontal view displays anterior extensions of the mastoid air cells. (These views are courtesy of the Radiology Department, Brookwood Medical Center, Birmingham, Alabama)

able pertaining to the articular eminence. The mandibular (glenoid fossa), the petrotympanic fissure, the ear, the mastoid air cells and their extensions over the mandibular fossa and occasionally into the articular eminence, and, sometimes, the styloid process are seen.

Since 1975, we have used the following modification to view the condyle from a frontal perspective. The orientation of the patient and the central ray are established by drawing lines at right angles to the long axes of the mandibular condyles. This action produces the angle of the central ray to the sagittal plane of the patient that will display nondistorted frontal views of the mandibular condyles. At the usual 1-mm cuts, four or five anteroposterior or frontal images of the condyles are available. Arthritic and other deformities that may not be evident on lateral views often are visible on the frontal projections. The shapes of the condyles are known; the shapes of the condyles from the frontal views are useful when interpreting lateral

views and, also, for planning an arthroscopic examination.

We emphasize that the normal angles of the long axes of the condyles to the sagittal plane and the normal frontal shapes of the mandibular condyles may be different on the patient's left and right sides.

Heffez and associates observed that the corrected hypocycloidal tomographic techniques produced greater accuracy and clarity of views of the TMJ than do other tomographic methods, and they use the technique to classify measurements of the condyle-disk-fossa/eminence relationships.[14,15]

### Microfocus Technique

Delfino and Eppley described the microfocus technique in comparison to tomographic images.[16] They found the microfocus technique, which involves geometric magnification of hard structures,[17] and the tomographic techniques had an equal ability to detect osseous changes of the condyle and eminence.

## Arthrography

The arthrogram provides information about the position, size, and shape of the meniscus (Fig. 3–10). The clinician can determine whether the disk is subluxated or dislocated, and most commonly in an anterior medial position, can visualize displacement. Adhesion of the disk to the condyle or to the glenoid fossa can be noted and perforations of the meniscus or of the posterior attachment are demonstrated. In the event of perforation, which may be either an incidental finding, indicative of pathologic involvement, or iatrogenically produced, the contrast medium is injected into the inferior compartment, but it enters the superior compartment either immediately or with function. Instead of injecting about 1 ml of contrast media before sensing resistance, 1.5 to 2.5 ml are used as the fluid flows through the perforation and into

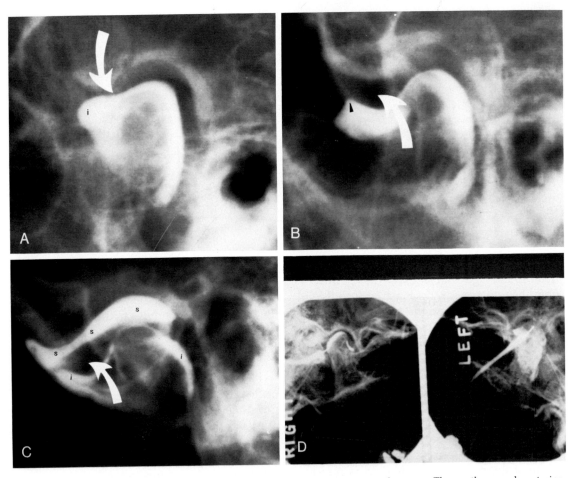

*Fig. 3–10.* TM joint arthrography. A. Normal TM joint inferior compartment arthrogram. The gently curved posterior band of the meniscus (white arrow) is seen just anterior to the dome of the mandibular condyle. In the closed position, there is a small amount of contrast material filling the anterior recess of the inferior TMJ compartment (i). B. The prominently rounded posterior band of an anteriorly displaced, thickened disk (white arrow) is seen anterior to the condyle. A point, or beak of contrast material (arrowhead), represents contrast material extending into the intermediate zone of the meniscus. The mouth is in the closed position. C. Inferior compartment arthrography in a patient with a perforation of the meniscus leads to filling of both inferior (i) and superior (s) compartments. The thickened meniscus (white arrow) is anterior to the head of the mandibular condyle in the closed position. (Figures 10A,B,C are courtesy of Dr. Eugene J. Messer.) D. Usual arthrographic examination of the inferior joint space in the patient's right TM joint. On the patient's left there was a misadventure with the extravasation outside of the joint space of the contrast media which resolved normally.

the superior joint space. Using the dynamic arthrogram, perforations are well documented and the exact location can often be noted. In general, however, the greatest value of an arthrogram is to confirm clinical impressions.

The difference between the static and dynamic arthrogram is the method of recording the study. The static arthrogram is recorded on radiographic film, and the dynamic is recorded on videotape. Frequently, abnormalities of meniscal motion, particularly early reductions and reciprocal disk motion, can be demonstrated only by utilization of a dynamic recording.

Although the injection of the contrast agent into both joint spaces is not always appropriate, each requires a separate approach. The joint spaces are small so the meticulous placement of the needle and the introduction of the contrast medium is usually monitored fluoroscopically. Also, the contrast medium remains in place for a short time, so the arthrograms must be made within a few minutes. To complicate the procedure even further, a thorough arthrographic examination necessitates obtaining several tomographs of the joint during the limited period to demonstrate the movement of the intra-articular soft tissues during various stages of function. The TM joint arthrographic techniques are now so refined, however, it is reasonable, with appropriate training, to produce arthrograms in an outpatient dental clinic without fluoroscopy.[18]

Although arthrography is relatively safe and effective, the procedure is contraindicated if the patient is hypersensitive to a component of the contrast agents or has a local skin or periarticular joint infection. In some cases, the patient experiences discomfort for 1 or 2 days after the procedure.

An arthrographic examination sometimes will relieve a patient of signs and symptoms of subluxation of the disk. The distension and flushing of the joint spaces with the fluid contrast media will have a beneficial effect on the mobility of the TM joint disk.

## Diagnostic Considerations

Kaplan and associates demonstrated that an arthrographic image of a concavity in the anterior recess of the inferior space may represent either a frequently occurring normal variation caused by the anterior ridge of the meniscus or an anterior displacement of the meniscus.[19] Correlation of the images with information from the physical evaluation help to explain the findings. Also, dynamic movements of the TMJ, as recorded on the videotapes, clarify the arthrographic views. A reliable diagnosis of an anteriorly displaced meniscus is possible on the basis of arthrographic findings without supplemental information from a videotape if the images reveal a double concavity of the superior margin of the recess produced by the meniscus being anteriorly displaced and folded at the thin central zone.

Other variations of normal included an observation that, with the mouth closed, the superior margin of the anterior recess was smooth and flat in 68% of the joints and in 32% it was concave; with the mouth in maximal opening, the anterior recess decreased to a crescent in 84% of the joints and in 16% it remained large. Also, the posterior recess was larger than the anterior recess, which was contrary to most previous reports. These findings in normal joints emphasize the need for continuing reliance on clinical evaluations and multiple imaging methods, as indicated, to establish probable diagnoses.

## History

Studies reported in the late 1960s and early 1970s focused on the correlations between presurgical arthrographic diagnoses and the conditions observed at the time of surgery.[20-23] In further arthrographic studies in the 1970s, investigators correlated the clinical signs and symptoms of TM joint disk subluxation and dislocation.[24-26] In 1978, Wilkes[27,28] described the arthrographic findings of the disk in clicking subluxation and locking dislocating positions of the TM joint disk. In 1979, Katzberg et al.[29] and Dolwick et al.[30] produced hallmark reports correlating internal derangements of the meniscus and arthrographic findings.

## Lateral Approach

The approach to the TM joint may be either laterally or through the anterior wall of the external auditory meatus. The lateral approach is through a puncture point located midway between the tragus and condyle with the mouth partially open to improve access into the joint space. The needle is guided to the posteriosuperior crest of the condyle, with the sensations of the needle tip transmitted through the shaft of a long needle that transmits vibrations better than a short needle. A soft tap is sensed when the needle tip touches the articular fibrocartilage at the condylar crest. Between 0.5 and 1.0 ml of contrast solution is injected into the inferior joint cavity. To inject contrast solution into the superior joint cavity, the patient's mouth is open wide to translate the condyle from the mandibular glenoid fossa. With the same initial puncture site, the needle tip is directed superiorly and slightly medially, until the superior aspect of the mandibular fossa is encountered. The needle is withdrawn slightly and 1.0 to 2.0 ml of the contrast medium is injected. If resistance to injection is encountered, the needle tip may be within the meniscus, the posterior ligament, or the periarticular soft tissue, and repositioning is necessary.

Lynch and Chase described the use of fluoroscopic guidance to aid in accurately injecting the joint spaces with contrast media.[31] Combined with fluoroscopic guidance, the use of angiocatheters was reported by Wilkes, Blaschke et al., and Westesson.[28,32,33]

### Aural Approach

Lynch and Chase developed an approach for needle entry to the TM joint through the anterior wall of the external auditory canal.[31] Irby[34] and Zetz et al.[35] wrote that this approach is "more exact, predictable and easier to accomplish" than the lateral approach. Fluoroscopy has been necessary to develop TM joint arthrography; however, the external auditory meatus approach is so anatomically logical and direct, it may be performed either as an outpatient survey examination, with given situations and patients, or with the use of fluoroscopy and medical radiographic equipment.

The contrast material is usually a 75% solution of sodium diatrizoate diluted 4/1 with a local anesthetic solution containing a va-

soconstrictor. The solution, with the local anesthetic and vasoconstrictor, is loaded into a 10- or 20-ml syringe. A 25-gauge needle with a plastic cannula for connection to the syringe is used to enter the joint spaces.

The patient is positioned convenient to the radiographic equipment to permit rapid acquisition of the images with no impediments to movements of the mandible. The periauricular and the external auditory meatus cutaneous tissues are prepared by surgical scrubbing and draping. Regional anesthesia is obtained by local anesthetic agents injected posteriorly and laterally to the TM joint and/ or by an auriculotemporal nerve block.

The needle puncture for the contrast material is made through the fibrous band of the tragohelicine incisure, 10 mm medial to the tragus of the ear. The shaft of the needle is parallel to the transverse plane and is directed 45° medially to the sagittal plane. The needle tip should encounter the posterior slope of the condyle, which can be confirmed by having the patient slightly move the mandible. After the needle tip is positioned on the posterior aspect of the condyle, positioning can be confirmed with lateral transcranial (for anteroposterior positioning) and anteroposterior skull or transorbital TM joint (for mediolateral positioning) radiographs. The preferred position of the needle tip is within the middle one third of the mediolateral width of the condyle.

When the proper position of the needle tip is confirmed, the patient protrudes the mandible 2 to 3 mm to enlarge the space in the posterior recess of the inferior joint space. The needle is withdrawn 1.0 to 2.0 mm and repositioned slightly medially. The syringe is aspirated; return of the sparse synovial fluid is rare. If blood is aspirated from the vascular bed or from incidental hemorrhage, the needle is moved to an area where blood is not aspirated. A 0.5-ml amount of the contrast solution is injected. The patient may feel pressure in the joint area and an alteration of the posterior occlusion.

The arthrographic studies may include transcranial plain radiographs, and fluoroscopic, panoramic, transorbital, anteroposterior, and tomographic views with the mouth in the closed, intermediate, and open positions. In normal intracapsular relations, the radiopaque lower joint space extends from the inferior aspect of the posterior recess superiorly to the crest of the condyle and anteriorly and inferiorly into the anterior recess. Arthrographic evaluation of the superior joint space displays the radiopacity below the mandibular fossa extending from the petrotympanic fissure posteriorly, to or past the crest of the articular eminence. Because the superior joint space extends laterally and inferiorly to the inferior joint space, the contrast solution tends to obliterate the features of diskal displacements best appreciated by inferior joint space arthrograms.

## Computerized Tomography

Computerized tomography (CT) is variously labeled computerized axial tomography, computer aided tomography, computerized transaxial tomography, computerized reconstruction tomography, and digital axial tomography. The method represents the successful combination of x-ray scanning and digital computer technology. The primary advantage of this system is that it eliminates the confusion caused by representing a three-dimensional object as a two-dimensional image—an image that superimposes all the structures within an object from superficial to deep. With CT, an internal structure can be seen clearly in spite of the structures of varying density superficial to and deep to it. The technique accomplishes this three-dimensionality by dividing the object to be examined into a series of slices, and each slice is scanned many times from many different angles. Typical slices for TM joint studies may be at 1 to 3 mm intervals and be 1.5 mm in thickness. The radiation is confined to the slices by using a collimated, fan-shaped beam. The radiation transmitted through the slices, from the edge, is detected by radiation detectors. By this cross-sectional imaging technique, the x-ray attenuation characteristic of a large number of tissue paths, at multiple angles through each slice of the object, is perceived by the detectors and sent to a digital computer. The computer processes the data and constructs the density profile morphology of each slice.

The one important single feature of CT scanning is its sensitivity for density discrimination. It can distinguish between tissues differing in slight densities. Normal blood, clotted blood, cerebrospinal fluid, grey and white matter, bone, normal soft tissues, and tumors appear as separate entities with proper adjustment.

CT is useful for evaluating intracranial and head and neck lesions of the paranasal sinuses, mandible,[36] salivary glands, nasopharynx, base of the skull, larynx, and cervical areas. In addition, CT provides information from the infratemporal and parapharyngeal spaces that cannot be imaged well or at all with conventional techniques.

An important consideration with any diagnostic procedure relates to the dose and distribution of radiation. Measurements show that the exposure from a series of complete transverse axial scans is roughly equivalent to a single conventional skull or abdominal radiograph. The typical conventional head and body procedure often involves a number of views. Therefore, the radiation dose from CT is frequently less than with plain film images because less tissue volume is irradiated with CT.

In CT scanning, a highly collimated x-ray beam passes through the patient, usually perpendicular to the long axis of the body. The transmissions are conveyed to a computer, which produces a series of radiologic images of planes of the body on both a video screen and for storage on magnetic tape. The images may be enhanced or diminished to help in distinguishing features. It is possible, for example, to produce an image that shows the meniscus of the TM joint and the small superior head of the lateral pterygoid muscle, also known as the sphenomeniscus muscle (Fig. 3–11).

Many different types of CT apparatus are available, but in general, all consist of passing the x-ray beam through the patient in a rotatory fashion, with the final image generated by computer manipulation of the signal from the x-ray beam. The image obtained represents a slice much like a conventional tomographic slice in that only one plane is studied at a time. The orientation of the slices are different (transverse to the part being exam-

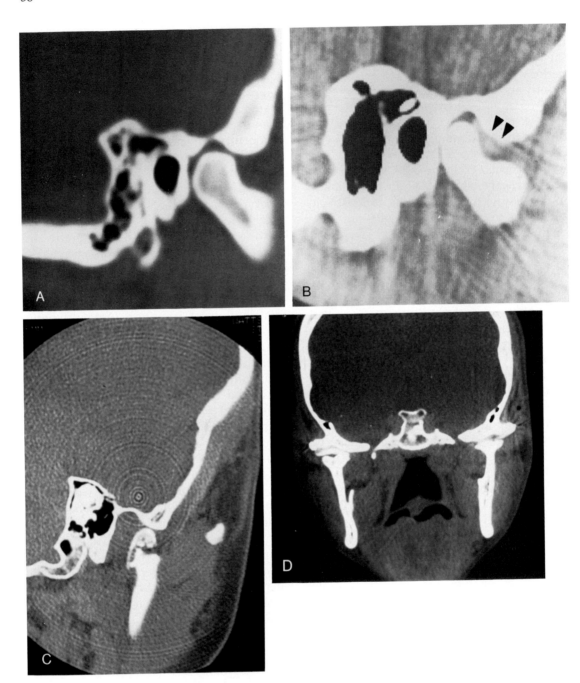

*Fig. 3–11.* Computed tomography (CT) of TM joint. A. CT image obtained through a normal TM joint at soft tissue windows. The luncency anterior to the mandibular condyle and condylar neck represents a normal finding of fat surrounding the pterygoid mucles and is probably indicative that the disk is in the normal position. B. CT image obtained at soft tissue settings in a patient with clinical evidence of an anterior displaced disk shows that the fat containing area normally found anterior to the condyle now contains a dense structure (arrowheads) which is the anteriorly displaced meniscus. (A and B courtesy of Steven E. Selzer, M.D.) C. CT image of an intracapsular fracture of the condyle. D. CT image of TM joint implants in a patient who had incurred bilateral condylar fractures several years prior to the placement of the glenoid fossae prostheses.

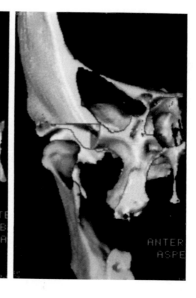

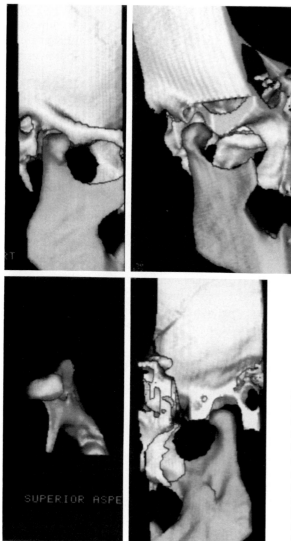

*Fig. 3–11.* Computed tomography (CT) of TM joint (continued). E. CT three dimensional reconstruction of a normal TM joint. Using the information stored from frontal CT 1 mm slices, reconstructions of any selected view of the ramus and TM joint are possible. The illustrations show mandibular ramus and TM joint in lateral, anterior oblique, anterior, superior, and medial views. (Appreciation is expressed to Dr. James Kamplain, Baptist Montclair Medical Center, Birmingham, Alabama, and to ISG (Innovative Systems Group) TECHNOLOGY, Mississauga, Ontario, Canada, for their cooperation in making these images available.)

ined rather than in a plane parallel to the tabletop), but CT is free of the obfuscating contiguous structures encountered in conventional tomography. The CT technique affords other interesting possibilities because an extremely thin (0.3 mm) slice can be obtained at fine resolution of less than 1 mm and with extreme contrast resolution, which allows examination of soft tissue as well as bony structures.

The use of CT images to study internal derangement has relative limitations. One limitation is a significant restriction of CT performance when the part being examined moves at all between slices, which essentially prevents any form of dynamic imaging. The TM joint, therefore, must be studied at fixed degrees of opening, and the position must be preserved at each degree of opening throughout the study. Thus, no direct control of the status of the meniscus at the time of imaging is possible, such as is achieveable with fluoroscopic arthrography. Another limitation is difficulty in resolving low-density soft tissue structures, such as the joint meniscus, when so closely surrounded by bone. Therefore, anteriorly displaced disks that do not reduce cannot be seen reliably with CT, because the density of a displaced disk may be difficult to discriminate from the adjacent density of musculature. The density of aponeurosis in the lateral pterygoid insertion into the condyle can also be confused for the disk.

Real-time evaluation of meniscus movements is not possible, and perforations of the meniscus are difficult to detect. Clinical indications of internal derangement of the TM joint have a high positive correlation with degenerative joint diseases;[37] in one study, 33% of patients with anterior nonreducing displacement of the disk had degenerative joint disease; 15.3% who had reduction of the disk had degenerative joint disease; and 5.0% of those with no identifiable meniscal abnormality had CT evidence of degenerative joint disease.

### Double Contrast Technique

Injection of air into the joint spaces after the injection and aspiration of contrast medium or, as described by Heffez and associates,[38] by having a small quantity of contrast medium in the needle of the syringe of air, help to produce exquisite images of the anatomy of joint spaces. After the introduction of the air under fluoroscopic visualization, the patient is positioned in a sagittal head holder for the production of sagittal CT planes. The air compresses the normal and the remodeled retrodiskal tissues and, without soft tissue interference from the meniscus, clear views of the lining structures of the cavities are produced; the structures are the condyle, the glenoid fossa, and the articular eminence.

The problems associated with double contrast arthroscopic techniques, whether accompanied by CT or other radiographic techniques, include the need to inject air into the enclosed space. Air escaping from the confinement of the joint capsule can produce a localized emphysema, yet the air will probably be resorbed without incident. A greater hazard is the possibility of injecting nonsterile air. The syringe containing the air, in place by withdrawing the plunger to the maximum without removing, should be autoclaved before use as an air injection syringe.

### Reconstruction in Different Planes

The basic problem with two-dimensional images for assisting in treatment regimens is that the usual two dimensions of CT are in a transverse plane, and the preferred views of TM joints are the sagittal and frontal planes.

Reconstruction of the CT information for viewing in the sagittal and frontal planes is performed with some loss of definition; this loss is minimal if the original CT transverse slices were thin.

### Three-Dimensional Reconstruction

The anatomy or pathology being examined may be displayed as a solid three-dimensional reconstruction of CT scans. Through the use of thin slices, masks, filters, and windows, selected tissues and structures of the TM joint may be visible on the reconstruction. These images are spectacular and accurate representations of the area being examined. The TM joint may be examined from any plane and selected surfaces and regions may be isolated in the views. This type of imagery, as it becomes available, will supplement and may supplant other techniques.

## Magnetic Resonance Imaging

Magnetic resonance imaging (MRI) is a refinement of nuclear magnetic resonance spectroscopy techniques that have been used in chemistry, physics, and biology for many years to study the structure of complex molecules. Both techniques are based on the fact that the nuclei of the atoms with an odd number of protons or neutrons are spinning and, therefore, they generate a magnetic field. These nuclei, of which hydrogen is most frequently used for MRI, are considered spinning magnets that are oriented randomly in most material, including the tissues of the body. Approximately 60% of the atoms in the body are hydrogen; most other atoms are too few in number or the MRI signal is too weak to be used for medical MRI.[39]

When tissue is subjected to a strong magnetic field, the nuclei align with the static magnetic field, like the needle of a compass aligns with the earth's magnetic field. When energy in the form of a radio signal of the proper frequency is added to the field, the nuclear magnets aligned with the magnetic field tip and become misaligned with the field. When the radio signal is terminated, the nuclear magnets tip back into alignment with the static magnetic field, and they transmit a radio signal that has a frequency unique to the element and a signal strength that is indicative of the element's relative abundance. These radio signals are the source from which the MR image is constructed by a computer and displayed on a screen.

The MRI system has the potential to produce images that are superior in contrast discrimination for detecting and diagnosing lesions not revealed by a CT scan. CT images are characterized by just one parameter, the x-ray attenuation coefficient of the tissues, but the MR images (strength of the radio frequency signals) are influenced by the density of the participating nuclei, the time it requires for them to realign with the magnetic field, and the effects of the interactions of the magnetic moments of the participating nuclei on one another. By varying the technique, any one of these MRI parameters can be emphasized over the other two, so that image contrasts can be tailored to a particular problem.[39] With these same parameters, MRI appears to have the potential to discriminate between normal and malignant tissue, measure blood flow even in the capillary beds, perform chemical analysis in the body to provide information on the processes occurring inside the cell, and even monitor intracellular pH.

## TM Joint

The advantages of MRI for TM joint evaluation are compelling. The patient is exposed to no ionizing radiation and, as with arthrography, no intracapsular injections of contrast materials are needed. Arthrography, however, may provide a dynamic evaluation of osseous and meniscal relationships during function and permit probable identification of meniscal perforations.[40] Because bone is relatively void of water, and therefore the hydrogen ions necessary to produce an MR image, the bone detail with CT scanning is better than that with MRI, but the soft tissue detail of the meniscus is superior with MRI. The imaging exposure time, measured in minutes, is relatively long, during which time the patient must remain immobile inside of a magnet that produces a claustrophobic reaction in some individuals.[41] With technical advances, shorter exposure times are anticipated and surface coils will be further perfected.

Katzberg and associates described the potential widespread clinical applications of MRI for TM joint diagnoses, especially with the use of TM joint surface coil technology rather than obtaining a photograph of a section of a total head scan.[42] The scanning times were reasonable, 52 seconds for a localizing fast scan and 256 seconds for the slow scan. Using surface coils, Wilk and associates[43] found that the accuracy of MRI was greater than arthroscopy, confirmed by operative findings, for displaying perforations of the meniscus and anterior dislocation of the disk. They noted that perforations of the retrodiskal tissues were difficult to identify with MRI unless there was the additional finding of bone to bone contact. Dolan and Moon compared MRI, arthrotomography, clinical and surgical findings in TM joint internal derangements; they found that MRI was as accurate as arthrography in confirming disk displacement, arthrography was best for disclosing perforations, and *the best correlations to surgical findings were the clinical evaluations.*[44] Dolan and associates evaluated preoperative MRI diagnoses of diskal perforations with findings at surgery and found only a 65% correlation.[45]

The MR images display meniscus positions and alterations, exquisite detail of the posterior attachment, and the position of muscular attachments. A report by Kircos and associates emphasized that MRI was the first imaging method that allows clear depiction of the demarcation between the disk and the posterior attachments to the bilaminar zone.[46] Sanchez-Woodworth and co-workers, in a prospective study of 211 patients with signs and symptoms of bilateral TM joint internal derangements, evaluated both TM joints with MRI.[47] They reported that 61 patients had normal findings, 45 had one side with meniscal displacement, and 105 had bilateral derangements. They noted the advantages of bilateral TM joint imaging with the noninvasive MRI techniques that, apparently, are biologically safe (Fig. 3–12).

## Nerve Tissues

Daniels and associates described the great clarity MRI provides for examinations of the

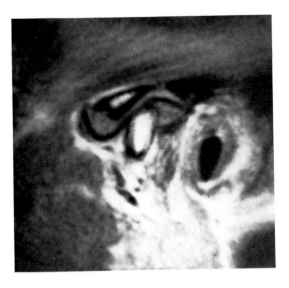

*Fig. 3–12.* Magnetic resonance image of a TM joint that has had a silicone rubber implant in place for 3 years. The implant is the dark S-shaped object; it is surrounded by a granular gray area that represents encapsulting fibrous connective tissue. The small lenticular-shaped white area is the temporal articular eminence; the larger white oval area is the lateral pole of the mandibular condyle. The external auditory meatus (EAM) is represented by the black oval area. The fan shape of the temporalis muscle is above and anterior to the TM joint, and the parotid gland is inferior to the TM joint and EAM.

trigeminal ganglion and the exit from the cranium of its three extracranial divisions and of the pterygopalation ganglion.[48] Because of the negligible signal returned from cortical bone, an MRI evaluation of a lesion of a nerve in the foramen rotundum, foramen ovale, or the pterygopalatine fossa, requires CT to demonstrate the osseous margins. Similarly, MRI is proving useful to produce views of lesions within the internal auditory canal.[49]

### Future Prospects

Relying on the physical phenomenon that produces magnetic resonance in tissues, MRI is producing an explosion of new information. Practicalities of cost containment, however, must be balanced against the expected gain in information that may be obtained from physical evaluation and less costly imaging techniques. Little doubt remains, however, that among the imaging techniques currently available, MRI, with its clarity of soft tissue imaging and its safety, may be the technique

of the future that will supplant many other imaging modalities. There will be technical advances that will produce thinner slices for greater clarity and for three-dimensional reconstructions of images without the biological hazards of radiation.

### Hazards

The strong magnetic field of MRI poses the greatest hazards. The absolute contraindications for MRI includes its use in patients with implant pacemakers, metal prostheses, and surgical clips.

## Arthroscopy

Arthroscopic examination of the TM joint spaces in human subjects began with Ohnishi.[50] The technique features the placement of a fiberoptic endoscope in the spaces of the TM joint. A light source passes illumination down the periphery of the viewing rod. The tip of the scope has varying contours and angles to permit a variety of viewing positions, ranging from wide angle, right angle, and various degrees, usually 30°, for forward viewing. A variety of devices may be attached to the viewing rod, including an ocular for direct vision, still camera, motion picture camera, and television camera. The latter permits transferring the highly magnified image to a screen, and the procedures are directed by the clinician monitoring the screen. The television accessory permits the production of video tapes of the procedure (Fig. 3–13).

The arthroscopic procedures of the superior joint space are usually accompanied by a flushing lavage of normal saline. The clarity of the solution is maintained by delivering the solution under enough pressure that incidental hemorrhages resulting from the penetration of the joint cavity are suppressed. Nitrogen gas instead of saline enhances the clarity and detail of the joint lining. Its use is associated with the danger of the gas escaping into the surrounding tissues, producing an emphysema, and an exudate is not obtained that may be centrifuged for biopsy analysis. Although the clarity with nitrogen gas is superb, the gases, as compared to irrigation with normal saline or Ringer's solution, may permit

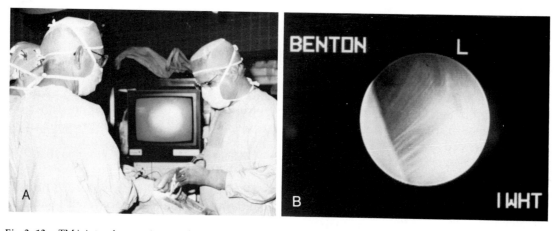

*Fig. 3–13.* TM joint arthroscopic procedures. A. Organization of the operating room during an arthroscopic procedure. B. Arthoscopic view of the left TM joint space. This view shows a normal disk and medial ligament. (Appreciation is expressed to Dr. Edward L. Mosby, Kansas City, Missouri, for this view of the TM joint.)

the collapse of adherences of the joint walls, which will obscure vision, and incidental hemorrhages are not suppressed.

An arthroscopic examination sometimes will relieve a patient of signs and symptoms of TM joint internal derangement. The distension and flushing of the superior joint space with irrigating fluid will have a beneficial effect on the mobility of the TM joint disk.

### Inferior Joint Space

Goss and Bosanquet described the inferior joint space as bell-shaped and small in terms of arthroscopic examinations.[51] Because of the potential for damage to the disk by the arthroscopic instrumentation, they recommended, " . . . arthroscopy of the inferior joint space be performed only in patients in whom surgical exploration is planned."

### Superior Joint Space

In the normal superior joint space, the articular eminence is a gently curved area covered with a grayish white, shiny, smooth cartilagenous appearing tissue. The edge of the articular eminence is tinged red. The disk, as viewed in the superior joint space, is gentle convex curving tissue that has a smooth surface with occasional fine folds. The edge of the disk is tinged blue. The synovial membrane on the medial and lateral walls of the joint space is pink with a translucent surface through which capillaries may be observed. As the intrajoint pressure increases, the capillaries decrease in size and may disappear.

### Divisions of the Superior Joint Space

Heffez and Blaustein proposed a regional anatomic classification to aid in the description of arthroscopic findings of the superior joint space.[52] They wrote, "Osseous landmarks are used to subdivide this space into a posterior or glenoid and an anterior or preeminence region. The boundary for these two regions is the apex of the articular eminence, recognized arthroscopically by noting the change in curvature of the glenoid fossa posterior-anteriorly (from concave to convex). The superior joint space is further divided into anterior and posterior glenoid regions by an imaginary vertical line dropped from the height of contour of the glenoid fossa.

Conventional anatomic nomenclature of the TM joint disk is supplemented by the following terms: (1) posterior incline of the posterior band defined as the posterior slope of the posterior band and (2) anterior incline of the posterior band defined as the anterior slope of the posterior band; (3) medial sulcus defined as the groove formed by the reflection of the medial capsule onto the medial-superior edge of the disk . . . ; and (4) lateral sulcus defined as the groove formed by the reflection of the lateral capsule onto the latero-superior edge of the disk . . . . Synovial plicae are defined as smooth reflections or folds of the capsule lining.''

## Technique

The Heffez and Blaustein examination technique is as follows.[51] The examination is performed with the patient under sedation and local anesthesia or under general anesthesia. The patient's head is stabilized in a cloth or plastic holder. The periauricular and external auditory meatus are prepared and the field is draped. The external auditory meatus is packed with a sponge or gauze carrying a topical antibiotic with care to avoid hydraulic pressure on the ear drum. A local anesthetic is infiltrated over the lateral and posterior aspects of the TMJ and/or an auriculotemporal block is used. The lateral lip of the articular eminence and the lateral aspect of the condyle are palpated and marked. A modified towel clamp is inserted at the mandibular angle to provide movement of the mandible.

The superior joint space is next dilated with 1.0 to 1.5 ml of 1/200,000 epinephrine solution using a 19-gauge needle to contact the lateral lip of the glenoid fossa. The needle is then guided medially until the concavity of the glenoid fossa is palpated, and the epinephrine solution is deposited. A 3-mm stab incision is made vertically over the lateral aspect of the mandibular fossa at its point of highest concavity. The cutaneous margins are undermined to assist in rapid access into the surgical site if necessary to control a hemorrhage. The capsule overlying the mandibular condyle is exposed with blunt dissection using a small curved hemostat. The position of the hemostat is verified by having the mandible moved while the hemostat contacts the condyle through the lateral capsule.

The sharp trocar is locked into the 2.0-mm sheath, and the unit is grasped between the index finger, the middle finger, and thumb, to permit optimum control of the instrument. The trocar is inserted into the superior joint space while the mandible is gently distracted anteroinferiorly. After entering the concavity of the mandibular fossa, the instrument is held gently against the roof of the fossa, and the sharp trocar is removed. The opposite hand maintains the sheath against the bone. Usually, the first intracapsular views are with the 2.4-mm 30° viewing telescope, which is inserted through the sheath. Constant irrigation is performed throughout the procedure to provide joint distention and hemostasis. Generally, 30 to 50 ml of fluid are injected per examination. The examination is performed in a systematic manner either directly through the arthroscope or on the video monitor.

## Examination Protocol

Heffez and Blaustein described a logical standard examination procedure.[52] Initially, the arthroscope moves with a sweeping anteroposterior motion to orient the clinician. The principal orientation landmark that is confirmed by gentle movements of the mandible to ensure the orientation of the image is the junction of the flexure of vascular retrodiskal tissue with the avascular posterior band in the case of the normal disk relationship; in the case of a displaced disk, the principal orientation is the junction of the vascular retrodiskal tissue with the slightly vascular remodeled retrodiskal tissue.

The examination has three distinct phases: the transverse phase, the longitudinal phase, and the dynamic transverse phase. The arthroscopic findings in the phases are recorded according to the field of view in which they are observed. For this purpose, the glenoid fossa is divided into a grid system consisting of nine components, each corresponding to an arthroscopic field of view. The grid system is arbitrarily composed of three equal transverse regions, anterior, middle, posterior, and three equal sagittal regions, lateral, central, and medial. An arthroscopic field is located geographically by using the name of the corresponding anteroposterior region followed by the name of the lateromedial region. The middle fields correspond to the regions directly under the highest convexity of the glenoid fossa, a convenient arthroscopic landmark. Arthroscopic findings are described in terms of shape, color, orientation (angulation), joint space configuration, and topographic relationships.

The transverse phase of the examination of the anterior and posterior glenoid regions is performed by holding the arthroscope along the transverse axis of the space while the condyle is gently distracted. The second phase of the arthroscopic examination is termed the longitudinal phase because the arthroscope is oriented in a plane that parallels the sagittal axis of the superior joint space. The mandibular condyle is not purposefully distracted except by fluid distention and horizontal positioning of the condyle. Arthroscopic findings are recorded according to three fields oriented transversely, called the lateral, central, and medial fields. The dynamic transverse phase features a gentle movement of the mandible while the arthroscope is held at the region of highest contour of the mandibular fossa. In this way, the clinician can observe the region where the superior surface of the condyle contacts the disk.

The postoperative phase begins with removal of the remaining fluid in the superior joint space by suctioning with a small tip passed through the telescope shaft. Skin closure is possible with one or two sutures. Antibiotics are not routinely prescribed, and corticosteroids are not routinely injected. The findings of the examination are logged on an arthroscopic map, which becomes a part of the patient's record. The experienced clinician usually performs a unilateral arthroscopic examination within 10 to 15 minutes. Postoperatively, the patient experiences minimal to moderate pain, which may be controlled adequately with a simple analgesic and codeine agent. A program of home physiotherapeutic exercises is prescribed, and a normal joint regains its preoperative range of motion within 7 to 14 days.

## Anatomic Limitations

The entire TM joint is not accessible to arthroscopic examination, according to Heffez and Blaustein.[52] "The lateral capsule, anterior band, anterior and posterior aspect of the lateral sulcus and infratemporal articulating surface are inconsistently viewed in an arthroscopic examination. The size of the inferior joint space of condyle-disk component has precluded its regular examination. The risk of iatrogenic damage to the disk, disk-capsule attachment, and fibrocartilage surface of the condyle could be significant. Certain temporomandibular joints with considerable reduc-

tion in radiographic joint space and a severe decrease in range of motion may not be amenable to examination."

Blaustein and Heffez, in a report of arthroscopic findings of arthrographically diagnosed disk displacements, confirmed by direct observation the remodeling of the retrodiskal tissues, and noted osseous changes of the articular eminence.[53] Their report included observations of perforations of the retrodiskal tissues that were not observed arthrographically. They cautioned against confusing the medial capsular ligament with adhesions.

## Complications

Risks and complications of arthroscopy include an immediate, usually transient, postoperative decrease in range of motion of the mandible. The limitation in motion may persist if an anterior disk dislocation has occurred.

A postoperative transient inferior alveolar nerve dysfunction may occur owing to a clamp that is used for distraction of the mandibular condyle passing into the inferior alveolar canal. Temporary to persistent facial nerve weakness of the temporal or zygomatic branches may result from infiltrations of local anesthetic solutions, resulting in facial nerve neuropraxia, or from damage to a branch of the facial nerve during the stab incision.

Hemorrhage may occur because of laceration of a vessel superficial to the lateral capsule when approaching the superior joint space with the sharp trocar. This bleeding may be controlled with pressure and application of hemostatic clamps, clips, or staples through the incision. The undermining of the tissues greatly facilitates the entry of instruments to achieve hemostasis.

Other potential complications include infection, penetration of the external auditory canal or the middle ear with loss of hearing, distraction of the sphenomandibular-anterior malleolar ligament with a resultant hearing loss, penetration into the middle cranial fossa, hemorrhage from the laceration of structures deep to the medial capsule, postoperative hemorrhage, permanent facial nerve injuries, traumatic entry into the ear or other retrodiskal tissue,[53,54] and auriculotemporal syndrome.

## Nuclear Medicine Techniques

Nuclear medicine, scintigraphy, nuclear imaging, or bone scan radionuclide scanning are synonymous terms for a diagnostic imaging technique. The technique exploits the fact that certain atoms or compounds have affinities for particular tissues and concentrate in "target" tissues. If one of these compounds is made radioactive by substituting a radioactive isotope for one of its constituent atoms, its location and relative concentration in a body can be determined by detecting the areas emitting gamma rays and measuring the intensity of the radiation. The procedure is similar to conventional radiography in that it uses a source of ionizing radiation to generate an image, but in contrast, the patient is the source of the radiation, and the image receptor is a so-called gamma camera or scintillation camera. The gamma camera utilizes a sodium iodide screen that produces a flash of light (a scintillation) when it absorbs a photon of (gamma) radiation. The flashes of light, generated by the radiation from a concentration of radioactive isotopes in a body, are amplified and are relayed to a display system that organizes them into an image that is in turn placed on a cathode ray tube and photographed for study and record. The image may also be stored in a computer for subsequent recall and display.[55]

### Conventional Scans

Technetium 99m-labeled compounds are widely used. They emit only gamma radiation, they have a half-life of only 6 hours, which minimizes patient exposure, and its gamma energy is a range that is about optimum for the gamma camera. This technique, however, only demonstrates altered tissue function, either an increased or decreased metabolism. Therefore, delineating the cause of a change necessitates coupling the information from tissue scans with clinical evaluation and, perhaps, other tests. At the same time, one of the most attractive features of such an examination is that it demonstrates abnormalities in tissue, as well as the extent of such changes, even before they are demonstrable on routine radiographs.

A radionuclide scan of a normal facial skeleton shows uniform uptake in the jaws, with the mandible imaged somewhat less intensely than the maxilla.[56] Both positive (increased uptake) and negative (decreased uptake) scans have proved useful for the detection of pathoses in and about the maxillofacial complex. Positive scans are found in cases involving fibro-osseous lesions,[57,58] neoplastic diseases,[59] odontogenic cysts,[60] inflammatory dental diseases,[61] and bone regeneration after a graft.[62] Negative scans are obtained in patients with traumatic bone cysts, idiopathic osteosclerosis, giant cell lesions, and slow-growing tumors.

### TM Joint

A joint involved in an abnormal mechanical or inflammatory disease process by necessity has abnormal regional blood flow (Fig. 3–14). Abnormal stresses are placed on the bones,

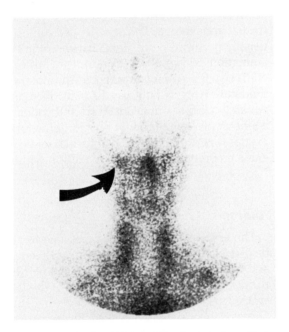

*Fig. 3–14.* Blood-pool image following injection of technetium 99-m labeled bone scanning agent, a sensitive indicator of increased metabolic activity, shows an area of increased activity in the extreme medial aspect of the right TM joint (arrow). In this early phase of the bone scan, the isotope is accumulating in areas of hyperemia presumably because of synovitis. (Courtesy of Dr. Eugene J. Messer.)

and these joints show increased deposition of bone-seeking radioisotope. By conducting a radioisotope scan of the TM joint in both closed and open positions of the mandible, the separation of the potential image delineates whether the lesion is in the mandibular or the temporal portion of the joint. Keller and associates reported positive indications of increased radiotracer accumulation within the TMJ of a small sample of patients in whom internal derangements were diagnosed arthrographically.[63]

## Emission Computed Tomography

Because the small TM joint is surrounded by the dense mass of bony skull, conventional bone scanning is not sufficiently sensitive to detect the subtle early changes of TM joint anomalies. The advent of single photon emission computed tomography (SPECT) and positron emission tomography (PET) have brought a new dimension to the application of radioisotope scanning in the detection of TMJ disease.[64,65] Using a rotating gamma ray detector and computer processing of emission data from the injected bone-seeking radio-

isotopes, tomographic images are generated (Fig. 3–15).

The radiation exposure of the patient resulting from SPECT and PET is lower than that resulting from conventional nuclear medicine techniques. This contrast is the result of the difference in labels used and because of the more efficient utilization of the image-forming photons. The cross-sectional technique delineates internal structure and permits the measurement of local biochemical processes, and has been called physiologic tomography.[66] Clinically useful applications are providing PET of the brain and pituitary, liver, heart, thyroid, adrenal glands, and bones; of special interest are the bones of the face and neck.[67,68] The radiation dose resulting from the administration of the radiopharmaceuticals labeled with so-called physiologic positron-emitting radionuclides is low.

### TM Joint

SPECT is a sensitive indicator of TM joint dysfunction and differentiates active, organic TM joint disease from both an arrested disease state and a healthy TMJ, according to studies reported by Kircos and associates.[69] Osterreich and associates[70] described bone

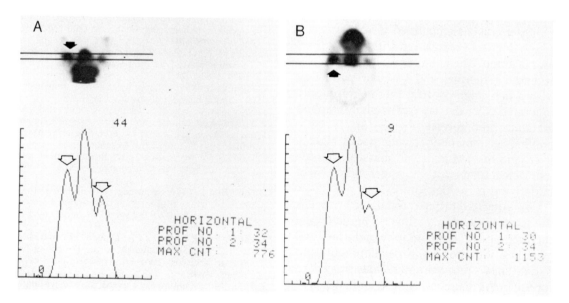

*Fig. 3–15.* Single photon emission computed tomograph (SPECT) images, in the coronal plane, A, and transaxial plane, B, shows an intense area of increased uptake in the right TM joint (arrow). The tomographic nature of SPECT imaging allows focal areas of increased uptake to be accentuated and quantitated by a computer program. Activity graph under the SPECT image shows an increased accumulation of radioisotope in the right TM joint compared to the left (open arrows). (Courtesy of Dr. Eugene J. Messer.)

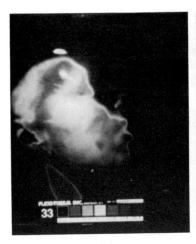 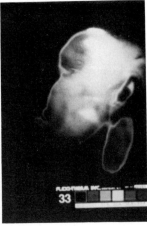

*Fig. 3–16.* Thermographic representation, actually in color, of topographic temperature variances of the facial soft tissues.

scanning and SPECT as providing information about functional disturbances in affected TMJ; their study included the use of SPECT to evaluate the effectiveness of bite splint treatment.

## Thermography

Liquid crystals, cholesterol derivatives, that selectively reflect polarized light in a narrow region of wavelengths have a specific color-temperature response and are used in color thermography. A cost-effective application of the thermographic technique involves the use of liquid crystals embedded in elastic sheet; a high degree of correlation with clinical findings is noted. The liquid crystals dramatically accentuate thermal and vascular pathology with a rich, high-contrast thermographically calibrated color display that is photographed for study and record (Fig. 3–16). Thermographic examinations of the facial tissues overlying the TM joint and masseter muscle may detect temperature changes indicative of underlying pathologic processes.[71]

Computerized infrared tomography avoids the surface irregularity artifact of liquid crystal thermography. Thermography of the face and neck is under study and development, and to date shows promise as a reliable procedure for use in the diagnosis of head and neck pain syndromes.

## References

1. Preti G., Bruscagin C., Scotti R., and Cardesi E.: Statistical study of the angle formed by the lateral part of the mandibular condyle and the horizontal plane. J Prosthet Dent, 50:571, 1983.
2. Lindblom C.: Technique for roentgen-photographic registration of the different condyle positions in the temporomandibular joint. Dent Cosmos, 78:1227, 1936.
3. Aquilino S.A., Matteson S.R., Holland G.A., and Phillips, C.: Evaluation of condylar position from temporomandibular joint radiographs. J Prosthet Dent, 53:88, 1985.
4. Chilvarquer I., et al.: A new technique for imaging the temporomandibular joint with a panoramic x-ray machine. Oral Surg Oral Med Oral Pathol, 65:626, 1988.
5. Southard T.E., Harris F.F., Walter R.G.: Image enhancement of the mandibular condyle through digital subtraction. Oral Surg Oral Med Oral Pathol, 64:645, 1986.
6. Fujita M., et al.: Digital imaging processing of dentomaxillary radiographs. Oral Surg Oral Med Oral Pathol, 64:485, 1987.
7. Fujita M., et al.: Digital image processing of periapical radiographs. Oral Surg Oral Med Oral Pathol, 65:490, 1988.
8. McNulty B.: Xeroradiography adds new dimensions to intraoral imaging. Quint Int, 11:91, 1980.
9. Nakasima A., Nakata S., Shimizu K., and Takahama Y.: Radiologic exposure and conditions and resultant skin doses in application of xeroradiography to the orthodontic diagnosis. Am J Orthod, 78:646, 1980.
10. Worfe J.N.: Xeroradiography: Image content and comparison with film roentgenograms. AJR, 117:690, 1973.
11. Gratt B.M., et al.: Xeroradiography of dental structures. IV. Image properties of a dedicated intraoral system. Oral Surg Oral Med Oral Pathol, 50:572, 1980.
12. Christensen E.E., Curry T.S., Dowdey J.E., and Murray R.G. Jr.: An Introduction to the Physics of Diagnostic Radiology. 3rd Ed. Philadelphia, Lea & Febiger, 1984.
13. Dunn M.J., Rabinov K., Hayens K., and Jennings, S.: Polycycloidal corrected tomography of the temporomandibular joint. Oral Surg Oral Med Oral Pathol, 51:375, 1981.
14. Heffez L., Jordan S., Rosenberg H., and Miescke K.: Accuracy of temporomandibular joint measurements using corrected hypocycloidal tomographs. J Oral Maxillofac Surg, 45:137, 1987.

15. Heffez L., Jordan S., and Going R. Jr.: Determination of the radiographic position of the temporomandibular disc. Oral Surg Oral Med Oral Pathol, 65:272, 1988.

16. Delfino J.J. and Eppley B.L.: Radiographic and surgical evaluation of internal derangements of the temporomandibular joints. J Oral Maxillofac Surg, 44:260, 1986.

17. Murphy W.A., et al.: Magnification radiography of the temporomandibular joint: Technical considerations. Radiology, 123:49, 1977.

18. Abramovitch K., Dolwick M.F., and Langlais R.P.: Temporomandibular joint arthrography without fluoroscopy. Oral Surg Oral Med Oral Pathol, 65:387, 1988.

19. Kaplan P.A., et al.: Inferior joint space arthrography of normal temporomandibular joints: Reassessment of diagnostic criteria. Radiology, 159:585, 1986.

20. Takaku S.: On the ten cases of the TMJ disorders comparing the arthrographical findings with the operative findings. Jpn Soc Dent Radiol, 7–8, 14–34, 1967.

21. Chao-chu C., et al.: Evaluation of temporomandibular arthrography in TMJ dysfunction. An analysis of 60 cases. Chin Med J (Engl), 10:132,601, 1973.

22. Carlsson G.E., Oberg T., Bergman F., and Fajers C.M.: Morphological changes in the mandibular joint disk in the temporomandibular joint pain dysfunction syndrome. Acta Odontol Scand, 25:163, 1967.

23. Agerberg G. and Lundberg M.: Changes in the temporomandibular joint after surgical treatment. Oral Surg Oral Med Oral Pathol, 32:865, 1971.

24. Nanthaviorj S., Omnell K.A., Randow K., and Obert T.: Clicking and temporary locking in the temporomandibular joint. A clinical, radiographical, and electromyographical study. Dentomaxillofac Radiol, 5:33, 1976.

25. Farrar W.B.: Characteristics of the condylar path in internal derangements of the temporomandibular joint. J Prosthet Dent, 39:319, 1978.

26. Van Willigan J.: The sagittal condylar movements of the clicking temporomandibular joint. J Oral Rehabil, 6:167, 1979.

27. Wilkes C.H.: Structural and functional alterations of the temporomandibular joint. Northwest Dent, 57:287, 1978.

28. Wilkes C.H.: Arthrography of the temporomandibular joint. Minn Med, 61:645, 1978.

29. Katzberg R.W., Dolwick M.F., Bales D.J., and Helms C.A.: Arthrotomography of the temporomandibular joint: New technique and preliminary observations. AJR, 132:949, 1979.

30. Dolwick M.F., Katzberg R.W., Helms C.A., and Bales D.J.: Arthrotomographic evaluation of the temporomandibular joint. J Oral Maxillofac Surg, 37:793, 1979.

31. Lynch T.P. and Chase D.C.: Arthrography in the evaluation of the temporomandibular joint. Radiology, 126:667, 1978.

32. Blaschke D.D., Solberg W.K., and Sanders B.: Arthrography of the temporomandibular joint: Review of current status. J Am Dent Assoc, 100:388, 1980.

33. Westesson P.L.: Double-contrast arthrotomography of the temporomandibular joint. Introduction of an arthrographic technique for visualization of the disk and articular surfaces. J Oral Maxillofac Surg, 41:1643, 1983.

34. Irby W.B.: Surgical treatment of TMJ problems. Vol. III. Edited by W.B. Irby. Current advances in oral surgery. St. Louis, C.V. Mosby, 1980.

35. Zetz M.R., Irby W.B., and Doles L.R.: A simplified method for injection of aspiration of the temporomandibular joint. J Am Dent Assoc, 194:855, 1982.

36. Osborn A.G., Hanafee W.H., and Mancuso A.A.: CT of the mandible: Normal and pathologic anatomy. AJR, 139:555, 1982.

37. Manco L.G., et al.: Internal derangements of the temporomandibular joint evaluated with direct sagittal CT: A prospective study. Radiology, 157:407, 1985.

38. Heffez L., Mafee M.F., and Langer B.: Double contrast arthrography of the temporomandibular joint: Role of direct sagittal CT imaging. Oral Surg Oral Med Oral Pathol, 65:511, 1988.

39. Morgan C.J. and Hendee W.R.: Introduction of Magnetic Resonance Imaging. Denver, Multi-Media Publishing, 1984.

40. Manzione J.V., et al.: Magnetic resonance imaging of the temporomandibular joint. J Am Dent Assoc, 113:398, 1986.

41. Vannier M.W.: Nuclear magnetic resonance imaging. Postgrad Med, 76:159, 1984.

42. Katzberg R.W., et al.: Magnetic imaging of the temporomandibular joint meniscus. Oral Surg Oral Med Oral Pathol, 59:332, 1985.

43. Wilk R.M., Harms S.E., and Wolford L.M.: Magnetic resonance imaging of the temporomandibular joint using a surface coil. J Oral Maxillofac Surg, 44:935, 1986.

44. Donlan W.C. and Moon K.L.: Comparison of magnetic resonance imaging, arthrotomography and clinical and surgical findings in temporomandibular joint internal derangements. Oral Surg Oral Med Oral Pathol, 64:2, 1987.

45. Donlan E.A., et al.: Correlation of magnetic resonance imaging and surgical findings in patients with meniscal perforation. J Craniomandib Disord Facial Oral Pain, 3:174, 1989.

46. Kircos L.T., et al.: Magnetic resonance imaging of the TMJ disc in asymptomatic volunteers. J Oral Maxillofac Surg, 45:852, 1987.

47. Sanchez-Woodworth R.E., Tallents R.H., Katzberg R.W., and Guay J.A.: Bilateral internal derangements of the temporomandibular joint: Evaluation by magnetic resonance imaging. Oral Surg Oral Med Oral Pathol, 65:281, 1988.

48. Daniels D.L., et al.: Trigeminal nerve: Anatomic correlation with MR imaging. Radiology, 159:577, 1986.

49. House M.D., Waluch V., and Jackler R.K.: Magnetic resonance imaging in acoustic neuroma diagnosis. Ann Otol Rhinol Laryngol, 95:16, 1985.

50. Ohnishi M.: Clinical application of arthroscopy in the temporomandibular joint diseases. Bull Tokyo Med Dent Univ, 27:141, 1980.

51. Goss A.N. and Bosanquet A.C.: Temporomandibular joint arthroscopy. J Oral Maxillofac Surg, 44:614, 1986.

52. Heffez L. and Blaustein D.: Diagnostic arthroscopy of the temporomandibular joint. Part I. Normal arthroscopic findings. Oral Surg Oral Med Oral Pathol, 64:653, 1987.

53. Blaustein D. and Heffez L.: Diagnostic arthroscopy of the temporomandibular joint. Part II. Arthroscopic findings of arthrographically diagnosed disk displacements. Oral Surg Oral Med Oral Pathol, 65:135, 1988.

54. Van Sickel J.E., Nishioka G.J., Hegewald M.D., and Neal G.D.: Middle ear injury resulting from tem-

poromandibular joint arthroscopy. J Oral Maxillofac Surg, *45*:967, 1987.

55. Barrett H.H. and Swindell S.: Radiological Imaging. Vol. 2. New York, Academic Press, 1981.

56. Alexander J.M.: Radionuclide bone scanning in the diagnosis of lesions of the maxillofacial region. J Oral Maxillofac Surg, *34*:249, 1976.

57. Higashi R., et al.: Technetium 99m bone imaging in the evaluation of cancer of the maxillofacial region. J Oral Maxillofac Surg, *37*:254, 1979.

58. Epstein J.B., Hatcher D.C., and Graham K.: Bone scintigraphy of fibro-osseous lesions of the jaw. Oral Surg Oral Med Oral Pathol, *51*:346, 1981.

59. Higashi T., Iguchi M., Shimura A., and Kruglik G.D.: Computed tomography and bone scintigraphy in polyostotic fibrous dysplasia. Oral Surg Oral Med Oral Pathol, *50*:580, 1980.

60. Lurie A.G., Puri S., James R.B., and Jensen T.H.W.: Radionuclide bone imaging in the surgical treatment planning of odontogenic keratocysts. Oral Surg Oral Med Oral Pathol, *42*:726, 1976.

61. Tow D.E., Garcia D.S., Jansons D., and Sullivan T.M.: Bone scan in dental disease. J Nucl Med, *19*:845, 1976.

62. Lee H.K. and Markowitz J.: 99m Technetium diphosphonate bone scanning of the mandibular bone graft. Oral Surg Oral Med Oral Pathol, *49*:471, 1980.

63. Keller D.C., Jackson R.F., Cusumano J.V., and Cook M.A.: Quantitative radionuclide scanning of the temporomandibular joint. J Craniomandib Pract, *5*:152, 1987.

64. Collier B.D., et al.: Internal derangement of the temporomandibular joint: Detection by single photon emission computed tomography. Radiology, *149*:557, 1983.

65. Katzberg R.W., O'Mara R.E., and Weber D.A.: Radionuclide skeletal imaging and single photon emission computed tomography in suspected internal derangements of the temporomandibular joint. J Oral Maxillofac Surg, *42*:782, 1984.

66. Phelps M.E. and Mazziotta J.C.: Cerebral positron computed tomography. *In* Advanced Imaging Techniques. Edited by T.H. Newton and D.G. Potts. San Anselmo, CA, Clavadel Press, 1983.

67. Ell P.J. and Khan O.: Emission computerized tomography: Clinical application. Semin Nucl Med, *11*:50, 1981.

68. Britton K.E.: Quantitation: Clinical applications. *In* Computed Emission Tomography. Edited by P.J. Ell and B.J. Holman. Oxford, University Press, 1982.

69. Kircos L.T., et al.: Emission imaging in patients with craniomandibular dysfunction. Oral Surg Oral Med Oral Pathol, *65*:249, 1988.

70. Osterreich F.-V., Jend-Rossman I., Jend H.-H., Triebel H.J.: Semiquantitative SPECT imaging for assessment of bone reactions in internal derangements of the temporomandibular joint. J Oral Maxillofac Surg, *45*:1022, 1987.

71. Pogrel M.A., et al.: Liquid crystal thermography as a diagnostic aid and objective monitor for TMJ dysfunction and myogenic facial pain. J Craniomandib Disord Facial Oral Pain, *3*:65, 1989.

# Diagnostic
# Anesthetic Methods

Local anesthetic agents are used in the oral regions primarily to block the transmission of pain that accompanies operations. Local infiltrations and anesthetic blocks are useful for differential diagnoses between pains of the soma and the psyche and, especially, of referred pains, neurologic pains, and atypical facial pains. Learning and relearning of anatomy is necessary to ensure delivery of appropriate amounts of anesthetic agents to given anatomic points when dealing with craniofacial pains with obscure etiologies.

Local anesthetic blocks may be used to identify the etiologic area in patients with peripheral neurologic and inflammatory disorders and to assist in discriminating between pains that may originate from two different structures. Also, referral of pain may be identified with anesthetic blocks; i.e., pain sensed in the temporal region may originate from a pulpitis in a maxillary molar tooth. An anesthetic blocking of the tooth will completely relieve the temporal pain; however, anesthetic infiltration in the temporal region will not clearly relieve the pain being sensed. As another example, blocking of specific trigeminal peripheral nerves may help in establishing the triggering area of tic douloureux. Likewise, discriminating between adjacent teeth as potential sources of noxious stimuli is possible with periodontal ligament infiltration of local anesthetic agents.

One may observe, when evaluating a chronic pain patient, that an anesthetic block produces immediate relief of pain. This success may lead to the assumption that the etiology of the pain is peripheral and originated in either muscular spasms, in a neurologic malady, or in the temporomandibular joint (TMJ). If, however, the pain relief lasts for a matter of minutes, for a period that is shorter than the expected duration of the anesthesia, one must not assume that the anesthetized area is the origin of the pain. In this situation, the placebo effect, including an endogenous opioid release, is likely responsible for the brief relief. With the hydrolysis of the endorphins dynorphin and enkephalin in the patient's blood plasma, the pain relief ends and the central mechanisms then again sustain the pain. Therefore, the results of peripheral anesthetic blocks should be considered in concert with all other available diagnostic data. As an example, a middle-aged patient who has had a diffuse unilateral facial pain for years with radiologic evidence of minimal bony changes in the TMJ of the affected side may have immediate and complete relief after an auriculotemporal nerve block. The relief lasts for only 7 to 8 minutes rather than the expected 30 minutes or more. One may not assume the etiology of the pain is principally peripheral in origin and that peripheral treatments, including an operation involving the TM joint would likely relieve the patient's pain. The direction of treatment should be toward controlling central pain mechanisms, usually with psychiatric or psychologic methods.

## Biochemical and Anatomical Considerations

The chemical structures of local anesthetic agents feature either an ester or an amide linkage. Blood plasma is the primary site of metabolism of degradation for all agents with an ester linkage; an example of these agents is procaine (Novacaine). The liver is the primary site for degradation and metabolism of agents with an amide linkage; examples of these anesthetic agents are lidocaine (Xylocaine), mepivacaine (Carbocaine), and bupivacaine (Maracaine).

The known chemistry of local anesthetic agents indicates that both the ester and the amide bond will break down into an alcohol through metabolic hydrolysis. This event could occur while the anesthetic is in the vicinity of the nerve fibers resulting in a persistent neurologic deficit.[1,2,3] In vitro studies of neuroreceptors have shown that a local anesthetic agent is capable of bonding noncovalently to the mammalian receptor.[4] A persistent neurologic deficit may be associated with the technique employed, total dose of local anesthetic agent administered, particular agent used, route of administration, and the physical condition of the patient.[5]

The peripheral sensory nervous system includes nerves composed of fibers with different thicknesses of myelin. The greater the thickness, the faster the nerve fiber will conduct. The least myelinated fibers, 0.1—1.0 microns, are the slowest transmitting fibers and conduct pain sensations. The more myelinated fibers, 1—4 microns, conduct cold and heat sensations; touch 4—8 microns; and pressure and proprioceptive functions 8—13 microns. Therefore, the type of sensations being reported will indicate which fibers within the nerve have not been affected by either anesthetic agents or other factors. The taste fibers of the chorda tympani nerve which joins the lingual branch are slow conducting fibers with some degree of myelination but less than those of the fibers of touch, pressure, and proprioception.[6]

## Terminology

When using a block type of anesthesia, the nerve to be anesthetized names the type of injection. The term *posterior-superior alveolar block* is preferable to zygomatic block or tuberosity block, because no zygomatic or tuberosity nerve exists. Also, the term *inferior alveolar block* is preferable to mandibular block, unless the block involves the entire third division of the trigeminal nerve, with the local anesthetic agent delivered at the foramen ovale.

An infiltration anesthetic is named by the region, the structure, or the area being anesthetized. Masseter muscle infiltration describes an injection one might use into a myospastic or trigger point in the muscle. An infiltration of the periodontal ligament of the left mandibular second molar is an exact description of anesthetizing a structure.

## Instruments, Materials and Anesthetic Agents

The materials needed to perform intraoral and extraoral diagnostic injection series include the following:

1. 3 × 3 inch or 4 × 4 inch cotton gauze sponges to dry an intraoral injection site and surrounding tissues. For extraoral injections, surgical scrub soaps, antiseptic solutions, and gauze sponges are required.
2. Cotton applicators to apply antiseptic solution for intraoral injections.
3. A selection of anesthetic agents without vasoconstrictors: 3% mepivacaine, 2% lidocaine, and 2% procaine.
4. Disposable needles, no smaller than 25 gauge.
5. An aspirating syringe.
6. Emergency equipment and agents.

If the stopper in the anesthetic cartridge does not travel smoothly down the lumen, the aspirating syringe should be withdrawn. The procedure is then reinstituted with a new anesthetic cartridge. In an effort to overcome this irregular movement, the dentist could apply extra force and cause the stopper to turn, which would permit the plunger on the syringe to drive forward, shattering the glass cartridge.

Mepivacaine, 3% (54 mg) is supplied in 1.8-ml anesthetic cartridges, produces a rapid onset and 20- to 40-minute duration regional anesthesia, and is most useful for diagnostic blocks and infiltrations. The maximum recommended amount of 3% mepivacaine solution is 270 mg in adults (five anesthetic cartridges). Mepivacaine 2% (36 mg) is supplied in 1.8-ml anesthetic cartridges with 1:30,000 concentration of a vasoconstrictor, levonordefrin (Neo-Cobefrin), and produces regional anesthesia of 2 to 4 hours duration. In equal concentrations, levonordefrin causes slightly less hypertension than epinephrine. The maximum recommended amount of the 2% mepivacaine with levonordefrin is 180 mg in adults (five anesthetic cartridges).

Lidocaine, 2% (36 mg), without the addition of epinephrine is supplied in 1.8-ml anesthetic cartridges, provides a rapid onset and 30 to 60 minutes duration regional anesthesia, and is useful for diagnostic blocks and infiltrations. The amount of lidocaine at 4.5 mg/kg should not exceed 300 mg in adults (about eight anesthetic cartridges). The addition of 1:100,000 epinephrine prolongs anesthesia to 2 to 4 hours; the addition of epinephrine slows the absorption rate and 7 mg/kg (500 mg) should be the maximum dosage in adults (about 13 anesthetic cartridges).

Bupivacaine, 0.25% and 0.50%, is supplied in multiple-dose vials and 1.8-ml anesthetic cartridges with and without 1:200,000 epinephrine. The regional anesthesia is rapid in onset and is prolonged to 4 to 8 hours without epinephrine and 4 to 10 with epinephrine. The onset is slightly more rapid with the 0.50% solution. Each milliliter of the 0.25% solution contains 25 mg of bupivacaine; each milliliter of the 0.50% solution contains 50 mg. The total daily dose in adults should not exceed 400 mg. The 0.25% and the 0.50% agents, with or without epinephrine, are recommended for peripheral nerve injections. Only the 0.25% solution, with or without epinephrine, is recommended for infiltration procedures; only the 0.25% without epinephrine for sympathetic nerve injections; and neither concentration for children under 12 years of age.

The dose required of any of the agents to produce regional analgesia or anesthesia varies depending on the area to be anesthetized, local vascularity, individual variations of age, tolerance, and technique. In all instances, the lowest dose needed to provide anesthesia is preferred.

The agents used for intramuscular injections of myospastic muscles and muscular trigger points and diagnostic blocks produce an area of destruction of the muscle. Procaine is the least destructive and toxic to muscular tissue. The availability of procaine and its relative short shelf life mitigate against the routine use of the agent. Marcaine has a destructive onset within 15 minutes; repair of the muscle takes 3 weeks. The usual agents are 2% lidocaine and 3% carbocaine, with mepivacaine being less destructive than lidocaine.[7,8]

For diagnostic purposes, these agents should be used without vasoconstrictors, which also are destructive to muscles. A severe hypertensive episode may occur in a patient who is receiving monoamine oxidase (MAO) inhibitors or antidepressant agents of the imipramine or amytriptyline types when a vasoconstrictor is injected. Therefore, anesthetic solutions containing either norepinephrine or epinephrine are used with extreme caution. Patients who are not taking MAO inhibitors have an endogenous release of catecholamines from fear and stress of dental therapy that is greater than that of the vasoconstrictor in a typical regional anesthetic injection. When MAO is inhibited in a patient, however, the exogenous amount of an anesthetic injection may become critical and lead to a cardiac crisis, as we have observed in two patients during the past 30 years.

Surface vapocoolants provide transient topical anesthesia for myospastic trigger points accessible to the spray. The usual topical vapocoolants are fluoromethane and ethyl chloride. Three or four puffs of the spray produce transient profound cooling of the cutaneous tissues and transient surface anesthesia, as well as apparent anesthesia of the immediately underlying muscular and subcutaneous tissues.

## Appointment for Diagnostic Injections

An appointment for diagnostic injections may last for several hours, and short action anesthetics without vasoconstrictors of either 3% mepivacaine or 2% lidocaine are usually used. In general, the most peripheral of the structures to be investigated are anesthetized first. The series of injections are planned to permit cessation of the series at the point at which a positive diagnosis is made. As an example, to identify a pain problem in the left nasolabial fold area, a likely diagnostic injection plan is as follows: (1) periodontal ligament infiltrations of suspected teeth; (2) nasopalatine canal infiltration; (3) infiltration over the anterior wall of the maxillary sinus; (4) infraorbital nerve block; and (5) maxillary division block. A pain problem in the temporal muscle could promote a diagnostic injection plan that begins with injection into the site of the perceived pain. If the problem is related to referred pain, some short-term relief may be noted owing to the release of endogenous opioids and the relaxation of the possible accompanying myalgia. These findings are then compared with the relief obtained from further diagnostic injections performed in the following order: periodontal ligament infiltrations of suspected teeth, posterior-superior alveolar nerve block, and a maxillary division block. If further injections are necessary, these include: periodontal ligament infiltrations of suspected mandibular teeth, mental nerve block, lingual nerve block, inferior alveolar nerve block, TMJ ligament infiltration, intracapsular infiltration, auriculotemporal nerve block, mandibular division block, and cervical sympathetic nerve block.

Most patients dread injections. A patient's fears are best allayed with a skillful operating team led by a dentist in whom the patient has confidence. If psychologic support is necessary, the operating team may use a high level of conscious sedation with inhalation of nitrous oxide and oxygen. The short duration of nitrous oxide and oxygen psychosedation is admirably suited to these diagnostic procedures.

## Injection Techniques

The anesthetic cartridge is loaded into the aspirating syringe and, if the anesthetic equipment permits, the rubber stopper in the anesthetic cartridge is engaged by the harpoon-equipped plunger in the aspirating syringe; a sharp slapping motion engages the stopper and the plunger. A small amount of anesthetic solution is expressed to ascertain that the solution can flow freely.

For transoral injections, the site of the injection is prepared by wiping and blotting with 7.5 × 7.5 cm or 10 × 10 cm cotton gauze sponges and applying an antiseptic solution. The antiseptic solution does not sterilize the injection site, although it decreases the number of micro-organisms that can be introduced into deeper structures by the needle. The soft tissues of the injection site are pulled taut by the dentist; the doctor should reassure the patient as the injection proceeds. The needle is introduced rapidly through the mucosa, and a few drops of anesthetic solution are deposited submucosally. As the needle is advanced to the point for deposition of the solution, the plunger is depressed; this action creates a flow of anesthetic solution ahead of the needle that may deflect blood vessels out of the path of the needle. When the needle reaches the site for injection, an aspiration is performed. A return of blood into the anesthetic cartridge does not indicate the unlikely event that the lumen of the needle is in a blood vessel; it probably indicates that vessels have been inadvertently lacerated and that blood is pooled in the tissues (Fig. 4–1).[9] Normally, the anesthetic solution is injected in a steady motion over a 15- to 30-second period per 1.0 ml.

For extraoral injections, the preceding techniques are followed with appropriate changes for cutaneous preparation; scrubbing with surgical soap, painting with antiseptic solutions, and use of sterile drapes around the injection site.

### Periodontal Ligament and Intraosseous Anesthetic Injections

The periodontal ligament has been used for decades as the pathway for introduction of anesthetic solutions, with the anesthesia primarily affecting a single tooth. Various injection instruments are now available for this purpose.[10] Although introduced into the ligament, the anesthetic solution diffuses through the osseous alveolar wall and its adjacent medullary spaces.[11] Thus, the effectiveness of the technique in producing reliable anesthesia varies considerably depending on the physical and physiologic characteristics of the periodontal ligament, the density of the cortex of the alveolus, the length of the root, the physical and physiologic characteristics of the medullary spaces, and the pressures used to introduce the anesthetic solution.

Effective anesthesia may be produced with a standard anesthetic dental syringe and a 25- or 26-gauge or smaller needle. After application of a topical anesthetic agent, the needle is inserted firmly, with the bevel toward the tooth, into the crevice between the gingival cuff and the tooth. If properly placed, only a few drops of the solution are expressed into the dense periodontal ligament by a pumping movement of the plunger. Blanching of the surrounding gingival cuff may be noted. The procedure may be repeated in two sites around single rooted teeth and at three or four sites around a molar tooth.

The mode of anesthetic production is not clear. Moore and associates compared lidocaine with 1:100,000 epinephrine and normal saline, and found the anesthesia was related to biochemical activity of the lidocaine and epinephrine.[12] Handler and Moore compared 2% lidocaine, with and without epinephrine, and 1:100,000 epinephrine;[13] surprisingly, the most effective agent was lidocaine, with a du-

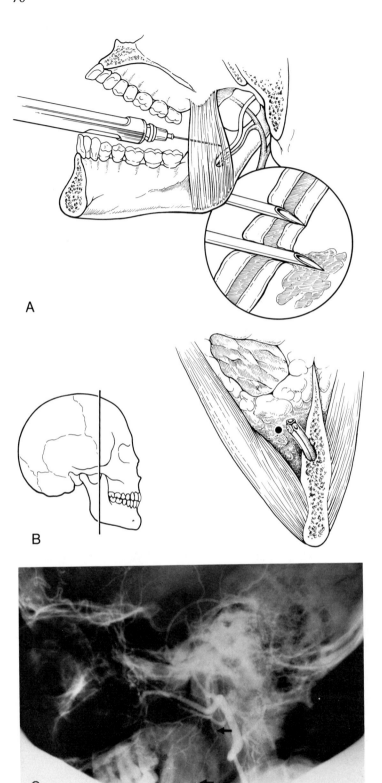

*Fig. 4–1.* Blood aspiration prior to an inferior alveolar nerve block. Blood aspirated when performing an inferior alveolar block anesthetic injection arises from blood spillages due to inadvertent lacerations by the injection syringe of blood vessels in the area. The longitudinal opening of the tip of the needle is longer than the cross section diameter of the inferior alveolar artery. A. Position of the needle advancing towards the pterygomandibular fossa, and proportionate approximation of the lumen of needle, and the cross-section of a large inferior alveolar artery. Blood spillage could arise from the inferior alveolar artery, vein, muscle, and facial tissues. B. Coronal section from a posterior view indicating the relationship of the internal (medial) pterygoid muscle and mandibular ramus that form a pocket for accumulating spilled blood in the intermuscular fascia. C. Arteriogram of the external carotid artery and its branches, including the inferior alveolar artery (two arrows).

ration of anesthesia of 35.7 minutes; second was 1:100,000 epinephrine, 26 minutes; third was lidocaine with 1:50,000 epinephrine, 25.5 minutes; and fourth was lidocaine with 1:100,000 epinephrine, 22.1 minutes. They concluded that the anesthesia may have been caused by pressure or ischema rather than the pharmacologic action of the anesthetic agent.

Regardless of the pharmacology or the physiology, the onset of anesthesia is prompt and profound and reliably lasts for approximately 30 minutes. Contiguous structures may be anesthetized, and the agent may spread into adjacent areas.[14] The potential for distribution of the solution to adjacent teeth must be considered when using this technique for diagnostic anesthetic testing of individual teeth.

Intraosseous anesthesia is produced by direct penetration into the medullary bone spaces and then injection of an anesthetic solution directly into the medullary spaces. Profound anesthesia of associated dentition follows intraosseous introduction of anesthetic agents.[15,16]

## Mandibular Division

**Mandibular Incisor Teeth Infiltration.** Anesthetic solution is deposited over the thin cortical bone adjacent to the apices of the four mandibular incisors, producing anesthesia of the incisor teeth and the labial gingiva. A patient with a painful pathologic process at the midline of the mandible or the incisor teeth requires anesthesia for possible anastomosing nerve fibers from the contralateral side.

**Mental Nerve Block.** This procedure is performed at or through the mental foramen, which lies just below the mandibular premolar apices or beneath the second premolar. It is located 10 to 12 mm above the inferior border of the mandible in most anatomic situations regardless of the overall height of the mandible. Although this and other descriptions involve a single foramen and nerve, we have observed during operations on the anterior lateral aspect of the body of the mandible that several trunks of the nerve may emerge from one or more foramina. The mental nerve exits through the mental foramen after traversing the short mental canal from the inferior alveolar canal. The lower lip and the chin can be anesthetized by deposition of approximately 1.5 ml of anesthetic solution into or lateral to the mental foramen. To anesthetize the incisors, the canine, the premolar teeth, the labial gingiva, and the inferior lip effectively, the needle must enter the mental canal for its entire distance of 3 to 6 mm. The canal projects laterally, posteriorly, and superiorly in the adult; thus, the needle must be directed inward, downward, and forward. The mental nerve block may be delivered intraorally or extraorally (Fig. 4–2). The mental nerve block injection techniques, to be completely effective, require that the needle enter the canal, which may require palpating with the needle point.

**Long Buccal Nerve Block.** A 0.3 to 0.5-ml amount of anesthetic solution is deposited into the vestibular mucosa just distal to the tooth or the area being investigated. Anesthesia of the buccal mucosa anterior to the injection site is produced. The long buccal innervation terminates in the area of the mental nerve.

**Lingual Nerve Block.** The clinician deposits 0.5 ml of anesthetic solution in the lateral posterior floor of the mouth, thereby producing discrete anesthetization of the lingual nerve. The lingual nerve has several normal positions in the posterior floor of the mouth: above and below the mylohyoid muscle and in various positions in the mucosa medial to the third molar. We have observed that the lingual nerve may have a trunk varying in size from 2 to 4 mm in diameter, and it may have more than one trunk. These observations were made during operations when, on the recommendation of a neurologist or a neurosurgeon, the lingual nerve was permanently sectioned. In the posterior floor of the mouth, the lingual nerve may be located just medial to the mandibular third molar (Fig. 4–3).[17] When an inferior alveolar nerve block is performed, the lingual nerve is usually affected by the deposition of the anesthetic solution. The sensory distribution of the lingual nerve includes the mucous membrane on the floor of the mouth, the lingual gingiva, and the mucous membrane of the anterior two thirds of the tongue.

**Inferior Alveolar Nerve Block.** This block

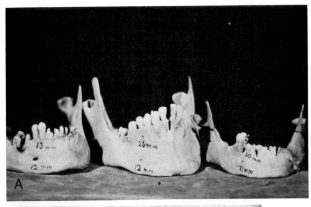

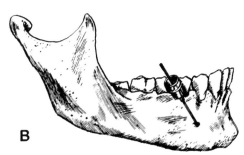

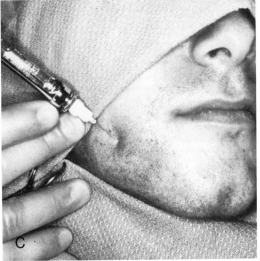

*Fig. 4–2.* The mental nerve block. The mental foramen is located at different levels below the height of the alveolar ridge, which is highly variable. However, the foramen is located approximately 10 to 14 mm above the anatomically stable base of the mandible, and it has an orifice directed posteriorly and superiorly. A. Variations of the distance to the superior margin of the alveolar ridge. Distance to the inferior base of the mandible is fairly constant. (Courtesy of the University of Michigan School of Dentistry and Clinical Dentistry.) B. The injection needle needs to be projected inferiorly and anteriorly to enter the foramen from either a transoral or C. an extraoral approach.

is performed with the bidigital palpation technique, which takes into account the variability of size and contours of the rami of the mandible in different individuals. Some of the variations are in the total anterior-posterior width, which may range from 20 to 45 mm; in the alignment of the ramus with the body of the mandible, which may range from straight extension of the body of the mandible to lateral flaring by as much as 25°; and in the placement of the interior alveolar foramen, which may be at, below, or above the general occlusal plane of the mandibular dentition. In a study at the University of Michigan performed several decades ago, Cook noted that the mandibular foramen and the sulcus are in a line between the narrowest anterior-posterior dimension of the ramus and two thirds the distance from the anterior to the posterior border.[18] The location of the center of the sulcus, two thirds of the distance from the an-

terior to the posterior border, was constant within 2-mm limits. With these anatomic facts established, a precise injection technique is possible wherein the sulcus is located in a line determined by the middle of the thumb and the middle finger. For a right inferior alveolar injection, the center of the palmar surface of the thumb is set at the innermost point of the indentation of the external oblique line, the center of the palmar surface of the third finger is set at the innermost point of the indentation of the external oblique line, and the center of the palmar surface of the third finger is set at the innermost point of the indentation on the posterior border. With the thumb and the third finger in these positions, the center of the sulcus is in a line between the fingers (Fig. 4–4). A straight line is more easily established with the thumb and the third finger than with any other finger, and this straight line is the essence of this injection. With the width of

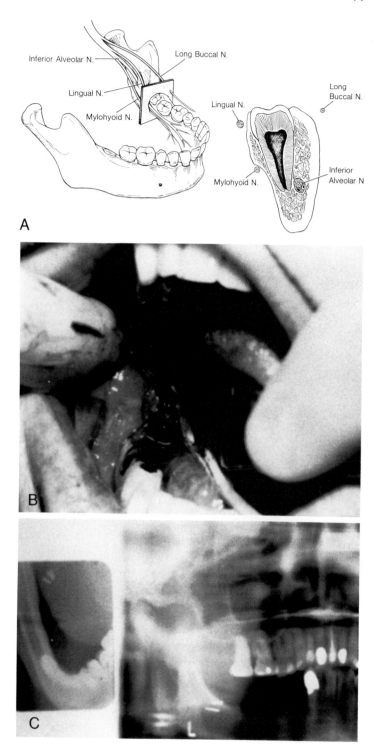

*Fig. 4–3.* A pathway of the lingual nerve; wide variations are the rule. (Courtesy of Alling, C.C., Dysesthesia of the lingual and inferior alveolar nerves following third molar surgery. J Oral Maxillofac Surg *44*:454, 1986.) A. The path of the nerve in the third molar region is in the proportion described by Kiesselbach and Chamberlain;[11] the proportions of the mandible, lingual plate, and third molar are as described by Wheeler. (Wheeler, R.C. Dental anatomy, physiology, and occlusion. Philadelphia, W.B. Saunders, 1974.) B. View of a lingual nerve trunk prior removing a 10 mm section. C. View of vascular clips on two trunks of a lingual nerve following sectioning.

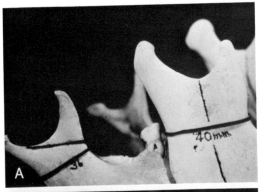

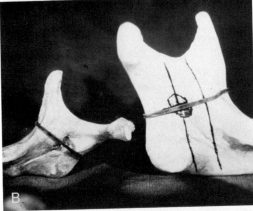

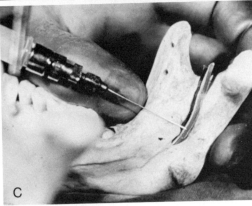

*Fig. 4-4.* Inferior alveolar nerve injection. A. There are variations in the angle and the width of the ramus to the body of the mandible. B. A line passing through the depth of the contour of the anterior and posterior borders also passes through the pterygomandibular fossa which contains, at its base, the inferior alveolar foramen. C. This anatomic fact is used in clinical applications by palpating the narrowest portion and letting the needle guide in on the plane between the fingers. (Courtesy of Clinical Dentistry; photographs courtesy of the University of Michigan School of Dentistry.)

the ramus established by palpation, the needle is inserted directly toward the inferior alveolar sulcus, which is located two thirds the distance from the anterior to the posterior border of the ramus. For the left inferior alveolar nerve block, the right-handed doctor may either place the fingers of the right hand on the left ramus and proceed as described, using the left hand to control the injection syringe, or place the left middle finger at the posterior margin of the ramus and use the left thumb both to retract the lips and to palpate the anterior border of the left ramus; the right hand manages the injection syringe.

A second advantage of this technique of bidigital palpation of the ramus is the physical control the dentist has of the patient. Because the doctor is supporting the mandible, the patient is not able to move it unexpectedly. Positive psychologic support of the patient is gained by the physical control employed by the doctor. In the past, these controls were necessary to avoid fracturing of injection needles; however, with the advent of disposable needles, needle breakage is exceedingly rare.[9]

The area anesthetized by an inferior alveolar nerve block includes, on the same side as the block, the mandibular teeth, the facial gingiva adjacent to the incisors, canine, and premolar teeth, the mucous membrane, the vermilion, and the skin of the lower lip, and the chin.

The inferior alveolar nerve has many aberrant pathways and extra trunks. A branch may separate from the mandibular nerve superior to the alveolar foramen, enter the mandibular ramus superior and anterior to the inferior alveolar foramen, and pass directly to one or more posterior teeth. The practical significance of the aberrant nerve structures may explain why the usual inferior alveolar nerve block, on rare occasion, is not completely effective. Occasionally, during ostectomy procedures performed in the first molar region, we noted the absence of an inferior alveolar canal, and the inferior alveolar neurovascular bundle was a matter of strands of soft tissue passing through the medullary bone. The great variability of the inferior alveolar nerve has also been reported by Carter and Keen.[19]

**Modified Trigeminal Third Division Block.** The anesthetic solutions are deposited near the foramen ovale through an intraoral approach described by Gow-Gates as follows:[20]

1. Place the head so that the intertragic notch assumes an upward inclination.
2. Open the mouth as widely as possible.
3. Palpate the anterior border of the ramus with the forefinger.
4. Dry the puncture point on the lateral margin of the pterygomandibular depression and just medial to the medial tendon of the temporal muscle, and paint with the antiseptic solution and topical anesthetic.
5. Align the needle with the plane that extends from the lower borders of the intertragic notches through the corners of the mouth, keeping it parallel to the angulation of the ear to the face.
6. Aim the needle at the posterior border of the tragus and advance it. The depth of penetration will be approximately 25 mm.
7. When the point of the needle reaches bone at the base of the neck of the condyle, withdraw the needle 1 mm.
8. Perform aspiration and deposit the anesthetic solution rapidly.
9. Keep the mouth open for another 20 seconds to permit diffusion of the anesthetic solution.

The advantages of the technique include one penetration of the needle to produce anesthesia of all the sensory branches of the third division of the trigeminal nerve. In a discussion of the anatomic aspects of this technique, Watson mentioned a decreased tendency to penetrate the temporalis or medial pterygoid muscles, avoiding a complication of postinjection muscle tenderness.[21]

Disadvantages of this technique for diagnostic injections are the necessity of opening the mouth widely, thus dislocating the TMJ in some individuals; the delayed onset of anesthesia (5 to 15 minutes); the necessity of using soft tissue landmarks not associated with the osseous anatomy of the mandible, as with the digital technique described previously; and the necessity to touch the bone with the needle point, thus possibly deforming the needle tip in the area of the maxillary

artery and its muscular branches. Likewise, a barb on the needle tip could damage the trigeminal nerve branches.

Because of anomalous innervations, anesthesia of the mandibular teeth does not occur in some patients, even though other areas of distribution of the inferior alveolar nerve are clearly anesthetized.[22]

**Extraoral Approach to the Trigeminal Third Division Block.** This form of anesthesia is initiated by palpation of the zygomatic arch and the mandibular notch.[23] A point is marked below the arch and a skin wheal of local anesthetic agent is raised (Fig. 4–5). A 5-cm, 22-gauge needle is inserted through the wheal perpendicular to the skin and is advanced slowly until either a peripheral nerve response is elicited or bone is encountered. The latter usually occurs at a depth of 38 to 45 mm, but may be 50 mm in a large patient. If bone is contacted, it is usually the lateral pterygoid plate of the sphenoid and the needle therefore is positioned too far anteriorly. It must be withdrawn and reinserted posteriorly and to a depth no more than 6 mm deeper than that at which the pterygoid plate was contacted. From 2 to 3 ml of anesthetic

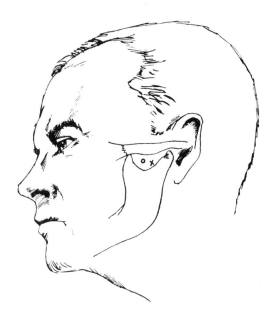

*Fig. 4–5.* Sites of injection for extraoral maxillary and mandibular division nerve blocks: x indicates maxillary site; o indicates mandibular site. (From Alling, C.C. and Mahan, P.E., Facial Pain, 2nd Ed, Philadelphia, Lea & Febiger, 1977, p. 251.)

solution gives profound anesthesia to the distribution of the mandibular nerve.

Two possible complications are: (1) penetration of either the internal maxillary or middle meningeal arteries, and (2) if the needle penetrates deeper medially than 2 or 3 mm beyond the lateral pterygoid plate, it may penetrate the thin membranous wall of the auditory tube.

**TMJ and Related Structures.** These structures may be discretely and independently anesthetized with judicious use of small amounts of short-acting local anesthetic agents. Differential diagnostic blocks are made by injections of local anesthetic agents in the lateral (temporomandibular) ligament of the TM joint, the intracapsular regions of the inferior joint compartment and the superior compartment of the TM joint, and a block of the auriculotemporal nerve.

The temporomandibular ligament block is performed as follows. After cutaneous preparations, the lateral pole of the condyle is palpated and the ball of a palpating finger is placed posteriorly and superiorly to the condyle to help in its stabilization. The anesthetic solution is infiltrated laterally and inferiorly to the bulge of the condylar process to anesthetize the lower attachments of the ligament, and a few drops are placed at the estimated location of the superior attachment of the ligament on the zygomatic process of the temporal bone.

To infiltrate the TM joint spaces in the lateral approach technique, the injection syringe needle is directed through the skin about 5 mm anterior to the tragus of the ear in a medial and superior direction that is calculated to intersect the posterior and superior slope of the condyle (Fig. 4–6). The bevel, not the tip of the needle, should engage the condyle. Aspiration usually produces no synovial fluid because the inferior compartment is a potential space with little free synovial fluid. A 0.25-ml amount of anesthetic solution, however, is easily injected if the tip of the needle is in the space and is not caught in the periosteum or in the meniscus. To infiltrate the superior cavity of the joint when necessary, the needle is advanced along the path of insertion just described for an additional 5 to 10 mm, and 0.50 ml of anesthetic solution is infiltrated into

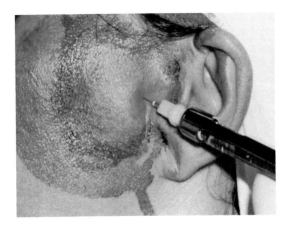

**Fig. 4–6.** Intracapsular injections. Position for the anesthetic injection needle for infiltration into the inferior joint space and, by advancing on the same path, infiltration into the superior joint space.

the superior cavity; if the needle tip is in the superior cavity, the solution flows easily from the syringe.

Zetz and associates described an alternative approach of introducing local anesthetic agents and radiopaque solutions into the joint spaces.[24] With the objective of entering the inferior joint space, the tragus of the ear is retracted anteriorly and the injection anesthetic needle is introduced into the external auditory canal in the tragohelicine incisure to avoid the cartilages of the ear. As the needle is advanced, local anesthetic solutions are infiltrated. The needle is directed superiorly at approximately a 20° angle and inward at a 30° angle until the posterior slope of the condyle is encountered, whereupon 1 ml of anesthetic solution is deposited.

The auriculotemporal nerve block is performed extraorally. The cutaneous surface anterior to the external ear is prepared with scrubs and anesthetic solutions. The lateral pole of the condyle is palpated as the mandible resides in the rest position. The cutaneous tissues overlying the head and neck of the condyle are anesthetized with a few drops of a short-acting local anesthetic agent. The needle is inserted just anterior to the tragus; for most individuals, the path of the needle is on an inclination anteriorly 30° to the frontal (coronal) plane and inferiorly 30°. The needle passes through the anesthetized zone to the posteriolateral surface of the condylar neck with the bevel of the needle staying against the mandible. The patient is then instructed to open 10 to 15 mm, the needle is withdrawn 2 mm, and the syringe is brought forward into the frontal plane and inserted immediately posterior to the condylar neck for an additional 6 mm. At this point, 0.50 ml of anesthetic solution is deposited to produce a block of the auriculotemporal nerve near the posterior center of the condylar neck. Diffusion of the anesthetic solution interrupts the motor activity of the frontal branch of the facial nerve in about 75% of the patients and the zygomatic branch in about 30%. Patients should be informed that the forehead may feel wooden or puffy and both eyes may tear for the duration of the anesthesia. Placement of a 10 × 10 cm warm damp gauze over the eye(s) both protects as well as comforts the patient. The facial nerve function returns as the anesthetic solution metabolizes.

Donlon and associates described an auriculotemporal nerve block in which the anesthetic needle is inserted through the cutaneous tissues anterior to the junction of the tragus and the lobule of the ear, and 0.2 ml of anesthetic solution is deposited.[25] Without additional injections, the needle passes through the parotid gland until the posterior surface of the mandibular neck is contacted. It is then directed 1 cm anteriorly and medially to the posterior neck of the condyle and 1.5 ml of the anesthetic solution is deposited, thus producing a block anesthetic of the auriculotemporal nerve.

## Maxillary Division

**Nasopalatine Nerve Block.** The mucosa overlying the premaxillary area on the palatal side of the dental arch is anesthetized. In some cases, a deep block, as indicated in the section on anterior-superior alveolar nerve block, causes an anesthetic effect in the incisor dentition. The needle is inserted just lateral to the incisive papilla and parallel to the long axis of the maxillary incisor to a distance of approximately 5 to 19 mm. The injection of 0.25 to 0.5 ml of solution anesthetizes the palatal tissue adjacent to the four incisor teeth and perhaps the canine teeth. Some fibers

may also participate in innervation of the maxillary central and lateral incisor (Fig. 4–7).

**Anterior Superior Alveolar Nerve Block (Fig. 4–8).** The maxillary incisor teeth and the canine teeth are anesthetized, unless the incisor teeth are innervated by the nasopalatine nerve. Deposition of 0.5 to 1.0 ml of anesthetic solution over the apices of the maxillary incisors produces anesthesia of the affected teeth and the associated labial soft tissues. In some patients, the clinician may need to give deep injections into the nasopalatine canal and/or intranasal injections to introduce 0.5 ml of anesthetic solution at the superior end of the nasopalatine canal to produce profound anesthesia of the incisor dentition.

**Maxillary Canine Tooth Infiltration (Fig. 4–8).** This technique is performed specifically for the canine tooth because of the possibility of separate and direct innervation from the infraorbital nerve. Deposition of 0.5 to 1.0 ml of anesthetic solution over the apex should produce anesthesia of the canine and the associated labial gingival tissues.

**Middle Superior Alveolar Nerve Block (Fig. 4–8).** Approximately 1 ml of anesthetic solution deposited supraperiosteally through tautly drawn mucosa overlying the second premolar tooth produces anesthesia of the premolars, the mesiobuccal root of the first molar, and the associated buccal soft tissues.

**Posterior Superior Alveolar Nerve Block (Fig. 4–8).** The anesthetic solution is delivered with the patient's mouth partially closed to prevent the coronoid process from traversing forward and obscuring the space lateral to the maxillary tuberosity. With the index finger, the clinician palpates the zygomatic process of the maxilla and retracts the cheek. The needle is inserted at a 45° angle to the sagittal plane and at a 45° angle to the occlusal plane, to a depth of 12 to 18 mm. If preanesthetic palpation reveals a great curvature to the tuberosity, a curve may be placed in the needle before the injection is made. The molar teeth and the associated buccal gingiva, with the exception of the mesiobuccal root of the first molar, are anesthetized by this injection in most patients. As with other nerves, the extent of innervation varies greatly; the dentition and the adjacent structures innervated by the posterior superior alveolar nerve

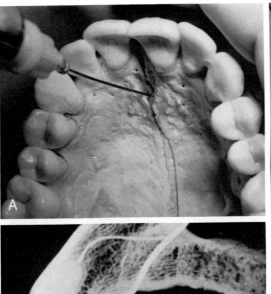

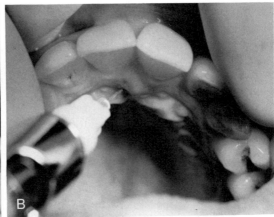

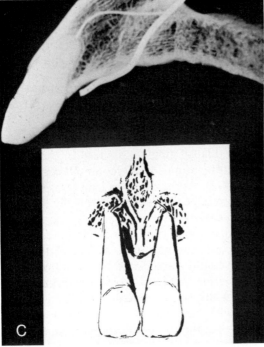

*Fig. 4–7.* The nasopalatine nerve block. A. Osseous anatomy. B. Position of the injection needle with the entry site just lateral to the incisive papilla. C. The nasopalatine nerve may bring sensory innervation to the dentition in the premaxilla, especially the central incisor teeth and possibly the lateral incisor teeth.

in different patients ranges from just the second or third molar to the usual situation just described, to even more anteriorly to the bicuspid teeth.

A hematoma may form rapidly if the needle inadvertently lacerates the posterior superior alveolar artery. This artery may be tightly bound to or grooved into the maxilla above the tuberosity, and it will not deflect away from the injection needle.

**Infraorbital Nerve Block (Fig. 4–9).** Structures innervated by the middle and anterior superior alveolar nerves are anesthetized. The infraorbital foramen is located directly below the center of the pupil of the eye as the patient gazes forward and 3 to 5 mm below the infraorbital rim. The infraorbital canal may be entered extraorally from an inferior and medial direction. Although this and other descriptions are of a single foramen and nerve, we observed during operations involving the midfacial skeleton that several trunks of the nerve may emerge from one or more foramina.

After sterile preparation of the skin, 0.3 ml of anesthetic solution is deposited over the area of the infraorbital foramen. The ball of the index finger of the hand that is not manipulating the syringe is placed on the orbital rim just superior to the foramen, the point of

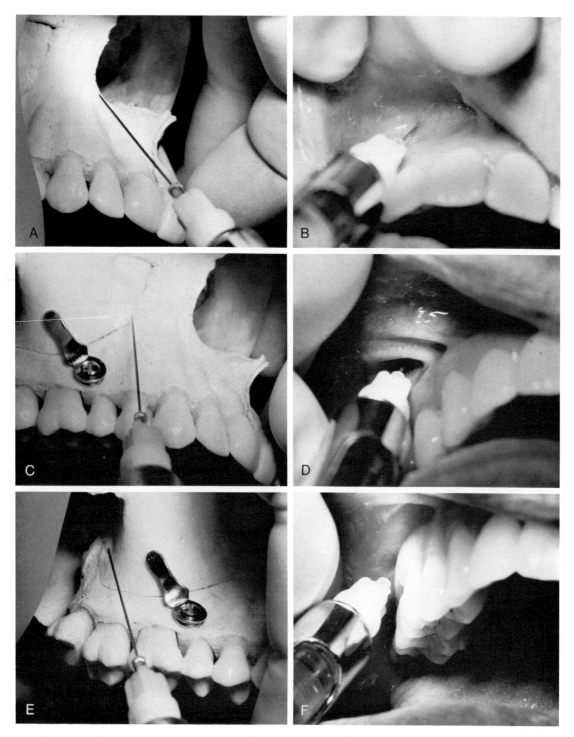

*Fig. 4–8.* The superior alveolar nerve blocks and infiltrations. A. The anterior superior alveolar nerve infiltration is anterior to the canine tooth. The canine is anesthetized by infiltrating the solution directly over the apex of the tooth. B. Position of the injection syringe to infiltrate the anterior superior alveolar nerve region. C. The middle superior alveolar nerve is in an area posterior to the canine and anterior to the first molar. D. Position of the injection syringe to infiltrate the middle superior alveolar nerve region. E. To anesthetize the posterior superior alveolar nerve, needle entry is in the vestibule lateral to the second molar, taking care to keep the tip of the needle away from bone lest the posterior superior alveolar artery be lacerated and produce a sudden onset hematoma. F. Position of the injection syringe to block the posterior superior alveolar nerve.

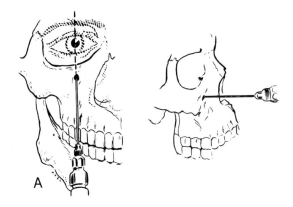

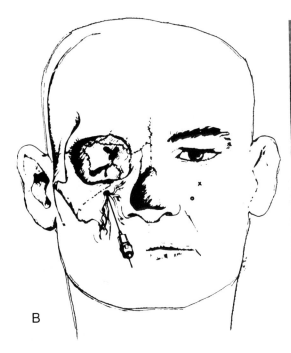

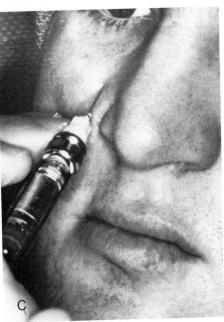

*Fig. 4–9.* Infraorbital nerve block. A. The infraorbital foramen is on a perpendicular line below the pupil, and the needle is directed medially. B. For an extraoral approach, the entry point, o, is medial and inferior to the foramen, x. C. Position of the syringe for an extraoral approach to the infraorbital foramen.

the needle is directed into the foramen approximately 5 mm, and 0.5 ml of solution is deposited in the canal. By retrograde flow, the other terminal nerves of the maxillary division of the trigeminal may be anesthetized.

**Anterior Palatine Nerve Block.** The palatal mucosa is anesthetized as far anteriorly as the canine teeth. The greater palatine foramen is located approximately at the junction of the alveolar process and the palatine process of the maxilla and approximately 3 to 4 mm anterior to the junction of hard and soft palates (Fig. 4–10). Thus, it lies approximately halfway between the second and the third molars

and approximately 10 mm from the bony palatal margin. The direction of the approach is from the opposite side of the mouth. Approximately 0.25 to 0.5 ml of anesthetic solution is used.

**Intraoral Maxillary Nerve Block (Fig. 4–11).** All branches of the maxillary division as well as the pterygopalatine ganglion are anesthetized. The maxillary nerve exits from the skull through the foramen rotundum and immediately enters the pterygopalatine fossa. The fossa is approached intraorally by passing the needle either through the greater palatine foramen and the pterygopalatine canal or pos-

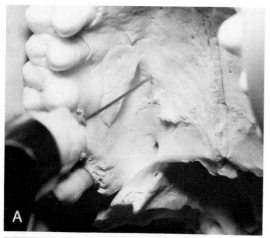

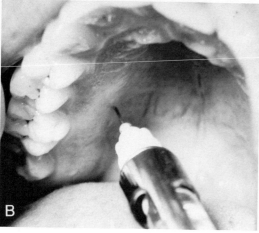

*Fig. 4–10.* The anterior palatine nerve block. A. The anterior palatine nerve exits from the greater palatine foramen and passes anteriorly to innervate the palatal mucosa. B. The nerve block and infiltrations are performed in the looser mucosa near the palatal vault posterior to the area being anesthetized.

terior to the maxillary tuberosity to the area of the fossa (a high tuberosity approach).

The maxillary division of the trigeminal nerve is blocked by using the pterygopalatine canal approach via the greater palatine foramen. A drop or two of local anesthetic is deposited in the mucosa overlying the greater palatine foramen at the junction of the alveolar process and the horizontal roof of the palate, approximately 3 to 4 mm anterior to the junction of the hard and soft palates. The resulting anesthesia permits probing with the point of the needle to find the orifice of the greater pterygopalatine canal. When the canal is located, the needle is advanced in a superior, posterior, and lateral direction. The max-

imum depth in the canal should not exceed 38 mm.[5] From 1 to 1.8 ml of local anesthetic solution is deposited in the pterygopalatine fossa and produces a block of the second division of the trigeminal nerve. In some instances, the foramen is too small or too inaccessible and a needle does not enter, and in others, the canal is too tortuous or too constricted to permit the safe passage of the needle. In these cases, the pterygopalatine canal approach is discontinued.

The high tuberosity approach is the same as the posterior-superior alveolar nerve block with the exception that the needle is inserted to a depth of about 30 mm and 1.8 ml of solution is slowly deposited. A slight curve of the needle facilitates this injection.

**Extraoral Maxillary Nerve Block (see Fig. 4–5).** A point below the zygomatic arch is marked that is lateral to the sigmoid notch of the mandible. A small wheal of local anesthesia is raised at the site. A 7.5-cm, 22-gauge, short-beveled needle is introduced through the wheal at a 45° angle to the frontal plane and slightly superiorly to the horizontal plane. If the needle contacts the lateral pterygoid plate at an approximate depth of 5 cm, it must be withdrawn slightly and redirected more anteriorly. A peripheral nerve response in the distribution of the infraorbital nerve should be elicited, and the needle is withdrawn 1 or 2 mm and 3 ml of solution is deposited. If no response is produced, and if the needle lies at a depth of not greater than 35 mm, then 3 to 5 ml of local anesthetic solution are deposited with the thought that the volume of solution produces the required anesthesia.

### Ophthalmic Division

The supraorbital nerve block (Fig. 4–12) is performed where the nerve emerges from the orbit through the supraorbital foramen or notch. The supratrochlear nerve emerges just medial to this foramen and usually is anesthetized by the injection. The supraorbital foramen, infraorbital foramen, and the mental foramen all lie on a straight line when viewed anteriorly. The patient is supine with the head stabilized. The skin is penetrated just medial to the supraorbital foramen, and 0.2 to 0.4 ml

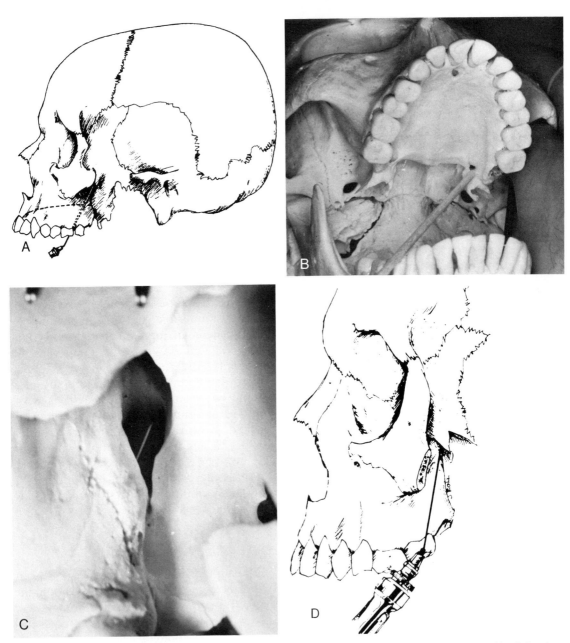

*Fig. 4–11.* The maxillary nerve block. V-2 (second division of the trigeminal nerve) may be anesthetized by delivering the anesthetic solution into the A, pterygopalatine fissure area just anterior to foramen rotundum via an injection needle passing up the B, greater palatine foramen and C, pterygomaxillary fissure. D. The pterygopalatine foramen and foramen rotundum area may be approached by a high maxillary tuberosity injection.

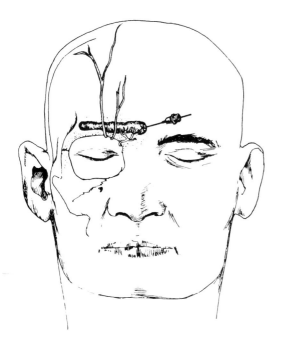

*Fig. 4–12.* Supraorbital and supratrochlear nerve blocks.

of solution is deposited as the needle advances to the foramen. The forehead and scalp are anesthetized posteriorly to the lamboidal suture area. Although this and other descriptions are of a single foramen or notch, we observed during operations that several trunks of the nerve may emerge from one or more foramina.

### Superficial Cervical Plexus Nerve Block

Anesthesia of the lesser occipital, greater auricular, cervical cutaneous, and supraclavicular nerves is produced by blocking the superficial cervical plexus. The patient is supine with the head turned to the side opposite that to be blocked. A skin wheal of a local anesthetic agent is raised on the posterior border of the sternocleidomastoid muscle at the junction of the upper and middle thirds of the muscle (Fig. 4–13). A total of 10 ml of anesthetic solution is injected both cephalad and caudad along the posterior border of the sternocleidomastoid muscle.

### Cervicothoracic Sympathetic Plexus Block (Stellate Ganglion Block)

This block has positive differential diagnostic value in differentiating pain sensations arising from the sympathetic autonomic system from pain sensations involving the trigeminal system. The pain of the sympathetic system is diffuse, has a constant burning character, and is classified as being of vascular etiology. The history usually includes a noxious event, e.g., the removal of a tooth followed by a routine alveolar osteitis, that leads, through modes not yet understood, to the autonomic reflex pain. The pain is promptly arrested by a successful "stellate ganglion" block. The block gives prompt relief and is diagnostic of causalgia of the oral region. When cervical injury is followed by diffuse, chronic pain in the regions of the ear, face, and teeth, this type of block sometimes provides relief. The first block may provide only 24 hours to several days of relief, and repeated blocks may result in permanent pain relief.

The cervicothoracic sympathetic block is administered by a clinician trained in its administration, often an anesthesiologist or a neurologist. The block is usually performed from an anterior approach, with the patient supine and the head in slight hyperextension. The cricoid cartilage is identified as a landmark overlying C-6. A local anesthetic agent is injected in the subcutaneous tissues lateral to the cricoid cartilage. The entire medial circumference of the sternocleidomastoid muscle is then retracted laterally with the fingers of the nonoperating hand, and the internal carotid artery and internal jugular vein, which are adherent to the posterior sheath of the muscle, are retracted laterally. The objective of the retraction is to remove all tissues anterior to the cervicothoracic ganglion with the exception of the skin, subcutaneous tissues, superficial fascia, and platysma muscle. The injection needle is inserted vertically through the anesthetized cutaneous tissues lateral to the cricoid cartilage and then advanced through the subcutaneous tissues, platysma muscle, prevertebral fascia, and possibly prevertebral muscles to touch the anterior tubercle of C-6.[26] The tubercle is a firm landmark, and additional pressure is uncomfortable to the patient. The needle is withdrawn slightly so the point resides anterior to the prevertebral fascia, and an aspiration is performed to ensure that the point of the needle

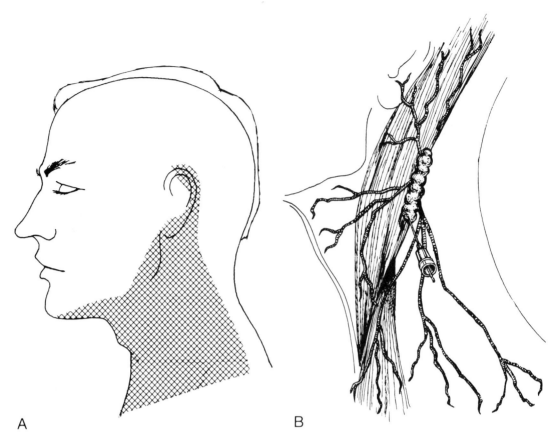

A    B

*Fig. 4–13.* Superficial cervical plexus nerve block and infiltration. A. Area anesthetized by a superficial cervical plexus nerve infiltration. B. Superficial cervical nerve infiltration is made along the posterior border of the sternocleidomastoid muscle.

is not in a vessel; of special concern is the vertebral artery, because a local anesthetic agent injected in the artery could cause convulsions. Before making the therapeutic or diagnostic injection, a test dose of no more than 0.25 ml is administered. If no contraindications are evident at this point in the procedure, a 10-ml bolus of the local anesthetic agent is deposited. The local anesthetic agent may be diluted with saline and an anti-inflammatory steroid preparation to provide a large volume of injection bolus, which aids in diffusion and reduces the inflammatory response to the injection. The anesthetic solution spreads superiorly and inferiorly, anesthetizing the ganglion. Proper placement of the solution is evident by ptosis, meiosis, enophthalmos, anhydrosis, and a rise in temperature of a finger. A sympathetic, autonomic nerve system causalgia of the oral cavity is relieved promptly by the block, thus differentiating, for example, between pains produced by local inflammatory processes and reflex sympathetic nervous system pains. Vital signs are monitored constantly during and after administration of the block. Resuscitation equipment must be available, because the possible complications include convulsions, phrenic nerve paralysis, hypotension, pneumothorax, paralysis of the intercostal muscles, and a minor inconvenience of transient hoarseness.

## Complications

**Prolonged Anesthesia.** This prolongation may result from incorporation of sterilizing solution or other material in the anesthetic cartridge, or from manipulating or interrupting the nerve during insertion or removal of the needle, especially if there is a barb on the point of the needle.

Prolonged anesthesia, or parethesia, may be a neurotoxicity secondary to an alcohol metabolite of the ester or amide local anesthetic agent. Observation of rare prolonged paresthesia following an injection of a local anesthetic agent can be explained by this chemistry of the metabolic hydrolysis of local anesthetic agents.[1]

**Incomplete Anesthesia.** A pool of anesthetic solution that is not close enough to the nerve does not produce anesthesia. Also, infection and acute inflammatory processes may render the local anesthetic ineffectual, because the low pH of the tissues prevents the liberation of the active free base of the anesthetic. Furthermore, increased circulation in an inflamed area rapidly removes the anesthetic from its area of injection.[27]

**Ischemia or Tissue Slough.** Loss of tissue may result from injecting too large a volume of anesthetic into confined tissues, producing local tissue damage. The dense, fixed palatal mucosa is especially vulnerable to sloughing from excessive quantities of anesthetics. Local anesthetic agents sensitize the oral mucosal proteins to denaturation by heat. Mucosal sloughing may occur if a patient takes hot food or beverage immediately after submucosal infiltration when the anesthetic has not been removed by local circulation (Fig.

4–14).[28] When large volumes of anesthetic solution are infiltrated into the mucosa, the patient should be instructed to avoid drinking or eating hot foods for 8 hours.

**Infection.** Infection usually results from the improper preparation of the injection sites.[29,30] Since the advent of disposable needles, infection from improper sterilization of injection equipment occurs only rarely (Fig. 4–15). Certainly if needles are re-used, contamination by the needles is possible.

**Eruptive Phenomenon.** Blisters, hives, or erythematous patches are indicative of an allergic reaction to the agent used.

**Angioedema.** This rare phenomenon is associated with an immediate response of sensitivity to a local anesthetic agent. It is usually self-limiting with painless swelling, but the patient should be observed closely to ensure no compromise of the respiratory system occurs. Depending on the severity of the attack, the dentist may administer antihistamines and/or epinephrine in addition to oxygen. The patient should be referred for allergy sensitivity studies.

**Broken Needles.**[9,31] This complication is rare today, probably because of the practice of using disposable needles, eliminating the problem of the needle undergoing repeated stresses. If this complication occurs, the re-

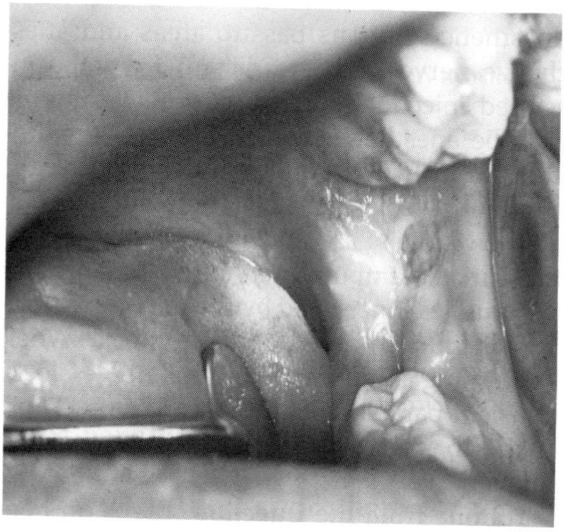

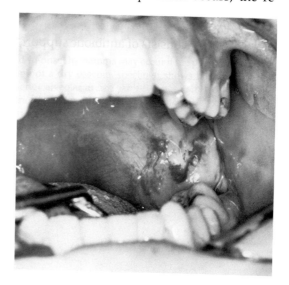

*Fig. 4–14.* Mucosal sloughing. Ulcerated loss of tissue may be observed in an area of anesthesia followed by the ingestion of hot liquids. Sloughing may also be due to surface infection caused by unsterile instruments or improper preparation of the injection site.

*Fig. 4–15.* Lateral pharyngeal abscess is an acute inflammatory condition, possibly life threatening, that may occur following an inferior alveolar nerve injection if there has not been appropriate preparation of the muscosal site of the injection.

pneumothorax, if a lobe of the lung projected into the neck in the area of the injection. If the agent spreads caudally, paralysis of the intercostal muscles may follow.

## References

1. Nickel A.A. Jr.: A retrospective study of paresthesia of the dental alveolar nerves. Anes Prog, 37:42, 1990.
2. Ritchie J.M. and Greene N.M.: In Pharmacologic Basis of Therapeutics, 7th ed., New York, Macmillan, 303–305, 1985.
3. Morrison R.T. and Boyd R.N.: In Organic Chemistry, 5th ed., Boston, Allyn and Bacon, Inc., 1987.
4. Nickel A.A.: Master's Thesis, Circular Dischroism of Acetylcholinesterase preparations from mammalian brain. Univ. of Calif. in San Francisco. 63–64, 1971.
5. Astra Pharmaceutical Products, Inc.: Information for Patients; Adverse Reactions. Xylocaine, Xylocaine Package Insert; Astra Pharmaceutical Products, Inc., Westborough, MA. 021561R14 rev. 4/87 (14).
6. Ganong W.F.: In Review of Medical Physiology. Los Altos, Lange Med Pub, 34–42, 140–142, 1981.
7. Hinton R.J., Dechow P.C., and Carlson D.S.: Recovery of jaw muscle function following injection of a myotoxic agent (lidocaine-epinephrine). Oral Surg Oral Med Oral Pathol, 59:247, 1985.
8. Benoit P.W.: Reversible skeletal muscle damage after administration of local anesthetic with and without epinephrine. J Oral Maxillofac Surg, 36:198, 1981.
9. Alling C.C. and Christopher A.: Status report on dental anesthetic needles and syringes. J Am Dent Assoc, 89:1171, 1974.
10. Malamed S.F.: The periodontal ligament (PDL) injection; an optional use of an alternative to inferior alveolar nerve block. Oral Surg Oral Med Oral Pathol, 53:117, 1982.
11. Smith G.N. and Walton R.E.: Periodontal ligament injection: Distribution of injected solutions. Oral Surg Oral Med Oral Pathol, 55:232, 1983.
12. Moore K.D. et al: A comparison of the periodontal injection using 2% lidocaine with 1:100,000 epinephrine and saline in human mandibular premolars. Anesth Prog, 34:181, 1987.
13. Handler L.E. and Albers D.D.: The effects of the vasoconstrictor epinephrine on the duration of pulpal anesthesia using the intraligamentary injection. J Am Dent Assoc, 114:807, 1987.
14. D'Souza J.E., Walton R.E., and Peterson L.C.: Periodontal ligament injection: An evaluation of the extent of anesthesia and postinfection discomfort. J Am Dent Assoc, 114:341, 1987.
15. Bennett D.R.: Monheim's Local Anesthesia and Pain Control in Dental Practice. St. Louis, Mosby, 1978.
16. Lilienthal B.: A clinical appraisal of intraosseous dental anesthesia. Oral Surg Oral Med Oral Pathol, 39:692, 697, 1975.
17. Kiesselbach J.E. and Chamberlain J.G.: Clinical and anatomic observations on the relationship of the lingual nerve to the mandibular third molar region. J Oral Maxillofac Surg, 42:565, 1984.
18. Cook W.A.: The mandibular field and its control with local anesthetics. Mod Dent, 22:11, 1955.
19. Carter R.B. and Keen E.N.: The intramandibular course of the inferior alveolar nerve. J Anat, 108:433, 1971.
20. Gow-Gates G.A.E.: Mandibular conduction anesthesia: A new technique using extraoral landmarks. Oral Surg Oral Med Oral Pathol, 36:321, 1973.
21. Watson J.E.: Appendix: Some anatomic aspects of the Gow-Gates technique for mandibular anesthesia. Oral Surg Oral Med Oral Pathol, 36:328, 1973.
22. Frommer J., Mele F.A., and Monroe C.W.: The possible role of the mylohyoid nerve in mandibular posterior tooth sensation. J Am Dent Assoc, 85:113, 1972.
23. Kramer H.S. and Schmidt W.H.: Local anesthetics and their use in pain control in oral-facial regions. In Alling C.C. and Mahan P.E. (eds): Facial Pain. 2nd Ed. Edited by C.C. Alling and P.E. Mahan, Philadelphia, Lea & Febiger, 1977.
24. Zetz M.R., Irby W.B., and Doles L.R.: A simplified method for injection or aspiration of the temporomandibular joint. J Am Dent Assoc, 104:855, 1982.
25. Donlon W.C., Truta M.P., and Eversole L.R.: A modified auriculotemporal nerve block for regional anesthesia of the temporomandibular joint. J Oral Maxillofac Surg, 42:544, 1984.
26. Murphy T.M.: Treatment of chronic pain. In Anesthesia, 2nd Ed, Edited by R.D. Miller. New York, Churchill Livingstone, 1986.
27. Kramer H.S. and Mitton V.A.: Complications of local anesthesia. Dent Clin North Am, 17:443, 1973.
28. Knapp D.C.: Local anesthetic-induced decrease in thermal stability of biological tissues. Abstracts of Papers. 45th General Meeting of the International Association for Dental Research, May, 1967.
29. Lovetto V.D. and Meador R.I.: Aseptic (if not sterile) technique. J Ala Dent Assoc, 63:20, 1979.
30. Connor J.P. and Edelson J.G.: Needle tract infection. Oral Surg Oral Med Oral Pathol, 65:401, 1988.
31. Thomas E.G.: Recovery of broken hypodermic needles in the throat. J Oral Maxillofac Surg, 1:1, 1953.

Appreciation is extended to Dr. Alfred A. Nickel, Jr., oral and maxillofacial surgeon of Walnut Creek, California, for his interest in this subject and his advice on the biochemistry of local anesthetic agents.

# *Background Milieu*

# Psychopathology of Pain

The clinician who treats patients in pain will be impressed by the wide range of patient responses to comparable levels of tissue damage or pathology. The responses can range from impassive stoic behavior to highly dramatic, hysterical behavior. These responses may even be observed in patients with no identified somatic pathology or pathofunction. Evidence indicates that the expression of pain is determined by the patient's personal background, the context in which pain is experienced, and its meaning to the individual, as well as the sensory phase of the pain experience.[1,2] The affective or emotional response phase of pain, therefore, is not directly related to the sensory aspect of pain in some patients.

Both the International Association for the Study of Pain and the American Psychiatric Association have classified orofacial pain of psychogenic origin. The International Association for the Study of Pain classifies orofacial pain as "pain of psychologic origin" only if no known physical cause or pathofunction can account for the pain and if contributing psychologic factors are undeniably present.[3] The American Psychiatric Association recently changed their classification of "psychogenic pain disorder"[4] to "somatoform pain disorder."[5]

A person is known by his or her facial characteristics, and many vital functions and pleasures of life are channeled through the face and mouth. The mouth has great emotional significance to the human. When pain and pathofunction affect the face, the patient is usually highly motivated to seek treatment and be restored to health. Patients with facial pain may pressure a clinician to treat them when the probability of a cure or restoration of function is minimal. They are willing to accept almost any diagnosis and treatment that promises relief. Some clinicians, facing the pressures and complexity of practice today, may be too ready to give the patient a diagnostic label without adequate examination and then refer them out of their office. The diagnosis of "TMJ" (temporomandibular joint) is often presented, and many patients believe they have a disease, "TMJ." They think they need only a clinician who treats such a disease and they will be cured.

Since TM joint syndrome, in its complexity of signs and symptoms, has many possible causes, a quick and simple cure is often not available. Because the etiology of TM joint syndrome is multifactional, the patient is often subjected to many reversible and irreversible, empiric treatment procedures. One clinician after another may subject the patient to a favorite treatment procedure that has successfully relieved pain in other patients. The attempts at treatment may become a series of worsening failures and mutilations when the primary problem is undiagnosed pain of psychologic origin. This oversight occurs when a clinician does not appreciate the power of the patient's mind over the body and the patient is not willing to discuss or admit to psychologic factors in their lives. Both the patient and the clinician are unwilling to either learn or expose the truth. Psychologic factors in the life of the clinician further complicate interaction with the patient during the examination and diagnosis process. Every clinician who treats pain patients has missed the diagnosis in certain patients with pain of psychologic origin. This chapter includes a discussion of the more common psychologic aspects of facial pain.

Most people accept the common pains and go about their lives treating themselves with over-the-counter medicines. The reasons are unclear why pain mentally and physically inactivates some people while others can carry on their lives in spite of pain. The severity of the pain is certainly one factor that explains the disparity. Severe pain may command the patient's total attention. The meaning of the pain, on the other hand, may be the factor that establishes the pain experience. When a patient believes a facial pain is caused by a tumor or a serious disease, the suffering aspect is typically amplified.

## Pain Behavior

Pain behavior refers to behaviors of the patient that are indicative of subjective pain or one attributed by the patient to the pain. They include grimacing, moaning, withdrawal, rubbing the painful part, splinting, guarding, taking medications, seeking medical-dental care, avoiding sex, staying home from work, and verbal communications of pain.

The words the chronic pain patient uses to describe the pain are divided into sensory, affective, and evaluative.[6,7] The sensory words describe the character of the pain in terms of temporal, spatial, pressure, thermal, or other properties. They include such words as: aching, stinging, burning, cutting, tingling, itchy, throbbing, and stabbing. Affective words describe the aversive feeling that accompanies pain. These words include: punishing, cruel, terrifying, sickening, vicious, blinding, and exhausting. Evaluative words describe the intensity of the pain. They include: mild, discomforting, unbearable, intense, horrible, miserable, and troublesome.

The words patients choose to describe pain provide clues to diagnosis and treatment. If a patient describes a pain as punishing, that patient may be revealing a sense of extreme guilt over some real or imagined terrible act for which the pain is punishment. A high percentage of chronic pain patients report physically abusive parents.[8] In patients with such a history, their pain may not be relieved by appropriate and well-executed treatment.

If a patient uses words like fearful or terrifying to describe an acute pain, the clinician may find that prescribing an anxiolytic drug in addition to an analgesic is required to relieve the pain completely.

## Hypochondriasis

Hypochondriasis is a pervasive preoccupation with somatic symptoms and a conviction that the signs and symptoms indicate impending, serious bodily disease despite repeated assurances from clinicians. Hypochondriacs are extremely vigilant with respect to their bodies, and they carefully monitor a variety of bodily sensations, such as minor aches and pains, itching, fatigue, heartbeat, bowel sounds, and dizziness. These bodily sensations are interpreted to mean serious illness, and hypochondriacs are either oblivious to the fact or do not accept the fact that these bodily sensations are common in healthy individuals who do not seek medical or dental care.[9] The concerns of the hypochondriac

about bodily sensations do not result in loss of bodily function.[4]

## Psychogenic Pain

Pain can occur in patients with psychiatric syndromes such as major depression, somatization disorder, conversion disorder, and hypochondriasis. Engle presented an hypothesis to explain how psychologic mechanisms can initiate and sustain pain.[10] According to this hypothesis, circumstances exist in which the experience of pain can reduce feelings that are even more unpleasant such as depression, guilt, and anxiety. Pain is better than the miserable conditions of daily existence for some patients, and it serves to reduce their level of suffering and becomes "pleasant" in a relative sense. Engle noted that guilt is the major factor in patients with psychogenic pain, and this pain is often localized in the head or face. The patient seems subject to painful injury and illness, and is attracted to situations that cause them to be exploited, injured, or defeated. Their pain is often exacerbated when their life situation improves, as though they have a need to suffer. Their pain increases when they indulge in aggressive or sexually gratifying behavior that is unacceptable to the patient, bringing on guilt feelings. These pain-prone patients seem to seek out situations that have negative or harmful consequences for them.[8] They can often be helped by psychiatric therapy; dental and surgical treatment procedures (even though they may be indicated) do not resolve their pain.

## Delusional or Hallucinatory Pain

Delusional or hallucinatory pain occurs in less than 2% of chronic pain patients.[3] These pains are typically associated with severe psychotic disorders. They are bizarre, having no known pathophysiologic mechanism to explain them, and no physical changes are apparent, except those of self-mutilation. The patient may describe worms crawling or electric wires inside their head and jaws, a ring around the head, or a crown of thorns (if they have messianic delusions). The pain is usually diffuse and vague (Fig. 5–1). It is often included as part of a delusional system reveal-

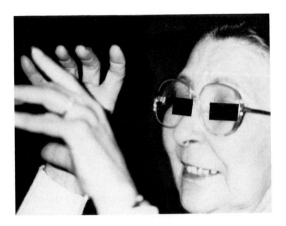

**Fig. 5–1.** A 54-year-old patient's attempt to describe her pain. Following referral for management of "TMJ," she was asked to point, with one finger, to the area where she was experiencing TMJ pain, but this was not possible because of the hallucinatory aspects of her pain.

ing grandiose expectations that cannot be fulfilled, a need for punishment, or other irrational behaviors. This pain does not occur before late adolescence. Other symptoms of psychosis such as agitation, sleeplessness, and hurried speech may accompany the pain report. These patients should be under the care of a psychiatrist.

## Suicide in the Chronic Pain Patient

The authors have experienced the tragic suicide of four patients in the past 9 years, three men and one woman. All but one of these patients had discussed suicide with us and/or family members. Three of them were being treated or had been treated by a psychiatrist. They killed themselves when a clinician informed them that their pain could not be cured and they would have to live with it. We admonished three of these patients to consult their psychiatrist and to stop seeing dentists for repeated tooth restoration or operations on their TM joint. These patients were resistant to the idea that their pain was not originating from the peripheral structure of the oral and maxillofacial areas, but that the pain was centralized. One coroner informed us that in suicide with a hand gun, the gun is usually placed on the mastoid process behind the ear; however, one of our patients placed the muzzle of the weapon, a hand gun, directly on the right TMJ, the painful joint. All

of these patients left notes stating that they could not stand the pain any longer.

When a nonalcoholic chronic pain patient calls the office at ten o'clock in the morning and is intoxicated, the danger of suicide is real. On the other hand, some patients threaten to commit suicide to get the attention of their treating clinicians. A question to pose the patient threatening suicide is, "How do you plan to kill yourself?" If the response is, "I just bought a box of shells for my husband's pistol," the patient is serious and should be referred immediately for supportive counseling. A detailed, highly lethal suicide plan is a serious risk factor. Eighty percent of individuals who commit suicide have attempted suicide at least once before. So, the most serious risk factor is a previous attempt.[11] Women attempt suicide three times more frequently than men, but men complete suicide three times more frequently than women. Suicide is now the second leading cause of death in adolescents.[12]

Clues that the patient is a serious suicidal risk are withdrawal of the patient from social interaction, giving away valuable gifts or family heirlooms, demonstrating inability to handle routine responsibilities, or showing preoccupation with death. Such a patient can be asked, "Mrs. Blank, you have been suffering this pain for many months (or years), have you ever felt that life is just not worth living?" The suicidal patient typically responds, "Oh yes, I have considered suicide many times!" Any suicidal patient who has made a serious suicide attempt needs to be hospitalized. A suicidal crisis typically lasts a few days to several weeks and, with proper therapy, resolution usually occurs within 6 weeks. These patients are not left with an irreversible desire to die. Even clinicians who are experienced in the management of suicidal crisis, however, have some patients who succeed in killing themselves. Direct questioning of the patient as just described, careful listening to the patient's comments, and timely intervention are the keys to the care of the suicidal patient.

Three fourths of all suicides are associated with depression or alcoholism; however, nondepressed patients can feel that death is the only way out of their suffering and may come to a "rational" conclusion that suicide is the answer. Approximately one in ten alcoholics die of suicide.

Suicide patients usually do not deny that they plan to kill themselves, but they rarely call or utilize suicide crisis centers. Most suicides by overdose are accomplished with prescription drugs, so when more than a lethal dose of a drug is prescribed, the drug should be entrusted to a family member or a trusted friend for safekeeping. Eight of every 10 patients who commit suicide have talked about it. Patients with chronic medical illness are more likely to commit suicide if the illness involves pain, loss of mobility, or disfigurement.

## Operant Conditioning in Chronic Pain

An operant is an action of the human organism that typically follows an antecedent stimulus. A twinge of pain in the lower first molar (the stimulus) may lead to the operant, "Oh Molly, I have a toothache!" If the concerned wife, Molly, immediately drops what she is doing and attends to her husband in pain, this attention reinforces or rewards the operant. The theory of operant conditioning states that operants are sensitive to the consequences to which they lead, irrespective of the antecedent stimulus. They may become controlled by environmental contingencies rather than the painful stimulus that initiated them.

A patient in pain for an extended period may become conditioned to hurt, regardless of the success of treatment or the healing that has occurred. The clinician often unwittingly contributes to this operant conditioning by writing pro re nato (prn) analgesics, prescribing rest for an inordinate period, and even by expressing immediate and automatic attention and concern for the patient.

When analgesics are prescribed on a prn basis, they may condition the patient to take pills.[13] If the patient gets relief of pain by taking an analgesic, the pain relief reinforces the operant, the pill taking. When the chronic pain patient is conditioned to take analgesics, prescribing agents on a time-contingent basis is often effective. The clinician should determine how long a pill controls the pain, such as 5 hours. The prescription should state "q4h," or every 4 hours, so each pill is taken while the patient is still painfree. The interval between medication can then be extended as painfree behavior is rewarded with praise or other supportive procedures. This procedure may decondition the patient from taking pills.

Direct punishment of well behavior should be avoided. The patient's family should be counseled to reward "well behavior" and to punish or not attend to "pain behavior." As the pain diminishes, the patient should not be admonished to avoid function for a period that exceeds healing of the injured part. Rest should be prescribed on a time-limited basis. The spouse of the patient with chronic pain may act as a potent reinforcer of pain behavior by providing desirable consequences such as sympathy and attention to the patient.[14]

Indirect reinforcers may also play a role in pain behavior. When a patient is on sick leave to recuperate after an operation, staying away from work is a means to avoid an oppressive job. (The medical directory of Workman's Compensation in Washington State reported that only 3 of 2000 claimants who had a second operation for back pain went back to work.[15]) Almost every aspect of the patient's environment is a potential contributor to pain behavior.[16] The clinician may not be aware of subtle, indirect reinforcers of pain behavior in the life of the patient. The patient's interface with his or her environment, not dental or medical pathologic processes, requires treatment to eliminate this patient's pain behavior.

The clinician should not ask a patient to do something the patient is not capable of doing. The chronic pain patient may have experienced pain behavior so long that well behavior is untenable. When the clinician changes the stimuli for chronic pain behavior, the patient is not only changed *from* something (pain behavior) but *to* something (well behavior). Chronic pain patients may have gaps in their well behavior repertoire. Fordyce noted that "people that have something better to do, don't hurt as much."[15] These patients need a coach to train them to live as "well persons." In counseling these patients, the authors often use the term coach when explaining the need for behavior modification by the clinical psychologist.

Unfortunately, all patients cannot be 100%

rehabilitated by dental and/or medical treatment. The patient with irreversible impairment of function postoperatively may not be able to return to work. When patients have been unemployed for years in chronic pain, many employers will not hire them. They are too high a risk in terms of medical liability. It may become the responsibility of the clinician to legitimatize retirement for the patient. We can sometimes reduce the patient's suffering so that the quality of life is acceptable or adequate even though the patient cannot function at work.

## Depression and Chronic Pain

Depression is defined as dysphoric mood accompanied by any four of the following signs and symptoms: insomnia or hypersomnia, loss of interest in sexual activities, fatigue or loss of energy, reduced appetite with weight loss, increased appetite with weight gain, feelings of worthlessness or guilt, recurrent thoughts of death, difficulty in thinking or decision making, psychomotor retardation, or agitation.

In an evaluation of the response of chronic pain patients to muscle relaxation training by a psychiatrist, about one half of the patients responded well to the therapy.[17] Psychiatric evaluation of the individuals that felt the pain was so severe that they had to stop therapy revealed the quitters were mildly to severely depressed.

Depression may be classified exogenous or endogenous. Exogenous or psychoneurotic depression occurs in response to external or environmental stress that overpowers the patient. Exogenous depression typically responds to psychotherapeutic intervention. Endogenous depression occurs in response to hormonal and biochemical abnormality affecting neurotransmitters in the brain and typically responds favorably to psychotropic medication, such as the tricyclic antidepressants. A reversal of response to treatment may occur, however, in which some endogenous depression responds to psychotherapy and some exogenous depression responds to antidepressant medication.

Authors have proposed that chronic pain is actually an expression of a muted depressive state.[8] In studies of a total of 900 chronic pain patients, signs of depression (anergia, anhedonia, insomnia, and depressive mood and despair) were prominent.[18–20] Women were affected more than men (1.7:1), and the age ranged from infancy to the seventies, with a mean age at onset of 39 years. The clinical features were hypochondriac preoccupation with their pain, desire for a surgical solution, denial of their difficulties with interpersonal relationships, a dislike of any scrutiny of their personal life, and a history of excessive work performance (egomania) since childhood until the onset of pain, after which all initiative and zeal for work is lost. They often have a history of submissiveness and of having been abused.

## Management of the Depressed Chronic Pain Patient

The depressed, chronic pain patient is difficult to treat. Use of narcotic analgesics is avoided and the aim of treatment should not be at the alleged peripheral source of pain. If the patient has a pathologic condition or pathofunction that needs treatment, the clinician should inform the patient that the treatment will not relieve the pain. A prudent measure may be to postpone needed treatment until behavioral therapy has had an effect. Antidepressant medication such as tricyclic antidepressants and sound behavioral management are most helpful in these patients. The patient should know that it may take 10 to 30 days before the antidepressants take effect. Traditional psychotherapy is usually not helpful in this group of patients.[8] Activity and continuation of work should be encouraged and the spouse or next of kin should be enlisted to help support this advice.

Exercise increases the input from muscle spindles and tendon organs that have input into the reticular activating system. The resulting state of arousal gives the depressed patient an endogenous elevation of mood from release of sympathomimetic amines. Therefore, exercise is usually indicated in the depressed patient and is therapeutic if they can be motivated to become active and exercise.

If the depression increases to the point that

the patient is suicidal, the patient should be referred immediately to a psychiatrist. The combination of behavior modification and antidepressant medication is the most effective program of treatment for depressed, pain-prone patients. These patients can remain at work if they are promptly and properly treated.

## Behavioral Management of Postoperative Pain

Postoperative pain can be reduced significantly by proper pre- and postoperative education and encouragement of the patient.

In a study of 97 surgical patients, 46 were given instructions and encouragement as special care patients.[21] They were told what would be done for postoperative pain, what causes the pain, and what they could do to minimize it. They were instructed to call for medication if they could not achieve a reasonable level of comfort. They were visited during the afternoon after their operation by the anesthetist to reiterate the instructions of the night before and to reassure them. Fifty one control patients received no instructions or encouragement regarding the postoperative pain. The narcotic requirements were the same for the two groups on the day of the operation, and they dropped to one half in the special care patients for the next 5 days. The patients who were educated and encouraged were ready for discharge 2.7 days before the control group.

Extremely frightened patients can become hysterical if the topic of postoperative pain is broached abruptly. We recommend building up to the discussion slowly and in an empathetic manner.

## Compensation Neurosis

A condition called compensation neurosis has been described in 25 to 33% of victims of auto or industrial accidents that: (1) were someone else's fault (in the patient's estimation), and (2) occurred under circumstances in which financial compensation is potentially available.[22] Patients with compensation neurosis fail to respond to therapy until the compensation issue is settled.

An inverse relationship exists between the severity of the injury and compensation neurosis in the patient. The incidence of compensation neurosis is related to social status. It occurs more frequently in unskilled workers and factory and office cleaners, not in skilled artisans who take pride in an important work. The patient tends to be dependent, insecure, and craving sympathy, and exhibits paranoid tendencies. The compensation neurotic often reports excellent physical and mental health until the accident, but their previous medical and work records do not corroborate this history.

Compensation neurosis may not develop until weeks or even months after the accident. Typical complaints include terrible, agonizing pain, dizziness, irritability, inability to concentrate, sleeplessness, hostility, restlessness, and an attitude of martyred gloom. The patient has an unshakable conviction of unfitness for work and absolutely no improvement of symptoms since the accident.

Most compensation neurosis patients no longer seek medical or dental supervision once the case is settled. Complete recovery is likely to follow settlement no matter which side wins the case. It is worthwhile to recall the words of H.M. Frost when considering compensation neurosis pain.

"In my time, I have seen for diagnosis and/or treatment, more than 10,000 patients with unresolved liability from a real or imagined injury. Yet in the same period, I have seen only 3 patients desiring help or advice for such injury after liability was closed."[23]

An unfortunate impasse occurs in many cases of compensation neurosis. The lawyers insist that no settlement is possible without clinical finality and the clinician insists that no clinical finality is possible until the case is settled. Some clinicians refuse to treat these patients until the case is settled in court. The policy of the authors is to explain compensation neurosis to the patient as a recognized human response to their situation (excluding the malingerer who plans to capitalize on the accident), and to initiate treatment, even though the probability of success is reduced.

The concept of compensation neurosis, as described above, has been questioned in recent years.[24,25] A controlled study of 47 patients with chronic low back pain involving personal injury litigation and 33 similar patients who were not involved in litigation, reported that the litigants described their pain as no more severe and had no greater psychological disturbance than the non-litigants.[26] Dworkin and others studied 454 chronic pain patients and reported that when unemployment and compensation were used to predict outcome, only unemployment was significant.[27] In a follow-up study of accident neurosis patients, Tarsh and Royston found that settlement of the claim does not lead to improvement in terms of return to work or symptom relief.[28] It has also been suggested that minor trauma to the skull may produce organic damage with psychological aftereffects that will not be alleviated by settlement of the case.[29] In an excellent review, Weighill and Buglass have pointed out that return to work does not indicate resolution of symptoms.[30] They concluded that trauma may cause psychological distress independent of compensation issues, that symptoms may not typically remit after settlement of the case, and that compensation neurosis may be more often conscious malingering than actual neurosis.

### Pain Laureates

Other chronic pain patients were described as "pain laureates" by Gessell.[17] They are often treated by a favorite clinician for many years without sufficient or continuous relief of pain. They are then referred to another clinician for a second opinion and possible new treatment. The laureates actually want to be certified "sick" so they continue to receive the advantages of the sick role that have accrued in the past. If the second clinician identifies an overlooked cause of pain and initiates therapy, the laureate immediately abandons the new clinician as soon as symptoms improve (Fig. 5–2). The laureate does not allow treatment to progress and is resistant to counseling by a clinical psychologist or psychiatrist.

A psychiatric diagnosis should not be made on the basis of lack of response to all known nonpsychiatric treatment procedures or to "diagnosis by exclusion." A psychiatric eval-

uation is time consuming and expensive, however, so a complete history, examination, and appropriate tests for all suspected pain etiologies are completed before referral for psychiatric evaluation.

### La Belle Indifference

The authors have observed patients with facial pain that have been diagnosed as La Belle Indifference by the psychiatrist. This most interesting patient usually appears for all appointments on time, dressed immaculately, with a most pleasant, confident, and contented manner, and describes the horror of excruciating pain in the face or TM joint. The patient does not grimace, frown, or display any sign of pain or discomfort, and seems quite satisfied with life in spite of the complaints of pain (Fig. 5–3). When asked, "On a scale of one to ten with ten being the maximum pain you can imagine, how much pain do you have right now?", the reply is, "I have a seven or perhaps a ten."

Psychiatric factors are prominent in this patient, who typically is resistant to therapy. Psychiatric theory states that this patient's symptom formation represents the solution of a conflict. The female patient grew up with an emotionally cold and rigid mother and weak, "hen-pecked" father. When as a young girl, she received no warmth or expression of love from her mother, she turned to her father for support. She soon learned that feminine behavior aroused her father's interest, but this soon led to alarming and forbidden interactions. She then withdrew from her father, somatosized this conflict, and became La Belle Indifference. She appears capable of dissociating from the pain and being objective in her reporting as if she were a bystander with insight into another person's pain. She should be referred for psychiatric evaluation after a complete history and examination reveals no pathologic condition or pathofunction to account for her pain.

### Psychogenic Headache

Pain symptoms that mimic muscle contraction headache may represent somatization of anxiety and depression.[31] These headaches

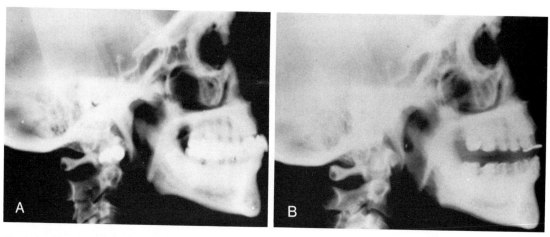

*Fig. 5–2.* Pre- (A) and postoperative (B) cephalometric x-rays of a 48-year-old female patient who, at the hands of several dentists, underwent treatments for "TMJ dysfunction" that included occlusal equilibrations, occlusal splints, and finally, full crown restoration of all teeth. Her pain problems associated with the major muscles of mastication persisted. She sought further somatic treatments, and because of her history of personal stress and conflict, was diagnosed a pain laureate.

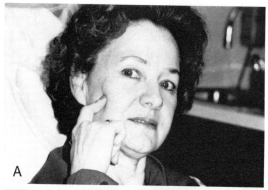

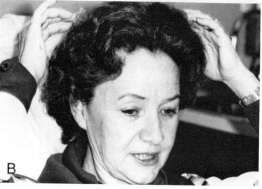

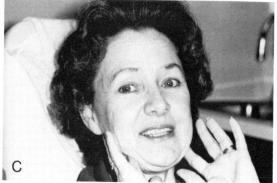

*Fig. 5–3.* A delightful 44-year-old lady who was referred for possible left TMJ surgery to correct TMJ pain was asked to point with one finger to the area of her chief complaint. She indicated sources of her pain in the (A) right masseter muscle, (B) bilateral posterior-superior cranial, and (C) bilateral submandibular regions. Her verbal description was of severe, chronic pains in these areas. A diagnosis of La Belle Indifference was made.

occur more frequently in young women, and typically begin as a mild aching that increases in intensity and duration. The pain is described as dull, aching, and throbbing, but it does not respond to medication for vascular headache (described in Chapter 13). After all reversible therapies for muscle contraction and vascular headache have failed to provide relief, these patients should be referred to the clinical psychologist for therapy.

## Psychiatric Evaluation of Dental Patients

The clinician who treats chronic facial pain should be aware of a psychiatric evaluation of dental patients who did not respond to conventional dental therapy that was published in 1955.[32] Moulton divided these patients into 6 groups of pain and dysfunction patients.

The first group included 14 glossodynia, idiopathic oral burning patients, all women. These patients had undergone vitamin and hormone therapy with no relief of their burning pain. They were classified as typically terror-stricken, menopausal women with a cancer phobia. All lacked sexual satisfaction in their lives. Six were frigid, five were widowed, and four had invalid husbands. Two dated the onset of symptoms to the death of their husband. One was cured when she moved in with her children.

The second group included 19 women and 1 man with neuralgia. They experienced radiating facial pain, flushing, edema, nasal swelling, and gastrointestinal symptoms. These patients seemed guilty and depressed and were happiest when they were convalescing from an illness or accident and were receiving care. They were polysurgical addicts. Fourteen of these individuals had a combined total of 52 operations. Moulton warned of a danger of suicide in these patients.

The third group was classified as having acute necrotizing, ulcerative gingivitis or Vincent's infection. Six patients were evaluated and all six had serious psychiatric problems. These patients were young (21 to 33 years of age), and they were living with tension, strain, and fatigue. They described their mouths as dirty, filthy, and odorous. They neglected their diet and oral hygiene. Two were young ladies just leaving their parents and starting sexual activity. One young man was impotent in relations with an older woman and later became a paranoid schizophrenic. One woman was beginning an extramarital affair. One young man would seek out homosexuals in bars, and the last man was attached to his wife, but would pick up women in bars and abandon them to go home with a bleeding mouth.

A fourth group included chronic periodontitis patients that did not respond to periodontal therapy. These individuals had less acute psychiatric problems. They demonstrated a need for dependency, and were often reared by older siblings after the death of their parents. The women in the group reported bleeding gums at menarche and then in other situations of anxiety.

A fifth group comprised periodontosis patients, who demonstrated advanced degeneration of the periodontium with a minimum of inflammation. All 10 women in this group had amazingly healthy emotional conditions.

The sixth group was identified as TMJ pain patients. In 16 of the 35 patients in this group, the pain was dental treatment initiated, and 18 were bruxists. Thirty-one of the 35 patients showed conspicuous psychiatric factors and 11 were classed as prepsychotic.

## Psychopathologic Assessment Methods

Many psychometric tests are often helpful and sometimes essential to the proper diagnosis of facial pain patients. Among these are the Minnesota Multiphasic Personality Inventory (MMPI),[33] the Symptom Checklist—90 Revised (SCL-90R),[34] Becks Depression Inventory,[35] TMJ Scale,[36] Sickness Impact Profile,[37] Chronic Illness Problem Inventory,[38] Illness Behavior Questionnaire,[39] Self-Rating Depression Scale (SDS),[40] and IMPATH:TMJ.[41,42]

### MMPI

The MMPI consists of 566 items, takes approximately 2 hours to complete, and provides 3 validity and 10 clinical scales. The clinical scales include: hypochondriasis, depression, hysteria, psychopathic deviance, masculinity-femininity, paranoid, psychasthenia, schizophrenia, hypomania, and social introversion. The 3 validity scales, listed as L, F, and K, help to indicate whether a patient tries to present fewer or more problems than may be true. An MMPI elevation of the first 3 clinical scales in a V pattern, with depression less elevated than hypochondriasis or hysteria, is called the conversion-V. Historically, it is associated with conversion hysteria and is characterized in a person who has adapted to the role of the invalid, focusing on a single pain symptom. The MMPI clinical scales are usually scored by the Roche Psychiatric Service Institute scoring program. The MMPI helps to identify maladaptive behavioral patterns, but it has not definitively succeeded in predicting response to treatment.[43] One of the main criticisms of the MMPI is that it was developed for a psychiatric population and not for a facial pain population.

## Symptom Checklist-90 Revised

The SCL-90 is a 90-item self-report inventory designed to assess psychologic symptoms in medical, dental, and psychiatric patients. Each item is rated on a 5-point scale from 0 to 4 (no distress to extreme distress). It provides measures of nine different symptom dimensions, including somatization, obsessive-compulsive, interpersonal sensitivity, depression, anxiety, hostility, phobic anxiety, paranoid ideation, and psychoticism. The SCL-90R also provides 3 summary scales of psychologic distress including global severity index (GSI), positive symptom distress index (PSDI), and the positive symptom total (PST). The SCL-90R is scored by the SCORE-90 computer program.

## TMJ Scale

The four page, self-report TMJ Scale contains 97 items. The first page collects demographic information. The patient is instructed in self-palpation of head and neck muscles and the TM joint and marks the pain 0 to 3 (no pain to extreme pain) on a drawing of the head. In the remaining parts of the TMJ Scale, the patient indicates the amount of time affected, on a 0 to 3 scale (none of the time to all of the time), by various signs and symptoms of facial pain. The TMJ Scale provides scores for the following: (1) pain report, (2) palpation pain, (3) perceived malocclusion, (4) joint dysfunction, (5) range-of-motion limitation, (6) non-TMJ disorder, (7) psychologic factors, (8) stress, (9) chronicity, and (10) global scale. The TMJ Scale shows significant elevations on all scales for TMJ patients relative to non-TMJ dental patients and normal subjects with acceptable reliability and internal consistency in all of the scales.[36]

## IMPATH:TMJ

This microcomputer-based assessment instrument is designed to identify efficiently the contributing factors in craniomandibular disorders. The patient interacts with the microcomputer and an immediate analysis and report of the results and storage of the data for clinical research is immediately available. With IMPATH, the patient cannot omit answering a question because the program does not continue until each question is answered. The software generates a medical and illness history, identifies biologic behavioral, and psychosocial contributing factors, and provides scores measuring symptom severity, illness impact, life functioning, and quality of life. The patient answers the questions in privacy at their own pace; about 1 to 2 hours are needed to complete the questions. Setting up the computer for the patient takes about 5 to 10 minutes of staff time.

Four major reports are generated by the IMPATH:TMJ. These include: (1) illness and medical history, (2) contributing factor list, (3) pre-post indices report, and (4) a patient summary report. The patient summary report may be given to the patient for their guidance during therapy, because it includes a review of contributing factors in understandable terms.

## Psychometric Evaluation of Chronic Pain Patients

Efforts to characterize the personality traits of facial pain patients have produced minimal amounts of evidence to indicate that facial pain is correlated with one specific personality trait.[44]

In a study in 1982, 240 patients completed a pain history questionnaire and took the MMPI.[45] These patients had been referred for psychologic evaluation for one of three reasons: (1) they had no organic basis for their pain, (2) they were unresponsive to traditional medical treatments, or (3) a presurgical evaluation was requested by a clinician. Of this group of 240 patients, 52% had low back pain, 10% had headache, 6% had shoulder/arm pain, 6% had chest pain, and 5% had stomach pain. The remaining patients had a variety of other pains.

A hierarchical clustering procedure was used to categorize the pain patients on the basis of MMPI. Three distinct MMPI profiles were identified, of which one group was essentially "normal." A second group showed the hypochondriasis configuration, and a third group had the highly elevated scales of the psychopathologic profile. Patients in the three groups did not differ in age, education, income, IQ, assertiveness, or duration of pain.

The patients in the third group showed the greatest restriction of physical activity, more dissatisfaction with life situation, poorer self-esteem, greater increase in anxiety since pain onset, more pessimism regarding the future, greater depression, more deterioration in social relationships, poorer sleep, and greater decrease in sexual frequency than patients in the other groups. In turn, individuals in the second group showed more distress from pain than those with the "normal" profile.

In another study, the MMPI was administered to 92 patients in a multimodal, inpatient low back-pain treatment program.[46] Their self-report of pain and response to treatment were statistically compared to a cluster analysis of the MMPI profiles. The cluster analysis yielded 4 groups of MMPI profiles in women and 3 groups in men, and these groups correlated with the subjects' pain histories but not with their response to treatment.

In 1985, three groups of patients with diagnoses of myogenic facial pain, TM joint internal derangement, or atypical facial pain, underwent a complete head and neck exam-

ination, psychiatric interview, and psychometric evaluation with the MMPI.[47] The atypical pain patients were older than the individuals in the other two groups. Certain MMPI scales were elevated in all three groups, but those of the myogenic and atypical facial pain patients were more dramatically elevated, particularly with regard to hypochondriasis, depression, and hysteria. Psychopathologic factors seemed to play a more dominant role among patients with myogenic and atypical facial pain than among TMJ internal derangement patients. The concept that myospasm progresses to jaw clicking was not substantiated by this report, because the myogenic pain patients were older than the internal derangement group.

In 1976, Derogatis and colleagues demonstrated that the then new SCL-90 showed high convergent validity with the MMPI when both tests were administered to 209 symptomatic volunteers in a clinical therapeutic drug trial.[48] The results of the SCL-90 and MMPI were consistent on all eight of the comparable scales. Then, in 1987, the psychologic characteristics of 100 craniomandibular patients were assessed by using the Symptom Checklist-90 Revised (SCL-90R).[49] Cluster analysis of the data revealed three discrete profiles that represented normal, moderately distressed, and severely distressed psychologic groups, just as were reported with the MMPI. The moderately distressed group showed elevations of T values, called the hypochondriasis profile, with elevations in somatization, depression, and anxiety scales. The severely distressed group had a psychopathologic profile, with extreme elevations in depression, somatization, obsessive-compulsive, interpersonal sensitivity, anxiety, hostility, phobia, and psychoticism. This group also showed significant elevations in the three summary scales of distress.

Despite the general replication of the three MMPI and SCL-90R pattern types across a number of studies of chronic pain patients, just how much the cases vary within each pattern type is not known.[50] MMPI scores of men and women may not be directly comparable. Demerol may cause delirium, dysphoria, disorientation, agitation, and transient hallucinations, which may alter the

MMPI profile of a pain patient. Patients with seizure disorders may also show altered MMPI profiles, and the patient who abuses alcohol and Demerol is usually labeled as a passive-dependent personality. These patients respond well to medical treatment. Therefore, elevated MMPI and SCL-90R profiles of chronic pain patients should be interpreted with caution.

Even though psychometric testing helps to identify the role of psychologic factors in pain behavior, the tests often do not identify the best type of treatment to be employed or predict the response to treatment. They help the clinician label the patient who does not respond to traditional treatment, but all too often, they offer little in the way of a more definitive treatment procedure. Perhaps future research in the psychopathology of pain will help to improve the management of chronic pain patients.

## Case Summaries Involving Psychogenic Aspects of Pain

### Patient 1: Psychogenic Headache

A 12-year-old girl had a chief complaint of "migraine headache." At onset, 1 month before examination, the headaches began with a sensation of temple pressure, nausea, and photophobia. She missed 18 days of school and attended school with a headache on the other days. She had been treated with ibuprofen (Motrin); butalbital with 30 mg codeine phosphate (Fiorinal #3); isometheptene mucate, dichloralphenazone, and acetaminophen (Midrin); and propranolol HCl (Inderal). None of these medications relieved her headaches.

Examination of the TM joints revealed slight tenderness to palpation of the capsule and moderate tenderness of neck muscles. She had first bicuspid rise occlusal function bilaterally, because her canines were not fully erupted. Light neck traction relieved the headache, but it returned immediately on release of the traction. She was referred to physical therapy for neck mobilization therapy. Her headaches continued to increase in intensity daily in a crescendo effect, and radiated into the frontal, masseter, and mastoid regions. She experienced no nausea, scotomata, or photophobia with the headaches at this time.

Baclofen (Lioresal) in an ascending dosage was prescribed, but the headaches became worse, so it was discontinued. After a 4-month course, the patient was attending school with headaches and would come home when it was unbearably intense. Midrin and oxycodone with aspirin controlled the headache temporarily, but adverse side effects prevented their use.

The patient was then referred to a clinical psychologist for evaluation and treatment. The patient and her parents were interviewed and the patient took the Childhood Depression Inventory (CDI), Fear Survey Schedule for Children (FSSC-R), Sentence Completion Test, and EMG muscle scanning. The patient reported having mild headaches at school for several weeks 3 years before this episode. She also had "chronic sinus headaches" that were relieved by pseudoephedrine HCl and chlorpheniramine maleate (Sudafed).

The patient's mother is a director of a Christian education program and her father is a college professor. She is a straight A student and a leader in her seventh grade class. A few days before the onset of headaches, the patient's father left the continent to work on a sabbatical. For 6 years before this time, the patient's parents had suffered marital problems and her father had undergone psychologic counseling for deep depression for about 1 year. The patient suffered from air sickness and had head pain when flying. She expressed a fear of flying or having her parents fly, and she did not like having her father fly out of the country.

The CDI score indicated the patient did not have a significant level of depression and the FSSC-R score indicated that she was not an abnormally anxious child. The Sentence Completion Test suggested the patient was concerned about her headaches, separations from her family, physical injury, and being embarrassed in front of other people. Her muscle tension was within normal limits. The conclusion was that the patient was experiencing continued vascular-muscle contraction headaches of psychogenic origin. She received training in progressive muscle relaxation and EMG biofeedback, but when her father returned from his sabbatical, the headaches slowly disappeared. She is now a high school student and a recent interview revealed she has remained free of headaches.

## Patient 2: Idiopathic Glossodynia and Self-Mutilation

A 35-year-old woman had initial complaints of burning in her tongue that changed to a complaint of pain as she interacted with us in a doctor-patient relationship. Evidence to justify these complaints could not be found and dietary treatment was to no avail. The patient seemed to look forward to her visits to the pain clinic every 2 or 3 weeks, having traveled from a university town about 90 miles away where she resided with her husband, an aggressive, status-conscious middle-level executive in the university administration. At our next-to-last visit with the patient, we remarked, "We cannot seem to find the reason for the pain in your tongue, but please try this (an alteration in her nutrition) and we will reappoint you in 3 weeks for observation."

The patient must have believed the doctor-patient relationship and the regular trips to the clinic were ending. On her next visit, before she protruded her tongue for examination she said, "Now, see if you can find something wrong with my tongue." Inspection of her tongue revealed it had been traumatized by her chewing on it (Fig. 5–4).

The patient was immediately referred for psychologic treatment, which was successful in removing the perceived pain from her tongue and in teaching her to manage her lifestyle.

## Patient 3: Delusional Pain

A 35-year-old female, basic-level government employee had few redeeming social graces as well as less than attractive physical attributes. She lived with her parents and her 18-year-old son who had been born out of wedlock. She had been subjected to two decades of criticism by her parents, which grew more intense as her son became more unmanageable. She came to us with a complaint

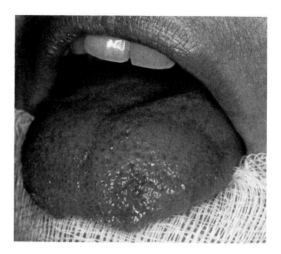

*Fig. 5–4.* A 35-year-old female patient with complaints of idiopathic glossodynia who, probably unknowingly, produced a self-inflicted injury to her tongue when she felt the doctor-patient relationship was ending.

of cranial pains and evidence of a painful subluxation of the left TM joint.

The patient had a severe malocclusion and her extensive and protracted treatment included a meniscus plication procedure and full mouth rehabilitation. After cessation of cranial pains and TM joint dysfunction for about 1 year, the pain and dysfunction returned to both areas.

The patient telephoned on the occasion of a scheduled visit to the pain clinic saying, "I have not been out of bed for 4 days because I feel so bad." In response to a question, she indicated she had not even left her bed to care for the requirements of normal body elimination. With our assurances that we cared for her as a fellow human being, she agreed to arise, bathe, and come to the clinic. When she arrived at the clinic, her face was garish because of a broad application of lipstick far beyond the normal vermilion margins, extending bilaterally past the nasolabial creases. She had applied sweeps of mascara that were at least 15 mm in width to her eyebrow regions, extending to the temporal sideburn hairlines.

We had witnessed the psychologic equivalent of a somatic suicide in our patient who had undergone a psychotic break. She was admitted to the hospital immediately by the psychiatric service. Her treatment included, as appropriate for the times, electric shock and other therapy. She recovered and learned to cope with her family by realizing she was basically a good person and that she had her own responsible contributions to make to society.

## Patient 4: Anxiety and Bruxism

A 40-year-old woman was referred for TM joint surgery because of a painful subluxation and intermittent dislocation of a left TM joint. The patient was the administrative secretary to a prominent leader of industry and the community who was being unjustly criticized. She remarked in the history phase of the treatment, "Did you know that the word secretary comes from the Latin and means the keeper of secrets?" We felt this remark and other findings in the history were indicative of a lady under pressures for responsibilities she had been assigned and had assumed.

Physical examination of her oral cavity revealed evidence of bruxism to the point the maxillary canine had worn a facet between the mandibular lateral incisor and canine, and had produced a hyperkeratosis in the labial mucosa (Fig. 5–5). She understood that the TMJ dysfunction was secondary to a somatic discharge of her energies by the unilateral grinding of her teeth. Subsequent therapy by a psychologist was only partially effective in behavior modification. Her loyal and under-

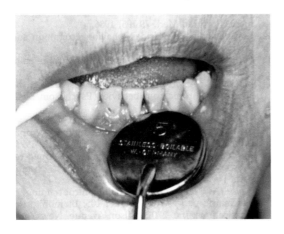

*Fig. 5–5.* A 40-year-old female with bruxism and clenching habits that were secondary to the stresses of her employment. She was referred for surgery to correct pain in the left TMJ. The bruxism and clenching produced an abraided area between the mandibular lateral incisor and the canine as well as a hyperkeratosis of her labial mucosa.

standing concerned services to her employer continued, and she had intermittent pains in her left TMJ for the next 2 years. The consensus of the treatment team during a recapitulation and review of the case was that the lady was a loyal employee in a protective mode regarding her position and her employer's activities.

## Patient 5: Psychogenic Muscle Pain

A 56-year-old physician, who was regarded as an authority on the clinical aspects of arthritic diseases, was invited to deliver a 2-day series of lectures before an august, learned body in a major metropolitan area of the United States. The lectures were to include reviews of applicable basic life sciences, which were somewhat afield of his main patient-care endeavors. He planned and invested 4 months of evenings and weekends toward the preparation of the lectures to be delivered in February. His preparations were particularly intense during the Christmas holidays, and on New Year's day, he was unable to occlude his posterior teeth because of bilateral capsulitis with edema of the TM joint. The TM joints were sensitive to palpation, and he experienced a trismus-like limitation of opening movements of his mouth.

The relation of facial musculature to psychic tension and anxiety were explained, and he had a splendid understanding of the effects of stress on musculature. With the knowledge that isometric contraction of the major muscles of mastication had produced the TM joint and musculature maladies, he was amenable to instruction in relaxation techniques. These efforts were successful, and he had normal occlusion and TMJ activity within 72 hours.

The authors now recommend that the patient who suffers from diurnal bruxism purchase a watch-sized repeat timer, set it for 15 minutes, and carry it or place it at their work station. When the alarm sounds, the patient immediately takes note of the position of the teeth. When they are clenched together, the patient is instructed to blow three times against the cheeks. This action causes the teeth to disclude and the muscles of facial expression are stretched. The patient then closes the lips together, keeping the teeth

# 6

# *Nutrition*

The subject of this chapter is nutrition as it pertains to head and neck pain and dysfunction. Basic nutritional and dietary principles are considered first, followed by clinical application of this information to the diagnosis and treatment of facial pain.

Most people choose their diet according to the dictates of taste, flavor, satiety, and habit (or familiarity), and do not consider nutrition when planning meals or selecting food at a restaurant. As a consequence, a typical modern diet contains excess fat, refined carbohydrates, calories, salt, caffeine, food preservatives, and artificial flavorings and coloring agents, and tends to be deficient in calcium, fiber, and magnesium. The average American consumes 140 pounds of sugar annually. Only one fourth of this amount is granulated sugar purchased by the pound in the grocery; the remainder is hidden in foods and beverages.

The human requires energy, carbohydrates, amino acids, lipids, vitamins, minerals, and water (approximately 40 essential nutrients) to maintain life processes. When these dietary components are digested and absorbed, they are synthesized into carbohydrates, proteins, and fats or are oxidized to release cellular energy. An adult human has approximately 81,000 calories stored in reserve. During times of fasting, the resting metabolism decreases from approximately 1700 to 1200 calories per day. Man can, therefore, survive approximately 67 days without food if water is available.

The biologic activities of carbohydrates, proteins, fats, vitamins, and minerals are so interdependent that an excess or deficit of any one likely affects most of the others. For example, the presence of vitamin C in the gastrointestinal tract enhances the absorption of iron and may correct an iron deficiency anemia.[1] Thus, everyone should eat a wide variety of foods at each meal and not segregate the various foods to be eaten at different meals.

A well-balanced diet includes foods from each of the four basic food groups (Table 6–1). The amount of these foods should be adjusted for age, weight, health status, and physical activity. Foods such as butter, margarine, salad oils, syrups, honey, jam, pastries, candy, and alcoholic drinks are not listed in the four food groups. These foods are not necessary and should be eaten only to adjust the calories needed. The well-balanced diet, as described in Table 6–1, contains all the nutrients necessary for total health, with the possible exception of fluoride.[2] If drinking water is not fluoridated, supplementation with fluoride is effective in reducing dental decay.

Processing and cooking foods reduces their nutritional value. Nourishing foods spoil quickly, whereas processed foods, depleted of their nutritional value, may keep on the shelf for years. Fresh peas lose 56% of their vitamin content when they are cooked.[3] If previously frozen, they lose 83% in cooking, and if previously canned, they lose 94%. As much as 50% of the lysine, arginine, tryptophan, and histidine content of protein is destroyed when it is cooked in moist heat with reducing sugars such as glucose.[4] Between the time food is harvested and the time it is eaten, its nutritional content is reduced 40 to

TABLE 6–1. *Four Food Groups*

| Group | Foods Included | Servings per Day |
|---|---|---|
| Fruits and vegetables | Dark green, leafy or orange vegetables and fruits | 4 |
| Breads and cereals | Whole grain, enriched or fortified cereals, breads, pasta, rice, oats, corn, and wheat products | 4 |
| Milk and dairy products | Milk (lowfat or skimmed), buttermilk, yogurt, cheeses, cottage cheese | 2 adults<br>4 teenagers and nursing mothers<br>3 children and pregnant mothers |
| Meat, fish, eggs, and legumes | Beef, veal, lamb, pork, liver, poultry, eggs, fish, shellfish, dried peas and beans, nuts, soybeans | 2 |

90%, depending on the type of food and how it is transported, processed, and prepared for consumption.

The recommended daily dietary allowances published by the Food and Nutritional Board of the National Academy of Sciences are intended for most healthy persons in the United States living under "usual environmental stresses." Extra nutrients may be needed to offset increased nutrient requirements caused by individual biochemistry, diseases, compromised mastication, physical inactivity, pollution, aging, medications, psychologic stress, trauma from accidents, and surgery. Several of these factors are discussed in detail in this chapter.

## Nutrition and Immune System Dysfunction

In recent studies, investigators have shown that multinutrient deficiencies lead to impaired immunocompetence.[5] Generalized malnutrition is common in patients with surgical and medical illnesses and in patients with chronic facial pain. Impaired immunocompetence increases susceptibility to respiratory, dermal, intestinal, and systemic infections, and may contribute to high morbidity and mortality rates in these patients. Single nutrient deficiencies, imbalances among individual nutrients, and excesses of single nutrients also affect immunocompetence. A deficiency of pyridoxine depresses both cellular and humoral immunity in animals. Human volunteers with short-term experimental pyridoxine deficiency show reduced antibody responses to vaccines. Experimentally induced, brief pantothenic acid deficiency in man also reduces antibody responses to immunization. Folic acid deficiency depresses immune function in both animals and man. Deficiencies of thiamine, riboflavin, niacin, and biotin have little effect on immunocompetence.

Vitamin C facilitates phagocytic cell migration and killing functions as well as the healing of wounds. Increases in dietary vitamin A enhance resistance to infection in animals and accelerate the rejection of skin grafts. Vitamin A deficiency in animals leads to depletion of thymic lymphocytes, depressed lymphocyte responses to various mitogens, and

an increased frequency and severity of bacterial, viral, and protozoal infections. Vitamin E deficiency depresses immunoglobulin responses to antigens, lymphocytic proliferative responses to mitogens and antigens, delayed dermal hypersensitivity reactions, and general host resistance.

Minerals also have important regulatory functions in the immune system. Iron deficiency is accompanied by lymphoid tissue atrophy and impaired in vitro lymphocyte responsiveness to mitogenic stimulation. On the other hand, iron excess can saturate plasma iron-binding proteins. This state increases the availability of iron for uptake by microorganisms and may lead to overwhelming sepsis. Zinc deficiency causes atrophy of lymphoid tissue and produces abnormalities in both cellular and humoral immunity. These abnormalities can be reversed by restoring zinc to normal levels. A modest increase in dietary selenium in combination with vitamin E enhances immune responsiveness to vaccine antigens in animals. Prolonged magnesium deficiency in animals is accompanied by thymic atrophy and reduced humoral immune response to a variety of antigens, but depletion in man is not known to produce immunologic impairment.

Dietary deficiencies of phenylalanine, tyrosine, valine, threonine, methionine, cystine, and tryptophan impair humoral antibody responses in mice but have no effect on cell-mediated immunity. Excessive intake of leucine reduces the antibody response to immunization in animals.

Abnormalities in lipid uptake and metabolism can initiate significant changes in immunity. Experimentally induced hypercholesterolemia in animals decreases resistance to bacterial and viral infections, suppresses inflammatory infiltrates, and impairs primary antibody responses. A deficiency of essential fatty acids depressed both primary and secondary antibody responses to both T cell-dependent and -independent antigens in mice. On the other hand, excess polyunsaturated fatty acids produce widespread immunologic defects in animals. Thus, immune dysfunction may be noted in every wasted or debilitated patient. Even obese persons may manifest micronutrient deficiencies, particularly of zinc and iron.

Drugs and other therapeutic measures, including the polypharmacy of many chronic pain patients, may induce single- or multiple-nutrient abnormalities. Food faddists with unusual diets may be immune suppressed, and all of these factors warrant consideration in the clinical history of a patient.

## Vitamins

The vitamins are classified water soluble (B complex and C) or fat soluble (A, D, E, and K). The water-soluble vitamins are easily absorbed, but fat-soluble vitamins require dietary fat, pancreatic lipase, and bile salts for absorption. The sources and uses of the major vitamins are summarized in Table 6–2.

The role of vitamin E in human nutrition has been the subject of much dispute. Find-

ings of recent studies, however, indicate that vitamin E has an important function in the maintenance of normal neurologic structure and function.[6] In 1950, a rare inherited condition, abetalipoproteinemia, was described in which the patients have total absence of beta (low density) lipoprotein and chylomicrons in their plasma. These patients show devastating ataxic neuropathy and pigmentary retinopathy by age 10 years. One postulate was that disordered fat absorption and transport caused the signs and symptoms, and vitamin A deficiency was suspected. Then, a total absence of vitamin E was noted in the plasma of these patients. Eight patients with abetalipoproteinemia have now been treated for as long as 19 years with massive oral doses of vitamin E to assure some absorption and transport of the vitamin. Five of these patients, who received the supplement before the age of 16 months, show no clinical

**TABLE 6–2.** *Vitamins*

| Vitamin | Source | Action | Deficiency |
|---------|--------|--------|------------|
| A | Yellow fruit, and vegetables | Epithelium, visual pigments | Keratosis, night blindness |
| $B_1$ (thiamine) | Liver, cereals | Pyruvate and alpha-ketoglutarate, decarboxylation cofactor | Neuritis, beri-beri, Wernicke's encephalopathy |
| $B_2$ (riboflavin) | Liver, milk | Flavoproteins | Glossitis, cheilosis |
| Niacin | Meat, yeast | NAD and NADP | Pellagra |
| $B_6$ (pyridoxine) | Wheat, corn, liver, yeasts | Prosthetic group on enzymes, transamination fatty acid metabolism | Seizures |
| Pantothenate | Yeast, liver, eggs | Coenzyme A energy release | Enteritis, dermatitis, alopecia, adrenal insufficiency |
| Biotin | Yeast, liver, eggs | $CO_2$ fixation in fatty acid synthesis | Enteritis, dermatitis |
| Folic acid | Green vegetables | Coenzyme for one carbon transfer synthesis of purines | Sprue, anemia |
| $B_{12}$ (cyanocobalamin) | Eggs, liver, meat, milk | Erythropoiesis coenzyme | Pernicious anemia |
| C | Citrus fruit | Collagen synthesis | Scurvy |
| D | Fish, liver | Calcium and phosphate absorption | Rickets |
| E | Milk, eggs, meat, vegetables | Red cell membrane, neuron structure and function | Fetal death, muscular dystrophy, ataxic neuropathy, pigmentary retinopathy |
| K | Green vegetables | Clotting factors | Bleeding |

abnormalities and retinal function remains normal. The other three patients who had developed clinical abnormalities before supplementation, show significant improvement in signs and symptoms of the disease. The absorption of vitamin E may differ from that of vitamins A, D, and K, because massive oral doses of vitamin E are required to maintain an adequate plasma level, whereas only conventional doses of vitamins A, D, and K are required.

Recently, patients with progressive ataxia, areflexia, and loss of proprioception by the teenage years were shown to have no vitamin E in their plasma, even though levels of low-density lipoprotein, triglycerides, and cholesterol were elevated. A good reason now exists to include serum vitamin E assays in the evaluation of spinocerebellar syndromes in children and young adults; degeneration of large myelinated neurons in the spinal cord dorsal columns and peripheral nerves is noted in these patients. Vitamin E supplementation is now recommended for all patients with chronic fat malabsorption who have reduced serum levels of the vitamin. The dosage varies from 200 mg/day as maintenance in cystic fibrosis patients to 11 mg/kg/day in abetalipoproteinemia patients.

## Pyridoxine Sensory Neuropathy

Recently, vitamin $B_6$ (pyridoxine) has been prescribed for such conditions as nausea of pregnancy, premenstrual syndrome, attention deficit disorder, carpal tunnel syndrome, depression associated with oral contraceptive use, asthma, autism, schizophrenia, atherosclerosis-associated thrombosis, and kidney stones.[7] Some of these patients as well as food faddists taking megavitamin doses of pyridoxine develop signs of neurotoxicity. One 27-year-old woman increased her dose to 5000 mg/day and maintained that dose for almost 1 year.[8] During this period, she noted a tingling sensation in her neck and feet when she flexed her neck. She became progressively ataxic, had difficulty handling small objects, needed a cane for walking, and then developed numbness in her lips and tongue. Two months after eliminating her pyridoxine intake, her symptoms improved significantly;

after 7 months she could walk without a cane. Her electrophysiologic sensory nerve status remains abnormal. This type of sensory neuropathy was noted in patients taking doses as low as 500 mg/day, which is 250 times the RDA. With a toxicity threshold at or below 500 mg/day, possibly thousands of individuals are potentially at risk.

Findings of a recent study in rats demonstrated the neuropathy produced by pyridoxine toxicity.[9] The rats received 600 mg/kg of pyridoxine by intraperitoneal injection twice daily. Ataxia began on day 3 of treatment, and by day 8, the rats were not able to walk. By day 3, degeneration was evident in the dorsal columns of the spinal cord. It progressed to loss of axoplasm and collapse of myelin sheaths. By day 8, the dorsal root ganglia showed significant loss of large cell bodies. Toxic doses of pyridoxine, therefore, produced a partial, chemical ganglionectomy, destroying the large neurons that subserve proprioception.

Pyridoxine is necessary for many metabolic functions. It plays a key role in the metabolism of neurotransmitters such as serotonin and dopamine. Clinical signs of pyridoxine deficiency are irritability and depression. Elderly people and women who use oral contraceptives are at a higher risk of having such deficiency. Pyridoxine intake warrants consideration in the differential diagnosis of a patient who complains of perioral numbness, has normal muscle strength, but cannot walk with eyes closed.

## Essential Minerals

The required dietary minerals include sodium, potassium, iron, copper, calcium, magnesium, lithium, manganese, cobalt, bromine, chloride, and zinc. Only trace amounts of some of these minerals are required. Because of its role in many functions, such as blood clotting, muscle contraction and relaxation, mineralization of bone, activation of enzyme systems, and nerve transmission, calcium may be involved in many head and neck pain syndromes. Calcium is the fifth most abundant element in the body, and 99% of it is stored in the bony skeleton. The RDA of calcium for adolescent, pregnant and lactating women, and persons with osteoporosis is 1200 mg/day. The typical woman loses three times more calcium from her skeleton during 6 months of breastfeeding than during 9 months of gestation. Calcium has been prescribed for many years for patients with hypoparathyroidism, postmenopausal and senile osteoporosis, achlorhydria, chronic diarrhea, vitamin D deficiency, pregnancy, lactation, and pancreatitis.[10] Inadequate dietary intake of calcium leads to increased risk of osteoporosis and osteomalacia. The daily calcium intake of individuals who do not drink milk regularly is typically only 200 to 300 mg/day.[11] This amount is well below the RDA. Intake of about 1½ pints of whole milk per day would be required to obtain the recommended daily requirement if milk were the only source ingested. About 20% of ingested calcium is absorbed in the small intestine. Absorption depends on an acidic gastric pH, presence of vitamin D, and relative absence of complexing or chelating compounds, such as oxalate. Of the 1% fraction of calcium in the blood, only 45% is ionized and physiologically active. Calcium is eliminated primarily in the stool as unabsorbed calcium. With adequate intake, urinary excretion ranges from 250 to 400 mg/day. Urinary excretion is reduced during pregnancy and during low calcium intake to a level of about 150 mg/day.

Hypercalcemia results in nausea, vomiting, anorexia, diarrhea, constipation, depression, apathy, fatigue, hypertension, myopathy, and renal stones. These conditions should be considered when calcium supplementation is contemplated, although hypercalcemia rarely develops with supplementation except in patients with renal failure. Calcium should not be prescribed for patients with hypercalcemia, sarcoidosis, renal failure, severe cardiac disease, and digitalis glycoside therapy. The administration of corticosteroids interferes with calcium absorption, and calcium interferes with tetracycline absorption. Cardiac irregularities may occur when patients receive calcium and cardiac glycosides concomitantly. Calcium supplements are commercially available as carbonate, gluconate, lactate, and phosphate.[12] The amount of calcium suppled by each salt varies greatly. Cal-

cium carbonate is 40% calcium, whereas calcium gluconate is only 9% calcium. The carbonate salts are better suited for calcium supplementation, because they contain more elemental calcium and are less expensive. In some patients, however, they cause increased intestinal gas. Some nonprescription antacids may be used as a calcium carbonate supplement.

## Nutrition in the Elderly

Institutionalized, chronically ill, elderly patients often have low concentration of vitamin C in their plasma and white blood cells. In a study of elderly women, those patients with intake of 30 mg/day or less had low plasma levels of vitamin C, whereas those with intake of 60 mg/day or more had plasma concentrations similar to those of young subjects.[13] In another study of elderly women receiving supplements as low as 30 and 50 mg per day for 12 weeks, plasma and leukocyte vitamin C levels rose to that of young, healthy women.[14] Therefore little evidence exists that elderly people with chronic disease require higher intakes of vitamin C than young people. The often reported low levels of vitamin C in elderly patients are probably related to low intake and can be corrected by small supplements of the vitamin.

## Diet and Headache

A relationship often exists between diet and migraine headache. Many migraine patients relate their headaches to ingestion of such foods as chocolate, alcohol, aged cheeses, histamine-containing wines, processed protein foods, and peanut butter. Foods that contain amines, nitrites, monosodium glutamate, and alcohol have a direct vasoactive effect that may precipitate a vascular headache.[15] The amines include serotonin, tryptamine, tyramine, dopamine, and norepinephrine. Many foods in a modern diet contain these amines and they generally produce no ill effects. Patients who take monamine oxidase inhibitors are not able to hydrolyze sympathomimetic amines at a normal rate, and they are especially sensitive to the tyramine in aged cheeses. A group of 17 patients with a history of migraine were tested with capsules containing 100 mg of tyramine or lactose placebo. In 26 trials with the placebo, two headaches occurred and in 49 trials with tyramine, 40 attacks occurred. Results of other studies show that some migraine sufferers are not sensitive to tyramine.

Phenylethylamine is believed to be the precipitating agent in chocolate. In a phenylethylamine and placebo study involving patients who related their headaches to chocolate ingestion, 18 reported attacks with phenylethylamine and 6 with placebo. These headaches occurred 12 hours after ingestion. This delay may occur because phenylethylamine releases vasoactive substances from the lungs that cause the vascular changes of headache.

When patients with angina pectoris ingest amyl nitrite, it typically causes a dull, aching headache and facial flushing. Nitrites are added to cured meats such as bacon, hot dogs, and salami, and many migraine patients experience a similar type of headache when they ingest these meats. Monosodium glutamate (MSG) is a food additive that enhances the taste of many foods. It is used generously in the preparation of Chinese food. The Chinese restaurant syndrome is well known and includes symptoms of pressure in the face, burning of the trunk, and headache. It typically occurs within 30 minutes of eating the food.

Alcohol has both central and direct vasodilator properties and is a well-known trigger for migraine headaches in sensitive patients. A sudden salt load also triggers headache in some patients. When these patients decide to have their drinks at a cocktail party and suffer the headache, they often ingest salty potato chips, pretzels, and peanuts, which magnify their triggering stimulus.

Many patients with migraines report that coffee tends to decrease the headache. Caffeine has a vasodilating effect on coronary arteries and a vasoconstricting effect on intracranial arteries, counteracting the vascular dilation associated with the headache. Excessive amounts of caffeine, however, may result in a rebound vasodilation and a late occurring headache. This effect may also manifest after excessive smoking as a rebound vasodilation from nicotine.

Treatment plans for patients with dietary migraine should include identifying the foods that trigger the headache and avoiding these foods. Other instructions emphasize keeping a regular schedule, eating and sleeping at regular times, even on the weekends.

### Ice Cream Headache

In a study of 108 persons, 31% of the 49 individuals who did not have migraine experienced headache after eating ice cream.[16] Ninety-three percent of 59 migraine patients experienced the ice cream headache. This headache likely results from the sudden cooling of the oral pharynx and the blood in the internal carotid artery. In the migraine-prone patient, this cooling causes the vascular dilation and headache that further demonstrates that the migraine patient suffers from instability of vasomotion.

## Alcohol Neuropathy

Ethanol is absorbed rapidly from the gastrointestinal tract into the circulation and 90% is oxidized in the liver. Because it is soluble in water, it passes into all fluid compartments of the body. It crosses the blood-brain barrier virtually without limitation. The body has a remarkable ability to develop tolerance to alcohol. After several hours of drinking, subjects can become sober at blood ethanol concentrations that are higher than those at which intoxication first developed. The adaptation to ethanol in alcoholics can be so successful that ordinarily lethal concentrations (500 mg/100 ml) no longer produce intoxication. Chronic alcoholics often have poor nutrition, and this combination of insults, after years, usually results in neuropathy and neurologic disorders such as Wernicke's encephalopathy, Korsakoff's amnestic syndrome, alcoholic dementia, cerebral atrophy, alcoholic myopathy, cerebellar degeneration, amblyopia, central pontine myelinolysis, Marchiafava-Bignami disease, and fetal alcohol syndrome.

Facial pain related to the ingestion of alcohol has been seen in chronic alcoholics. In a report of three cases, chronic alcoholics experienced mandibular and dental pain.[17] Two of the three patients had multiple root canals and extraction of teeth (in spite of clinical and normal radiographic findings) in attempts to eliminate pain. The pain was relieved only when the patients stopped drinking alcohol because of hospital treatment or because of taking of codeine and not wanting to mix alcohol and codeine. In each patient who resumed drinking, the pain returned. The clinician should consider the possibility of chronic alcoholism in patients with normal findings of radiographic and oral examinations but complaints of dental and jaw pain.

## Food-Induced Allergic Arthritis

The concept that allergy to foods could cause arthritis has been suggested but is difficult to prove. Recently, a 52-year-old woman with active rheumatoid-like arthritis was examined in a clinical research center in a blinded, controlled fashion.[18] The woman believed that ingestion of meat, milk, and beans caused exacerbations of her arthritis. Both the patient and the rheumatologist evaluated her arthritis as she fasted, took only a bland diet (Vivonex), or took Vivonex plus lyophilized foods in opaque capsules. The arthritic symptoms decreased significantly during fasting, ingestion of Vivonex alone, or Vivonex plus capsules of D-xylose or lyophilized lettuce and carrot. She suffered symptomatic deterioration on four different occasions when challenged with lyophilized milk equivalent to 8 ounces of milk per meal. Laboratory analyses showed the patient had marginally increased IgG-milk circulating immune complexes and high levels of IgG4 antibodies to milk. This single-patient study provides new insights into the pathogenesis of inflammatory joint disease. In patients with rheumatoid-like signs and symptoms involving the TMJ, the history should include questions about possible relation of flare-ups to diet.

## Tryptophan Supplementation and Facial Pain

An increase in plasma tryptophan levels increases brain levels of serotonin. Increase in brain serotonin levels is accompanied by improvement in sleep patterns, pain relief, and reduction in symptoms of depression. The focus of a recent study of chronic facial pain patients was to investigate the effects of the daily administration of 3 g of tryptophan in conjunction with a high carbohydrate, low fat, and low protein diet.[19] Forty-three patients with diagnoses of TMJ pain-dysfunction, atypical facial neuralgia, migrainous neuralgia, trigeminal neuralgia, phantom tooth pain, ciliary neuralgia, and cervical osteoarthritis were included in the study. Each patient rated their pain on a subjective scale of 0 to 100, with 100 representing maximum pain. They underwent a battery of psychologic tests. Their pain perception and tolerance thresholds were measured on an upper incisor with a digital pulp tester. They were told how to implement a high carbohydrate, low fat, and protein diet, and 250-mg capsules of either tryptophan or placebo were provided, with instructions to take two capsules six times a day. On the fourth week, psychologic tests, pain rating, and pulp-testing procedures were repeated and the patients described all possible side effects of the tryptophan. Thirteen patients violated the experimental protocol and were dropped from the study. The results revealed a significant reduction in pain rating, no difference in the psychologic measure for depression and anxiety, and significant increase in tooth pulpal pain tolerance, but not pain threshold, in the tryptophan group. The most common side effects were "rested feeling" and mood elevation, but some patients reported urinary changes, nausea, diarrhea, and skin itching. Because of the small number of patients, no breakdown of the data according to type of facial pain treated was provided.

The long-term efficacy of this treatment mode is not known. More research is needed before tryptophan supplementation can be considered as standard therapy for chronic pain. At the present time tryptophan has been taken off the market because of deaths from an eosinophilic myalgia syndrome. It is believed that a contaminant in the tryptophan causes the eosinophilia.

## Vitamin Status and Burning Mouth Syndrome

Painful burning of the tongue and oral mucosa affects many patients, especially those in the older age group. The burning may be constant or not present on waking, to begin immediately or build up during the day. The mucosa may be red and inflamed or may appear normal in color and texture. It is often relieved by eating, drinking, or denture removal. The condition may be related to hormonal status, chronic depression, denture irritation, and medications, such as cyclandelate (Cyclospasmol). The role of nutrition in burning mouth syndrome was studied recently in 70 patients.[20] A complete history included questions about depression, anxiety, recent bereavement, and cancerphobia. Oral and maxillofacial examinations were performed and dentures, if present, were evaluated. For a complete blood analysis, plasma vitamin $B_{12}$, folic acid, iron, and ferritin levels, as well as total iron-binding capacity, were determined for each patient. Plasma and urinary glucose and salivary candida tests were performed. Sixty-six of the patients were women. The results showed that of the 54 patients with dentures, 8 dated the onset of their burning with provision of new dentures. Ten of the patients tested positive for candida; 8 of these individuals responded promptly to topical antifungal therapy and were excluded from the study. Four patients were overtly depressed and required a psychiatric evaluation; in 2 of these patients, the burning persisted in spite of counseling and antidepressant therapy. Plasma vitamin levels were normal in these 3 patients. Twenty-eight patients were deficient in vitamins $B_1$, $B_2$, $B_6$, or a combination of these vitamins. They had normal plasma vitamin A, C, D, and E levels, normal hematologic findings, normal salivary flow rates, and no significant numbers of candida. The remaining 27 patients had normal vitamin and hematologic profiles. Forty percent of the burning mouth patients had a B vitamin deficiency. In 80 control subjects without burning mouth syndrome, only 7.5% had a B vitamin deficiency. For 4 weeks, the 28 patients with vitamin B deficiency received replacement therapy according to which B vitamin they lacked. The 27 non-vitamin-deficient patients were randomly treated with the same vitamin B replacement therapy. Of the 28 vitamin-deficient patients, 24 were pain-free after 1 month and remained so after 3 months. Only 8 of the non-vitamin-deficient patients improved after 1 month, but this number dropped to 2 at 3 months. Therefore, 88% of the patients with burning mouth syndrome and B vitamin deficiency were painfree at 3 months, and only 7% of the non-vitamin-deficient patients were improved (not painfree) at 3 months.

Results of this study seem to show that vitamin B complex deficiency is a possible cause of burning mouth syndrome. Commercial vitamin B complex preparations may not contain enough vitamin to treat this condition, and therapeutic single-vitamin doses may be required.

## Preoperative Nutritional Supplementation

When surgical intervention is indicated and optimum healing is desired, all the building blocks for tissue repair should logically be available at the site of the operation. Optimal nutrition pre- and postoperatively plays an important role in the success of the procedure. Many patients who seem to be well nourished may suffer significant nutritional deficiencies. In one report, 59% of randomly selected patients in a municipal hospital had vitamin deficiencies.[21] As many as 35% of medical patients have low serum albumin levels.[22] Patients often receive nothing by mouth from 8 hours preoperatively until several days postoperatively. A recent study involving 24 patients was performed to determine the efficacy of preoperative and postoperative high-calorie liquid supplementation in orthognathic surgery patients.[23] The patients, who require maxillomandibular fixation for 6 weeks postoperatively, were divided into three groups of eight patients each. A "postload group" received a nutritionally complete liquid supplement (Ensure Plus) at 50% of their calculated daily caloric requirements per day beginning 4 weeks before until 6 weeks after the operation. The preload group received an additional 236 ml of Ensure Plus per day to attempt to increase their weight by 5% before the procedure. The control group received no supplement either before or after the operation. The mean duration of hospitalization was 4.3 days, and fluid intake, hospitalization, and intravenous therapy were the same for all groups. The control group lost an average of 9.7% body weight over the 10-week study, and all groups lost weight during the first postoperative week. Nitrogen balance was significantly lower in the control group than in the supplemental groups. The average caloric intake of the control group decreased from 134% of the RDA on day 1 of the preoperative evaluation to 55% 6 weeks later. Caloric intake in the postload group decreased from 115% of the RDA on preoperative day 1 to 99% 6 weeks later. The preload group consumed a level of calories greater than 100% of the RDA throughout the study. The diet of the control group was deficient in iron, thiamine, and niacin throughout the postoperative period, but all three groups consumed adequate levels of protein. Results demonstrated that supplementation postoperatively at a level of 50% of estimated caloric requirements can result in improved nitrogen retention and protein sparing. Supplementation sufficient to achieve weight gain preoperatively does not increase these benefits.

Facial pain patients whose pain increases with mastication tend to limit their diet to mechanically soft foods. These foods often provide excessive refined carbohydrate and are deficient in fiber and vitamins. Several computerized nutritional programs are now available that quickly produce a nutritional profile of a patient. The software is compatible with most personal computers in dental and medical offices. These programs analyze the diet diary of a patient, indicate deficiencies and excesses, and make recommendations of types of foods needed to improve the patient's nutrition. The authors use the Nutrition Profile by Wellsource (15431 S.E. 82nd Dr., Clackamas, OR 97015) when a brief nutritional history reveals a potential problem in a patient.

## Counseling Patients in Nutrition

An excellent method of counseling patients regarding food selection for optimal nutrition was recommended by Ringsdorf and Cheraskin.[1] They categorized foods into three groups: foods to eat liberally (Table 6–3), foods to eat sparingly (Table 6–4), and foods to avoid (Table 6–5). If vitamin supplementation is indicated, the patient is instructed to read the label on the bottle. Some multivitamin-mineral preparations have large amounts of the inexpensive vitamins and limited

**TABLE 6–4.** *Foods to Eat Sparingly*

Animal flesh (trim off fat)
Low fat yogurt
Fats used for frying
Hydrogenated fats in margarine, peanut butter, shortening, and coffee whitener (coconut oil)
Salt (reduce salt intake and taste will acclimate)
Coffee, tea, cocoa, chocolate
Honey (can be used sparingly to replace table sugar)

**TABLE 6–5.** *Foods to Avoid*

Alcohol
Refined sugar foods (sweetened breakfast cereals, cakes, icings, cookies, pies, graham crackers, sweet rolls, coffee cakes, doughnuts, ice cream, ice milk, sherbet, canned or frozen fruit in syrup, sweetened applesauce, candied sweet potatoes, chocolate, syrups, candy, mints, cough drops, Instant Breakfast, Breakfast Squares, Pop Tarts, sweet pickles, sweetened yogurt, Jello, puddings, custards, milkshakes, Ovaltine, Kool-Aid, sweetened breakfast drink, frozen fruit drinks, soft drinks, popsicles, dessert wines and cordials)
Artificial flavorings and coloring agents and food preservatives (when reasonable to avoid)
Nitrite-preserved foods (bacon, hot dogs, luncheon meats, ham, sliced sandwich meats, salami, bologna, liverwurst, smoked fish, corned beef)

**TABLE 6–3.** *Foods to Eat Liberally*

| White cheese | Skimmed milk | Fish |
|---|---|---|
| Poultry | Fruit | Berries |
| Fresh vegetables | Legumes | Whole grains |
| Cereals | Pasta | Nuts |
| Seeds | Brown rice | Whole corn |
| Potatoes | Peas | meal |
| Corn | | Beans |

Fruits, vegetables, nuts, and seeds should be eaten as snacks instead of foods to be avoided. Do not peel the fruits and vegetables if the peel is edible. If vegetables are stir-fried, use safflower, sunflower seed, or corn oil.

amounts of the expensive ones. The patient should select the vitamin preparation that provides as close to 100% of the minimum daily requirement of all the vitamins as possible.

# References

1. Ringsdorf W.M. and Cheraskin E.: Optimal nutrition: A new prescription. J Pedodont, 8:123, 1984
2. Guide to Dental Health, Eating for Fitness. JADA, Special Issue, 1985
3. Marks J.: The Vitamins in Health and Disease; A Modern Reappraisal. Boston, Little, Brown, 1968
4. Editorial: Present status of heat processing damage to protein foods. Nutr Rev, 8:193, 1950
5. Beisel W.R., et al: Single-nutrient effects in immunologic functions. Report of a workshop sponsored by the Department of Food and Nutrition Advisory Group of the American Medical Association. JAMA, 245:53, 1981
6. Muller D.P.R.: Vitamin E—Its role in neurological function. Postgrad Med J, 62:107, 1986
7. Podell R.N.: Nutritional supplementation with megadoses of vitamin $B_6$, effective therapy, placebo, or potentiator of neuropathy? Postgrad Med, 77:113, 1985
8. Schaumburg H., et al: Sensory neuropathy from pyridoxine abuse. N Engl J Med, 309:445, 1983
9. Krinke G, et al: Pyridoxine megavitaminosis: An analysis of the early changes induced with massive doses of vitamin $B_6$ in rat primary sensory neurons. J Neuropathol Exp Neurol, 44:117, 1985
10. Replacement solutions: Calcium salts. In Drug Information-84: American Hospital Formulary Service. Edited by G.K. McEnvoy. Bethesda, American Society of Hospital Pharmacy, 1984
11. Jowsey J.: Osteoporosis: Dealing with a crippling bone disease of the elderly. Geriatrics, 32:41, 1977
12. Keyler D. and Peterson C.D.: Oral calcium supplements, how much of what for whom and why? Postgrad Med, 78:123, 1985
13. Newton H.M.V., et al: Relation between intake and plasma concentration of vitamin C in elderly women. Br Med J, 287:1429, 1983
14. Newton H.M.V., et al: The cause and correction of low blood vitamin C concentrations in the elderly. Am J Clin Nutr, 42:626, 1985
15. Diamond S, et al: Diet and headache, Is there a link? Postgrad Med, 79:279, 1986
16. Raskin N.H. and Knittle S.C.: Ice cream headache and orthostatic symptoms in patients with migraine. Headache, 16:22, 1976
17. Mulry J.T., et al: Alcoholic facial neuralgia: Report of three cases. J Am Dent Assoc, 112:847, 1986
18. Panush R.S., et al: Food-induced (allergic) arthritis, inflammatory arthritis exacerbated by milk. Arthritis Rheum, 29:220, 1986
19. Seltzer S., et al: The effects of dietary tryptophan on chronic maxillofacial pain and experimental pain tolerance. J Psychiatr Res, 17:181, 1982–1983
20. Lamey P.J., et al: Vitamin status of patients with burning mouth syndrome and the response to replacement therapy. Br Dent J, 160:81, 1986
21. Leevy C.M., et al: Incidence and significance of hypovitaminemia in randomly selected municipal hospital population. Am J Clin Nutr, 17:259, 1965
22. Bollet A.J. and Owens S.: Evaluation of nutritional status of selected hospitalized patients. Am J Clin Nutr, 26:931, 1973
23. Olejko T.D. and Fonseca R.J.: Preoperative nutritional supplementation for the orthognathic surgery patient. J Oral Maxillofac Surg, 42:573, 1984

# Part IV

# Musculoskeletal System

Many patients with facial pain are surprised to find that most or all of their head and neck muscles are tender to palpation on one or the other side. They were not aware of the role muscles play in their chief complaint. The identification of head and neck myalgia does not provide a diagnosis in many cases, but it helps to evaluate the involvement of myalgia in the problem and to establish the differential diagnosis.

## Skeletal Muscle Innervation

Skeletal muscle is innervated by small diameter neurons, A delta and C, that subserve pain, temperature, and vasomotion; large neurons, A alpha, that activate the contractile mechanism; intermediate neurons, A gamma (fusimotor), that activate the intrafusal muscle fibers in the muscle spindles; and large neurons, A alpha and beta, that subserve the primary and secondary endings in the muscle spindles and complex receptors on the muscle fibers and tendon organs (Fig. 7–1).

The free nerve endings that subserve pain, temperature, and vasomotion terminate mostly on the tendons, fat, connective tissue, blood vessels, and musculotendinous junctions, but a small number end on intrafusal and extrafusal muscle cells.[1] Dysfunction of any nerves that innervate muscle may ultimately initiate and/or maintain pain and dysfunction in head and neck muscles.

## Lability of Muscle Length

The concept that skeletal muscle length in the adult is fixed has been modified. For example, the common belief was that the vertical dimension of occlusion could not be changed. Even though this concept is still correct in the practical sense, the theory must be modified.

Under special conditions, the number of sarcomeres in mammalian muscle can be increased as much as 20% and decreased by as much as 40% in 4 weeks.[2] The hind limb of adult cats was fixed in a cast at stretched or foreshortened lengths for 4 weeks, and the sarcomeres in the fixed and control soleus muscles were counted. Another finding, when using tritiated adenosine, was that the

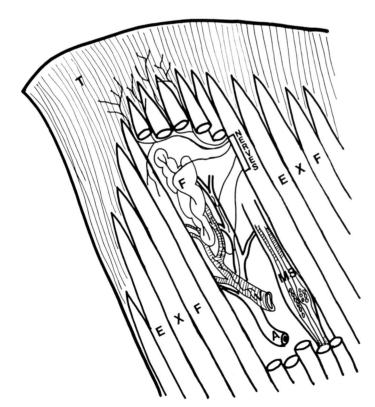

*Fig. 7–1.* Small fiber innervation to skeletal muscle in a window cut in the upper, anterior quadrant of the masseter muscle. Small fibers end on tendons, aponeuroses, fat, blood vessels, and musculotendinous junctions with very few on intrafusal and extrafusal muscle. T— tendon or aponeurosis, F—fat cells, V— vein, A—artery, MS—muscle spindle, EXF—extrafusal muscle fibers.

new sarcomeres were added at the ends of the muscle fibers. It seems that, when the actin and myosin filaments are pulled out from each other and fixed for 4 weeks, a force acts to interdigitate them at their resting length. Each sarcomere is shortened by the addition of new sarcomeres at each end of the muscle (Fig. 7–2).[3] (In these studies, when the foreshortened or lengthened muscles were removed from the casts for 4 weeks, the number of sarcomeres returned to the point at which they were equal on the two sides.)

This lability of muscle length may explain the adaptation of some pain patients to splints that have been inappropriately resurfaced repeatedly, increasing the vertical dimension by 10 and even 30 mm at the anterior teeth. These patients cannot be restored at such occlusal vertical dimensions, because the crown-root ratio is so great that the teeth could not function without compromising the integrity of the periodontium, even if the muscles would function at this excessive length. Because the change in the number of sarcomeres is reversible, the clinician can successfully close the opened bite slowly to a restorable vertical dimension.

A minimal electromyographic (EMG) potential in masseter and suprahyoid muscles occurs at 6.8 mm of opening in women and 10.4 mm in men.[4] This potential was measured even though the clinically determined

interocclusal distance (free way space) was 2.1 mm. The clinical significance of these minimal EMG potentials has yet to be determined.

### Occlusal Splint Thickness

A group of 75 head and neck pain patients were treated with splints of different thicknesses.[5] Twenty-five patients wore a splint opening the occlusal vertical dimension 1.0 mm between nose tip and menton. Twenty-five individuals wore a splint opening the occlusal vertical dimension 4.4 mm, and 25 wore a splint opening the occlusal vertical dimension 8.1 mm. The patients evaluated 21 signs and symptoms of temporomandibular (TM) joint pain and dysfunction for 3 weeks. Results showed that the 4.4-mm and 8.1-mm splints relieved signs and symptoms more quickly and more completely than the 1-mm splint. No difference in relief of symptoms was noted between the 4.4- and 8.1-mm splints. Because a 4.4-mm opening at nose tip and menton opens the second molars approximately 2 mm, it seems no additional benefit of lengthening mandibular muscles accrues after the second molars are opened approximately 2 mm.

## Muscle Trigger Points

Acute and chronic overload of skeletal muscle often leads to weakness and restriction in the stretch range of the muscle.[6] These muscles usually develop myofascial trigger points that are extremely tender to digital pressure. These trigger points are sometimes located in a taut band of fibers, and have been shown to contain accumulations of acid mucopolysaccharide between the muscle cells, degranulated mast cells, extravascular blood platelets, and giant myofilaments.[7] The degranulated mast cells release histamine and heparin into the muscle and the extravascular platelets release serotonin. Trigger points, therefore, may contain a vasodilator, histamine, a vasoconstrictor, serotonin, and an anticoagulant, heparin. Heparin counteracts the accumulation of platelets and their release of serotonin. Serotonin is a potent vasoconstrictor in the extracellular compartment that

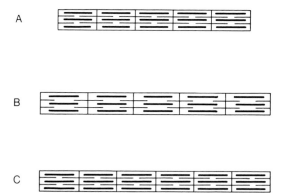

A

B

C

*Fig. 7–2.* Lengthening of skeletal muscle by addition of new sarcomeres. A. Five sarcomeres in a muscle fiber at resting length. B. Five sarcomeres lengthened by decreasing overlap of actin and myosin in each sarcomere. C. After 4 weeks of fixation at the increased length a sixth sarcomere has developed in the fiber bringing the overlap of actin and myosin back to normal at the new length.

tends to counteract the vasodilating effect of histamine.

Myofascial trigger points can be eliminated by injection of local anesthetic without vasoconstrictor into the site, by acupressure, and by vapocoolant spray-stretch followed by warming.[6] The muscle lengthens with these treatments and the patient is instructed to maintain stretching function. The acupressure procedure is painful at the time it is applied and the mechanism of action is not understood.

## Ischemic Muscle Pain

When skeletal muscle is forced to function during inadequate blood flow, a noxious, deep aching pain develops in the muscle.[8] This sensation is demonstrated by placing a blood pressure cuff around the upper arm and pumping the pressure to 180 mm Hg. When the subject squeezes to make a fist once per second for 1 minute or less, the arm begins to ache until it becomes unbearable. When the cuff pressure is released, the pain immediately vanishes. If the cuff is rapidly reinflated, the pain returns at a slightly lower intensity. These findings led to the conclusion that contracting muscle releases an algogenic substance into extracellular water that stimulates pain. This substance has not been definitely identified, but such agents as histamine, acetylcholine, phosphorylcreatine, serotonin, potassium, and bradykinin are possible chemical mediators of the pain.

## Electromyographic Recordings

Action potentials that pass along the sarcolemma of activated muscles may be recorded as the EMG potential. EMG recordings have been interpreted as indicators of muscle contraction via neuromuscular activation at the motor end-plate. Mandibular muscles demonstrate standard patterns of activity in healthy subjects during vertical and horizontal movement of the mandible.[9,10] The masseter and temporalis muscles usually act as "on-off" muscles (Fig. 7–3). These muscles produce power or crushing force when the teeth are clenched in intercuspal position (centric occlusion) or when a hard bolus of

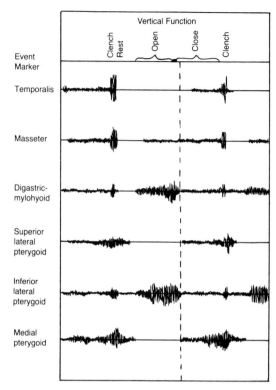

**Fig. 7–3.** Simultaneous EMG recording from the right mandibular muscles during a clench–rest–open–close–clench cycle. Note that the masseter and temporalis are active only when the teeth are in contact (or biting against a hard bolus of food). The medial pterygoid serves as a lateral positioner as well as an elevator and shows a graded response rather than on-off type of activity. The lateral pterygoid inferior head shows activity during opening while the superior head shows activity during closing.

food is interposed between the teeth. When the mouth is open, the masseter and temporalis show minimal activity.

The medial pterygoid, on the other hand, shows a graded response or gradual build up and drop off during opening and closing, respectively. The medial pterygoid is directed upward and medially from its insertion on the medial side of the mandibular angle. Therefore, it has a horizontal or lateral component to its function. Because it serves as a lateral positioner of the mandible, the medial pterygoid does not show an on-off activity like the more vertically positioned masseter and temporalis muscles. It continues to function in mouth-open positions to control lateral positions of the mandible, assisted by the lateral pterygoid muscle (Fig. 7–4).

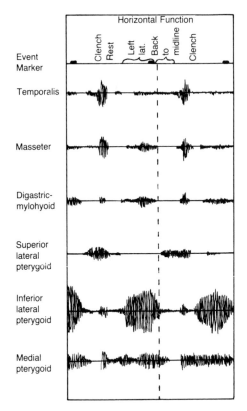

*Fig. 7–4.* Simultaneous EMG from the right mandibular muscles during a clench–rest–move to left lateral–back to midline–clench cycle. Note that the inferior head of the right lateral pterygoid is the major muscle moving the mandible contralaterally and the superior head functions reciprocally in horizontal movement, just as it does in vertical movement.

The lateral pterygoid muscle consists of a superior and an inferior head (Fig. 7–5). The superior head (sphenomeniscus muscle) is roughly one third the cross-sectional area of the inferior head. The inferior head originates from the lateral surface of the lateral pterygoid plate and inserts in the pterygoid fovea in the neck of the condylar process. The superior head originates from the orbital lip of the greater wing of the sphenoid bone and inserts into the anterior-medial margin of the disk and upper pterygoid fovea. The proportion of fibers that insert into the disk and into the condylar neck is variable. The typical cadaver dissection shows approximately 15% of the fibers attaching into the disk and 85% attaching into the condylar neck at the pterygoid fovea.

Results of EMG studies indicate that, in most subjects, the inferior head contracts on opening and the superior head is electrically active during closing.[9] Therefore, the superior head is contracting while it lengthens as the condyle translates back up into the fossa. These functional characteristics applied to the lateral pterygoid muscle (Fig. 7–6) keep the disk positioned between the condyle and temporal bone to best stabilize the condyle on the eminence. It also serves to close-pack the condyle against the posterior incline of the eminence during mouth closure.

## Eccentric or Negative Work

Muscles that are in the active state while lengthening act almost like transducers and perform eccentric or negative work.[11] They use minimal amounts of energy, activate few motor units, and produce high tensions.[12] Examples of these factors are seen in the young lady closing a car door when a strong gust of wind blows the door open rapidly. The tension in her arm flexors builds so rapidly that the biceps can tear from its insertion on the radial tuberosity and forearm fascia. Also, a nonathlete can fatigue a trained athlete to exhaustion on stationary bicycles facing in opposite directions with the sprockets connected by a chain. The nonathlete peddles backwards, resisting the athlete who peddles forward. The thigh muscles of the athlete are contracting while shortening and those of the nonathlete are in the active state while lengthening. Joggers are fatigued jogging uphill and are injured while jogging downhill when the anterior thigh muscles are instantaneously tensed during lengthening.

When skeletal muscle is lengthened by contraction of its antagonist, it resists the elongation even before it is activated at its motor end-plate by virtue of the stiffness that has developed in it.[13] This stiffening phenomenon, when applied to the function of the superior head of the lateral pterygoid, also keeps the disk in a functional position during mouth opening and closing.

Because the superior-lateral pterygoid routinely contracts, or is in the active state while lengthening, it is capable of producing high tensions and is more susceptible to injury than the inferior head.

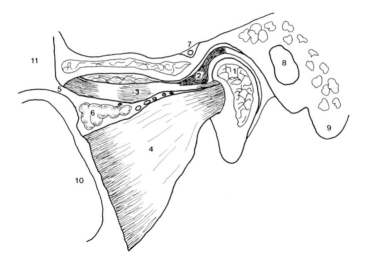

*Fig. 7–5.* Parasagittal section through the middle of the condyle directed 25 degrees medially through both heads of the lateral pterygoid muscle. 1. condyle; 2. TM joint disk; 3. superior head of lateral pterygoid muscle; 4. inferior head of lateral pterygoid muscle; 5. inferior orbital fissure; 6. fat; 7. middle meningeal artery overlaid by dura mater; 8. external auditory meatus; 9. mastoid process; 10. maxillary antrum; 11. orbit.

## Muscle Splinting

When a joint is opened in a laboratory animal and a noxious stimulus is applied to the exposed structures, the muscles that flex and extend the joint contract simultaneously, so the joint becomes fixed. These muscles, called splinting muscles, tend to serve as a protective reflex, limiting the movement of the painful joint. With prolonged splinting, the muscles may become the source of primary pain. Limited mouth opening may result from splinting of mandibular muscles. This phenomenon is seen often in association with de-

generative arthritis, when the patient can open only 20 to 25 mm. The stoic patient tells the clinician that the mouth will open wider but it will hurt!

## Muscle Contracture

Contracture of skeletal muscle is a painful condition that has a longer duration than a muscle cramp. Both of these conditions represent a powerful muscle contraction.[14]

Contracture and cramping differ in that the contracture is electrically silent and occurs under conditions in which energy metabolism

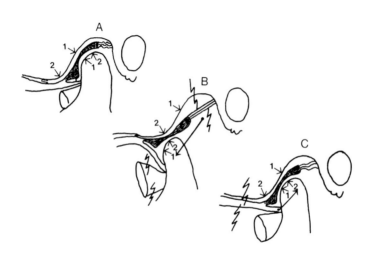

*Fig. 7–6.* Reciprocal activity of the two heads of the lateral pterygoid. A. the condyle is seated in the fossa with the teeth in occlusion. Arrows number 1 mark the narrowest joint space and thinnest zone in the disk. B. the condyle is translating as the mouth opens. The disk is carried forward by tight attachment to the condylar poles but rotates backward on the condyle. Now arrows number 2 mark the narrowest joint space and thinnest zone in the disk. Only the inferior head of the lateral pterygoid is active; the superior head is soft and elastic. C. the condyle-disk assembly is translating back into the fossa as the mouth is closing. The superior head of the lateral pterygoid becomes electrically active rotating the disk back onto the anterior-superior surface of the condyle and holding the condyle against the eminence as it translates up into the fossa. The inferior head is now relaxed.

is impaired, e.g., in McArdle's syndrome, which involves a deficiency of myophosphorylase.[15] These patients are not able to utilize muscle glycogen, so their muscles are filled with stored glycogen. They cannot run or walk long distances because of excruciating muscle cramps, and they cannot masticate hard or tough food without painful cramps in mandibular muscles. This condition is diagnosed by taking a blood sample from an arm vein for lactate assay. A second sample is taken from the vein after exercising the arm muscles with a blood pressure cuff around the arm to produce ischemic pain. Patients with McArdle's syndrome show no rise in postischemic exercise blood lactate levels, whereas normal subjects show an increase of 3 to 5 times normal levels. The plasma creatine kinase level in the patient with McArdle's syndrome is 5 to 100 times the normal value, depending on the presence or absence of painful contracture.

## Painful Myopathies

Muscle pain is rare in association with muscular dystrophies, myotonic disorders, and most forms of congenital myopathy.[16] Painful muscles are more likely in conditions that involve rapid destruction of muscle cells, the intramuscular blood vessels and connective tissue, or muscle energy metabolism, as described in association with McArdle's syndrome. The painful myopathies include inflammatory myopathies, polymyalgia rheumatica, acute alcoholic myopathy, drug-induced myopathies, and defects in muscle energy metabolism.

### Inflammatory Myopathies

These conditions include polymyositis and dermatomyositis, systemic lupus erythematosus, polyarteritis nodosa, Sjögren's syndrome, and viral polymyositis. In the acute inflammatory myopathies, myoglobin leaks into the plasma and filters into the renal tubules. Myoglobinemia and myoglobinuria, therefore, are usually associated with these diseases and may lead to renal impairment. Myoglobinuria, however, may occur in normal individuals after strenuous exercise. The muscle enzyme creatine kinase, which plays a significant role in muscle contraction, may also leak out into the plasma and indicate muscle damage.

### Polymyositis and Dermatomyositis

Myalgia is a prominent feature of both polymyositis and dermatomyositis, even though, in some cases, it may be absent. These diseases include inflammation of multiple muscles, predominantly those of the shoulders and pelvis.

Dysarthria and dysphagia are common in association with polymyositis, and painful mandibular muscles may prompt these patients to see the dentist for treatment of a suspected dental, TM joint or occlusal problem. If the disease is accompanied by skin inflammation, the diagnosis is dermatomyositis. These conditions affect young women twice as frequently as young men, but in older age groups, men predominantly are affected.[17]

Biopsies of muscle tissue from polymyositis and dermatomyositis patients reveal muscle cell necrosis, mononuclear cell infiltrate, variation in size of both fiber types, phagocytosis, and basophilic fibers. The creatine kinase level is elevated in 70% of patients and the erythrocyte sedimentation rate is elevated in 60% of cases.

These diseases are usually treated with high doses of anti-inflammatory steroids, even though this treatment has been questioned.[18] A high mortality rate is noted in association with polymyositis and dermatomyositis, but these diseases may disappear spontaneously after a few years. Polymyositis may occur in association with the connective tissue diseases such as systemic lupus erythematosus, rheumatoid arthritis, and Sjögren's syndrome.

### Systemic Lupus Erythematosus

Systemic lupus erythematosus (SLE) may result in inflamed and damaged connective tissue in any part of the body, and affects the joints and muscles of the stomatognathic system. Patients may have oral and throat ulcers, a butterfly-shaped rash or redness across the bridge of the nose, aseptic necrosis of the TM joint, and mandibular muscle tenderness.

Myalgia occurs in as many as 50% of cases, a symptom that may represent referred joint pain elicited by synovitis.[19] SLE most often affects young women and is a chronic illness with recurrent flare-ups that may be severe or, infrequently, fatal.

Medical management of SLE includes physical therapy, an adjustment of lifestyle, and medications that include nonsteroidal anti-inflammatory agents, steroids, antirheumatics, and immunosuppressives.

## Polyarteritis Nodosa

Polyarteritis nodosa is a disease of small and medium-sized arteries. Extensive involvement of skeletal muscle arteries may cause muscle pain, tenderness, and intermittent claudication.[20] The pain may be referred from joint synovitis or result from infarction of muscle because of arterial occlusion. Creatine kinase levels may be elevated. Treatment involves high doses of corticosteroids or immunosuppressive drugs.

## Sjögren's Syndrome

This disorder consists of the triad of dry eyes, dry mouth, and rheumatoid arthritis. Skeletal muscle is involved in 9% or less of cases, manifested by muscular weakness with focal interstitial myositis. The condition responds poorly to corticosteroids when myositis is involved.

## Viral Polymyositis

Commonly seen in childhood, viral polymyositis may affect adults. The pain and weakness is often confined to the calves and occurs after a systemic viral infection, usually the coxsackie or influenza virus. Recovery is usually complete within a few days or weeks.

## Polymyalgia Rheumatica

Polymyalgia rheumatica causes muscle pain and stiffness in the middle-aged and elderly patient.[21] The onset may be insidious or acute and the symptoms fluctuate in intensity. It responds dramatically to low doses of prednisone (10 to 20 mg/day). If it occurs with giant cell arteritis (temporal arteritis), the dosage is increased to 60 mg/day until the erythrocyte sedimentation rate (ESR) drops to the

normal range. In patients with polymyalgia rheumatica, the ESR is elevated and the creatine phosphokinase (CPK) level is normal.

## Acute Alcoholic Myopathy

This condition occurs in chronic alcoholics who enter into a heavy bout of drinking.[22] The muscles become painful, weak, and swollen. CPK levels are grossly elevated and myoglobinuria and renal failure may occur. The condition is usually reversible, but it can be fatal. After the immediate medical problem is under control, these patients should be referred to a psychiatrist or an alcoholic mutual support group, such as Alcoholics Anonymous, for help with their drinking problem.

## Drug-Induced Myopathies

Many drugs may produce painful myopathy that resembles that caused by alcohol.[23] Examples of such drugs are amphetamine, emetine, vincristine, cimetidine, heroin, amphotericin B, liquorice, and carbenoxalone.

Acute and subacute drug-induced myopathy presents with muscle pain and weakness that may progress to complete flaccid paralysis unless the drug is withdrawn. In severe cases, myoglobinuria and renal failure may occur. Certainly the most common drug-induced myopathy is related to steroid use, but it is invariably painless.

## Myopathy from Defects in Energy Metabolism

### McArdle's Syndrome

In patients with McArdle's syndrome, also discussed in the section concerning muscle contracture, myophosphorylase deficiency results in the lack of adenosine triphosphate (ATP), because the muscle cannot utilize glycogen. The energy for muscle contraction comes from the hydrolysis of ATP. Muscle relaxation involves the re-uptake of calcium ions into sarcoplasmic reticulum, which also requires the hydrolysis of ATP. In the absence of an energy supply, the muscles cramp painfully. In McArdle's syndrome, the muscles are filled with stored glycogen, resulting in a heavy muscled, mesomorphic appearance of the patient. These patients depend on oxidation of fatty acids and other nonglucose substrates for their energy requirements. This enzyme deficiency is recessively inherited. It usually begins in childhood, but it has been reported to begin later in life.

### Phosphofructokinase Deficiency

Deficiency of phosphofructokinase in muscle produces symptoms identical to those of McArdle's syndrome.[24] Both diseases have no cure, but patients can benefit from short-term therapy with diazepam (Valium) (5 mg/day) and low doses of the muscle relaxant baclofen (Lioresal) for a few weeks when a high level of muscle activity is required.

### Abnormal Muscle Mitochondria

A rare myopathy with exercise intolerance and muscle pain has been reported in patients with accumulation of abnormally shaped mitochondria within the muscle fibers.[25] Defects in muscle mitochondrial metabolism are believed to be responsible for these signs and symptoms. Thus, some painful myopathies are related to defects in muscle energy metabolism. If these patients are bruxists, they experience pain in the mandibular muscles and may seek help in a dental office.

## Volkman's Contracture

After a surgical procedure involving the temporal fossa, the probability is high that a contracture of the temporalis muscle will occur.[26] This condition may immobilize the mandible and should not be confused with a TM joint ankylosis. The condition may be the result of postincision scar contracture in the temporalis muscles, organization of a hematoma, and/or Volkman's contracture in the temporalis muscle.[27]

The Volkman's ischemic process follows interruption of the blood supply to the temporalis muscle, which may result from a surgical incision, the use of electrocautery, stripping of the temporalis muscle and periosteum from the temporal fossa, and sacrificing the main branches of the deep temporal arteries. The ischemia is progressive with time, but elongation and hypertrophy of nor-

mal remaining muscle may compensate for the contracture. The condition can be prevented by postoperative physical therapy, including active and passive mouth opening exercises.

## Fibromyalgia

A condition known as fibromyalgia, fibrositis syndrome, or nonarticular rheumatism is receiving a great deal of attention in the field of rheumatology.[28,29] It is considered to be the third most common disorder treated by the rheumatologist.[30] Patients with fibromyalgia demonstrate as many as 14 typical sites of deep tenderness on palpation (Fig. 7–7). Some sites are in muscle and others are in dense soft tissue. The painful trigger points include midpoint of the upper border of the trapezius, spinous processes of C4–C6, and the trapezius at the medial border of the scapula. The other tender points are below the

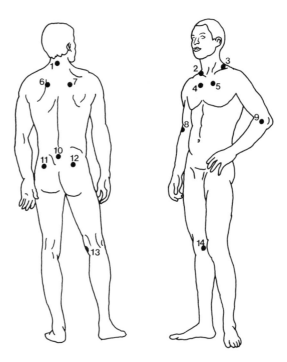

*Fig. 7–7.* Painful trigger points of fibromyalgia. 1. spinous processes of C4 to C6; 2. and 3. midpoints of upper border of trapezius muscles; 4. and 5. costochondral junctions of second ribs; 6. and 7. trapezius muscles at medial border of the scapulae; 8. and 9. brachioradialis muscles at the lateral epicondyles; 10. spinous process of L5; 11. and 12. gluteal aponeuroses; 13. and 14. fat pads medial to the knees.

head and neck and include the costochondral junction of the second ribs, brachioradialis muscle at the lateral epicondyle (tennis elbow), spinous process of L−5, gluteal aponeurosis, and the fat pads medial and just proximal to the knees. Most clinicians accept a minimum of 7 of these 14 points as pathognomonic of fibrositis syndrome.

Patients with fibromyalgia complain of sleep disturbance, stiffness, and fatigue on awakening, and usually are not aware of their classic deep tender sites. These patients have a normal ESR, CPK level, rheumatoid factor, antinuclear antibody factor, and thyroid stimulating hormone levels. Fibromyalgia may be caused and/or exaggerated by a disturbance of delta stage sleep. The patients show an alpha rhythm intrusion on their delta wave electroencephalogram during deep (delta) sleep. Fibromyalgia has been produced in healthy university students by keeping them awake for 48 hours, producing an abnormal alpha intrusion on their delta wave sleep. Interestingly, these patients show a normal REM (rapid eye movement) sleep pattern.

### Primary and Secondary Fibromyalgia

Primary fibromyalgia follows a triggering, stressful life situation, such as an auto accident, and anxiety evoking events that disturb sleep, such as insoluble domestic difficulties. Secondary fibromyalgia occurs in patients who have diseases or conditions that disturb normal sleep for about 30 days. These diseases and conditions include female hormone imbalance, facial pain, rheumatoid arthritis, osteoarthritis (degenerative arthritis), and neck-back pain syndrome.[31,32] Therefore, to diagnose primary fibromyalgia, the absence of joint signs and symptoms of disease must be determined.

Secondary fibromyalgia is more common than primary fibromyalgia. The authors have identified this syndrome in a high percentage of facial pain patients in whom the pain prevents normal sleep.

### Treatment

Chlorpromazine (Thorazine) facilitates slow wave (delta) sleep, and it has been used to treat fibromyalgia. In a double-blind, 9-week trial of amitriptyline and placebo in 70 fibromyalgia syndrome patients, 50 mg amitriptyline significantly reduced morning stiffness, improved sleep pattern, and pain analog scores over the baseline scores.[33] The fibrositic point tenderness did not improve significantly. Physical fitness also mitigates the symptoms. A patient who has not been physically active and is in poor physical condition should be referred to a clinician who can provide the proper exercise program.

The authors have successfully treated fibromyalgia patients by prescribing proper nutrition with nutrient supplementation if indicated (see Chapter 6); 12 minutes per day of aerobic exercise; and doxepin (Sinequan; 10 to 25 mg capsule) at bedtime or amitriptyline (Elavil; 25–50 mg tablet) at bedtime, unless contraindicated.

## Local Anesthetic-Induced Myopathy

Results of studies show that local anesthetics selectively and reversibly damage skeletal muscle.[34,35] The response is directly proportional to the potency of the anesthetic. Procaine is the least toxic anesthetic. Epinephrine, in concentrations greater than 1:200,000, also produces muscle necrosis. When epinephrine and anesthetic are administered together, the damage exceeds a simple additive effect. Repeated paramuscular injections of local anesthetic-vasoconstrictor combinations can lead to permanent microscarring of the muscles.[36] Destruction of muscle fibers begins within 15 minutes of the injection and is complete in 48 hours. The patient's creatine kinase level is elevated, and a serum muscle enzyme assay done at this time will not be valid.[37] The necrosis is typically completely restored with new tissue in 3 to 4 weeks. Lidocaine preferentially destroys white fibers and bupivacaine is more toxic to red fibers.[38] Blood vessels in the injected muscles are not affected and this factor facilitates regeneration.

The injection of a low potency anesthetic without vasoconstrictor is often used clinically to treat muscle trigger points. Clinical experience shows that the firm nodule in the muscle immediately softens and the pain is relieved.

The patient feels a stinging-like sensation when contracting the muscle for several days. The use of procaine or mepivacaine without vasoconstrictor is preferred, and the clinician should instruct the patient to avoid forceful biting for 2 weeks.

In a recent double-blind comparison of mepivacaine injection versus physiologic saline injection for myofascial pain, equal volumes of mepivacaine and saline were injected, and improvement during treatment was reported in 68% of saline-injected patients and 74% of mepivacaine-treated patients.[39] The authors postulate that pain relief by muscle injection is not related to local anesthesia but to reflex muscle relaxation stimulated by the irritant effect of the injection.

## Drug Side Effects

Drug side effects resulting in mandibular muscle spasm, dyskinesia, and pain may be a difficult and serious problem.

### Phenothiazines and Haloperidol

The phenothiazines, particularly prochlorperazine (Compazine), may produce a unilateral, preauricular pain that mimics myofascial pain dysfunction.[40–42] This pain can occur with low oral doses. Prochlorperazine injection may produce massive, bilateral spasms of mandibular depressor muscles so that the lateral pterygoid muscles subluxate the condyles and tear the retrodiskal connective tissues, resulting in a TM disk derangement

Haloperidol (Haldol) may produce acute dystonic reactions when given at low doses.[43] Some evidence exists that higher doses of phenothiazines and haloperidol are not as likely to produce extrapyramidal reactions.

### Tardive Dyskinesia

This condition is seen in elderly patients who discontinue phenothiazine medication after prolonged use. It appears that the phenothiazines block dopamine receptors in the striatum, effectively denervating the striatal cells.[44] When the medication is discontinued,

a "denervation hypersensitivity" occurs; endogenous dopamine function is relatively excessive and tardive dyskinesia ensues.

The fact that some patients develop mandibular dyskinesia while receiving neuroleptic agents is explained by the concept of two nerve cell populations in the striatum: small, dopamine-facilitated neurons and large, dopamine-inhibited neurons.[44,45] Tardive dyskinesia is a hyperactive response of the dopamine-facilitated neurons to dopamine when the neuroleptic is discontinued, whereas drug-induced dyskinesia (pseudoparkinsonism) is caused by the lack of response of the dopamine-inhibited receptors to dopamine. Dyskinesia affects the tongue and mandibular muscles early and does not respond to antiparkinsonian medication such as trihexyphenidyl (Artane) and diphenhydramine (Benadryl). The usual treatment for tardive dyskinesia involves the administration of dopamine receptor site blockers, such as chlorpromazine (Thorazine) or haloperidol (Haldol).[46] These patients should be referred to a physician who is familiar with these treatment procedures. Anticholinergic medication is contraindicated in these patients.

## Meige's Disease

Idiopathic orofacial dystonia (Meige's disease) is similar to tardive dyskinesia.[47] The symmetric dystonic contractions of the orofacial muscles produce bizarre facial contortions. They consist of repetitive, uncontrolled, unintentional movements of the tongue, orbital, oral, buccal, and mandibular muscles. Mouthing movements and slow or rapid, lateral and protruded movements of the tongue also occur. When the mouth is open, the tongue may appear to writhe. Repetitive sucking and smacking movements of the lips and repetitive eye blinking (blepharospasm) are common.

This disease affects adults 60 years of age and older, with a high incidence of mental depression. It is rarely familial. These patients can be differentiated from neuroleptic drug dyskinesia patients by the absence of a history of neuroleptic drug use. Physostigmine aggravates Meige's disease and levodopa has no effect. Meige's disease, therefore, is likely a result of striatal dopaminergic preponderance. This rare disease is treated with apomorphine, chlorpromazine (Thorazine), or haloperidol (Haldol), which attenuate striatal dopaminergic transmission.

## Muscle Fiber Types

A typical skeletal muscle contains two types of extrafusal muscle fibers. Type I are the red, slow-twitch fibers, which are rich in oxidative enzymes. Type II are the white, fast-twitch fibers, which are rich in the enzyme myophosphorylase. These fiber types are differentiated by staining frozen sections for ATPase preincubated at pH 9.4 or pH 4.3. Type I fibers stain after incubation at acid pH, and type II fibers stain after incubation at alkaline pH. These fiber types are typically intermingled in a muscle. An intermediate type II fiber has been reported in human mandibular muscles as described below.

When a muscle is partially denervated, the denervated fibers evoke a response from neighboring healthy nerve fibers that send out fine filaments to reinnervate them, the process of terminal sprouting. Because all the denervated muscle fibers in the vicinity of a surviving nerve are reinnervated by one nerve, they all become one metabolic type. Such a denervated muscle shows grouping of fiber types rather than intermingling of types in histochemically stained sections.[48]

Another abnormality seen in histochemical stains of muscle recovering from polyneuritis is target fibers. Cross sections of these fibers show a central zone devoid of enzyme activity and an intermediate zone of intense enzyme activity. These zones coincide with the presence of increased numbers of mitochondria in the intermediate zone.

Histochemical staining for ATPase in human masseter and temporalis muscles has demonstrated a third or intermediate type of muscle fiber when compared to only types I and II in the biceps brachii of the same subject.[49,50] The significance of this difference in mandibular muscles is not known. In one histochemical study of temporalis muscle in denture wearers and subjects with a natural dentition, comparison revealed no difference in the size of the fiber types.[51] The type II fibers

in subjects who rated their dentures as deficient were smaller than those in subjects who rated their dentures satisfactory. The authors postulated that this difference was attributed to altered functional demands on the muscle.

## Myasthenia Gravis

The progressive muscle weakness of myasthenia gravis is believed to result from the reduction in the number of acetylcholine receptors at the motor end-plate. Damage to the acetylcholine receptor may result from an autoimmune process. The myasthenia gravis patient may develop a severe anterior opened bite, with little or no pain.[52] In a complete denture patient, the dentist must guard against overextending the impression into flaccid muscle, which could result in a denture base that occludes salivary ducts.[53] Results of muscle biopsies in myasthenia gravis patients are not pathognomonic, but they may show groups of lymphocytes and plasma cells between muscle fibers and elongation of the end-plate.

## Chronic Steroid Therapy

Atrophy of type II fibers occurs in long-term treatment with the fluorinated steroids. In this myopathy there is absence of fiber necrosis, phagocytosis, cellular infiltration, or collagen infiltration.[48]

## Hormonal Factors in Myopathy

Hypothyroidism involves musculoskeletal stiffness that is worsened by cold weather and can be confused with primary fibromyalgia.[54] These patients also suffer from headache, constipation, and numbness. Myopathy can be detected in almost all hypothyroid patients. It is manifested by weakness, cramps, aching, and tender muscles. Acid maltase deficiency has been reported in hypothyroid muscle, and thyroid-deficient patients may require treatment for months before the response is significant.

Menopausal and amenorrheic women frequently experience chronic muscle stiffness, pain, spasm, and trigger points in mandibular muscles that respond to estrogen therapy, often taking the form of secondary fibromyalgia.

## Trismus

Painful or painless limited opening of the mouth may be caused by ankylosis of the TM joint, mechanical blockage of mandibular movement by synovial chondromatosis, meniscus abnormalities, tumors, fractures, elongate coronoid process, and scars, or by a lack of relaxation of mandibular elevator muscles. Factors that cause trismus due to a lack of muscle relaxation include radiation therapy,[55] injection of local anesthetic into the masticator space,[56] submandibular salivary duct calculi,[57] masticator space infection,[58] hysteria,[59] cancrum oris,[60] tetanus,[61] and idiopathic (postdental treatment) etiology.

### Radiation Therapy

When radiation therapy is administered through the mandibular muscles, they may slowly lose their ability to relax and typically become mildly to moderately painful. Patients usually respond to low-dose therapy with diazepam (Valium) (2 mg b.i.d.), daily stretching exercises, and moist heat therapy.

### Local Anesthetic Trismus

The trismus that follows injection of local anesthetic usually occurs with multiple injections and probably results from the destruction of muscle fibers by the local anesthetic and vasoconstrictor as described previously. The condition occurs within a few hours of the injection and is usually painful. The possibility of infection must be considered in this patient. In the absence of infection, the condition should be treated with analgesics, moist heat, muscle relaxants, and vigorous physical therapy.

### Submandibular Duct Blockage

Blockage of the submandibular salivary duct (Wharton's duct) often produces pain in the submaxillary triangle and limited opening of the mouth. Treatment involves surgical removal of the calculus and supportive therapy.

The trismus rapidly disappears after removal of the stone and control of any infection (Fig. 7–8).

### Masticator Space Infection

Such infection usually results in a painful trismus. It is typically caused by sinus tract formation from an infected molar. Treatment includes antibiotic medication, incision of the affected space with drainage, and extraction or endodontic treatment of the offending tooth (Fig. 7–9).

### Hysterical Trismus

Hysterical trismus is usually difficult to diagnose. The absence of all known physical causes and indications of emotional factors usually provide the diagnosis and indication for referral to a psychiatrist. Response to psychiatric therapy confirms the diagnosis.

### Cancrum Oris

In cases of noma or cancrum oris, massive tissue necrosis is accompanied by trismus and scarring of the elevator muscles. Physical therapy should accompany the antibiotic therapy, debridement, supportive care, and correction of malnutrition.

### Tetanus

Two hundred cases of tetanus occur per year in the United States. The incidence is highest in nonwhites of the southeastern states. The mortality rate is 45%. *Clostridium tetani* may enter the tissues through a trivial wound and release a toxin that acts at inhibitory synapses blocking spinal inhibition. The incubation period is usually 14 days, but it ranges from 2 to 56 days. Of special interest to dentists is the fact that a cranial nerve palsy may accompany the trismus in cephalic tetanus. It is typically a seventh nerve palsy. In this condition, no cervical or submandibular lymphadenopathy is evident. The patient should be referred immediately for medical treatment.

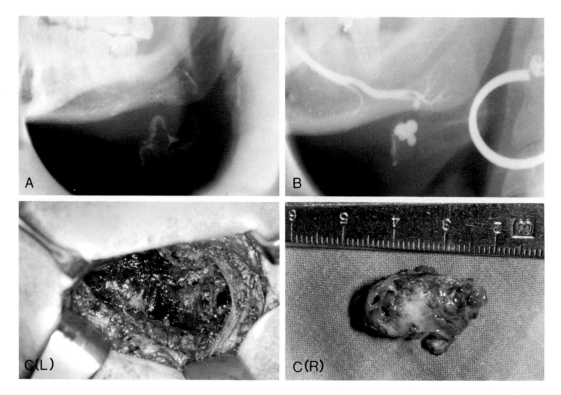

*Fig. 7–8.* A. Radiograph of a group of salivary stones in the submandibular gland. The patient suffered intermittent pain in the digastric triangle and muscle trismus for several years. B. Sialogram of the submandibular gland shows incomplete filling due to stone and sialodochitis with fibrosis. C, left. View of operative site of submandibular gland excision; C, right. Excised submandibular gland.

## Idiopathic Mandibular Muscle Trismus

This type of trismus typically occurs 3 to 5 days after a long dental appointment in heavy, short-muscled (mesomorphic) patients. It is usually painless but is incapacitating, because the maximum opening may be from 0 to only a few millimeters. Patients develop the condition after a dental procedure involving posterior teeth for which the mouth must be opened maximally. The muscles function normally for the first 3 to 5 days. This condition is not understood, but it seems to be a contracture of motor units in the elevator muscles.

Idiopathic mandibular muscle trismus can be treated acutely or chronically. The acute method involves intravenous sedation and analgesia, then slowly forcing the mouth open. The opening may be accompanied by cracking or tearing sounds, but the patient has little discomfort after the procedure. The chronic method involves mouth opening exercises using tongue blades or the patient's thumb and fingers in a lever action to open the mouth 3 minutes per session, three sessions per day. In some patients, the opening increases slowly at first and then rapidly opens; others may not begin opening for 2 or 3 weeks. Ultrasound therapy increases the flexibility of connective tissues and is an effective adjunct to the treatment of trismus.

## Myotonic Syndromes

Myotonia is the delayed relaxation of skeletal muscle after a voluntary contraction. It comprises diseases with different etiologies varying from a congenital condition to a reaction to several classes of drugs and chemicals.[62]

Patients complain of painless muscular stiffness on initiation of movement that slowly resolves within 5 to 15 seconds. They may have difficulty relaxing the grip when shaking hands, eyes may become momentarily "stuck" in one position, and they may

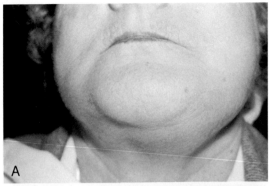

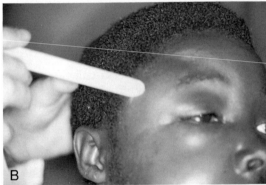

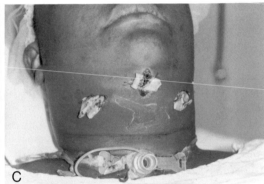

*Fig. 7–9.* A. Woman with mandibular third molar pericoronitis extending into the masseter muscle space. B. Young boy with a maxillary second molar periapical abscess extending into the temporalis muscle space. C. Ludwig's angina involving multiple spaces. Incision, drainage, and antibiotic measures are often indicated to preserve life.

have difficulty with speaking and swallowing. Repeated use of the muscles usually leads to increased mobility, but stiffness returns when the muscle is rested. Forceful contractions may cause the muscles to lock in the contracted state briefly. The condition is aggravated by fasting, cooling, menstruation, potassium ingestion, and sudden emotional shock. The muscles of the face and any muscle of the body may be affected. The patient usually has a "Herculean" muscle development, probably because of repeated, involuntary isometric exercise. The site of pathology in myotonia is in the sarcolemma.[63]

Congenital myotonia begins in childhood with onset of walking, but it is not progressive.[64] The male to female incidence is 3 to 1, life expectancy is not shortened, and the primary defect is in muscle membrane chloride conductance.

Myotonic dystrophy affects a variety of tissue, not just muscle, and is a progressive disease affecting facial, oropharyngeal, truncal, and limb musculature.[65] Death usually occurs in the fifth or sixth decade from cardiac arrhythmia, respiratory failure, or intercurrent infection. It is difficult to distinguish from congenital myotonia in the early stages.

The plant herbicide 2,4-D produces myotonia in humans after accidental ingestion.[66] The drug 20,25-diazocholesterol (20-25-D) is used to lower cholesterol levels in hypercholesteremic patients.[67] Some of these patients develop a myotonic syndrome that subsides several weeks after the drug is discontinued.

When patients with myotonia are examined by concentric needle EMG, they show insertional activity and prolonged, repetitive discharges of motor units that wax and wane in frequency and amplitude. This type of activity is also seen with needle movement, muscle percussion, or voluntary contraction, and leads to the diagnosis of myotonia. The disease usually responds well to diphenylhydantoin (Dilantin) therapy.

## Masseter Hypertrophy

Hypertrophy of the masseters may occur bilaterally or unilaterally for no apparent reason (Fig. 7–10). It may be accompanied by hypertrophy of the parotid gland, in which case it is the parotid-masseter hypertrophy-

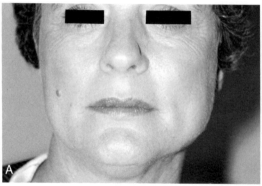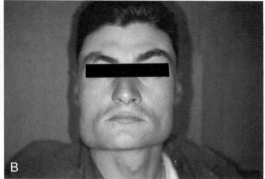

*Fig. 7–10.* A. Woman with unilateral masseter hypertrophy. The hypertrophy regressed following occlusal therapy. B. Man with bilateral masseter hypertrophy that did not respond to nonsurgical modalities. The patient's left side has been corrected by muscle and mandibular reduction.

traumatic occlusion syndrome.[68] These patients have a malocclusion that leads to noxious clenching and/or bruxing. This isometric exercise hypertrophies the masseters so they bulge outward on clenching, which causes tensing of the upper aponeurosis against the parotideomasseteric fascia, occluding the parotid duct. The duct obstruction leads to sialodochitis and swelling of the parotid gland. Occlusal therapy relieved the signs and symptoms of this syndrome in 15 patients.[68]

When masseter hypertrophy occurs without parotid involvement, patients report a slow, progressive, painless enlargement, with the enlarged masseter seeming larger on some days than on others. Patients may or may not have abrasive facets on the teeth, and most are young (under 25 years of age). Some patients are aware of chewing on one side habitually when the masseter hypertrophy is unilateral. Radiographs usually reveal flaring of the angle of the mandible and a bone spur at the angle.

The condition is not esthetic and most patients consult their dentist, oral and maxillofacial surgeon, or plastic surgeon regarding treatment. These patients should be evaluated for bruxism, clenching, unilateral mastication, or a habit of contracting the masseters as the mouth is opening (eccentric work). Most patients respond to occlusal therapy with masseter atrophy in a matter of a few weeks. The therapy may take the form of a muscle relaxation splint and occlusal adjustment when a malocclusion has been identified. Older patients develop a flabby skin appearance in the lower, preauricular area of the face when the muscles atrophy. When the occlusal therapy for bruxism and/or behavioral therapy with a repeat timer to prevent diurnal clenching does not reduce the hypertrophy within 4 weeks, surgical intervention is considered when the problem is incapacitating. Several procedures have been devised for removing a wedge of masseter muscle to correct this condition.[69]

## Masseter Tenomyositis

The upper anterior quadrant of the superficial masseter is an aponeurosis. It attaches to the zygoma and zygomatic arch. When this tendon becomes torn by rapidly applied tension, each subsequent masseter contraction reopens the tear and interrupts the healing process. This inflamed scar may persist for months and prompt a patient to consult a clinician for relief.[70] The history usually includes sudden pain from a minor trauma or biting down. The condition can be diagnosed by palpation during which the clinician identifies tenderness at the anterior margin of the masseter beneath the anterior zygomatic arch and absence of tenderness at the lower one half of the masseter. A provocation test elicits pain in the anterior masseter when the patient attempts to close as the clinician holds the mouth open with two fingers and supports the patient's head at the forehead (Fig. 7–11).

Treatment includes a soft or liquid diet, nonsteroidal anti-inflammatory medication, heat and cold application, and nutritional

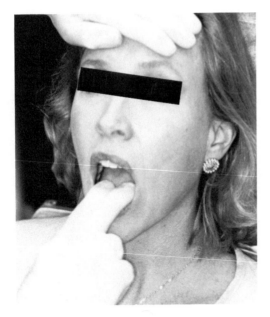

***Fig. 7–11.*** Test for masseter tenomyositis involves provocation of pain by holding the patient's head back against the head rest while pushing downward on the anterior mandible. Severe pain will be elicited if the condition exists.

counseling, if the history indicates less than optimal nutritional status for rapid healing. A 20-mg injection of methylprednisolone (DepoMedrol) into the area of tenderness may bring rapid relief.

## Myositis Ossificans

This rare condition of ossification in skeletal muscles usually involves the muscles of the arms and legs. The myositis ossificans patient may be displayed as the stone man at the circus side shows. Myositis ossificans usually begins in childhood and is a progressive disease.

A localized type of the disorder is believed to develop in areas of muscle injury. In a few cases, myositis ossificans was noted in the masseter muscle.[71] The process begins as a swelling that indurates and forms bony lumps. The overlying skin becomes red and rough and may become ulcerated. Articular surfaces in joints are usually not involved.

No treatment for the progressive type of myositis ossificans is known, but the localized type is treated surgically. The bony masses that are removed are surrounded by a periosteum-like tissue, so muscle cells are not attached directly to bone. To prevent recurrence, all surgical dead space must be eliminated. Because a postoperative hematoma is likely to organize and re-ossify, pressure dressings are applied. Rendering a diagnosis of myositis ossificans depends on biopsy findings, because sclerosing osteosarcoma and fibrous dysplasia may present physical and radiographic signs that are indistinguishable from those of myositis ossificans.

## Muscle Examination

To examine the head and neck muscles in a facial pain patient, the clinician should proceed in a systematic manner, with inspection for abnormal masses and atrophies. The examination then involves palpation of the muscles, bilaterally, and asking the patient if the two sides feel the same. This technique saves time, because the patient can easily compare the two sensations and answer yer or no. If the patient replies "No" (the two sides do not feel the same), the clinician asks, "How are they different?" Often the patient describes a soreness on one side. The clinician may note the sore muscle also feels more firm than the muscle on the opposite side.

### Muscle Pain Scale

A scale of zero to 3 is used to record the evaluation of muscular pain elicited from palpation of muscles and ligaments, with zero being no pain, 1 being mild pain, 2 being moderate pain, and 3 being maximum pain. The examiner should watch the patient's eyes as the muscles are palpated. If the patient squints the eyes and the pupils dilate, level 2 pain is indicated. If the patient rapidly pulls the face away from the palpating fingers, the jump sign, the pain is level 3.

### Masseter Muscles

To be systematic and efficient, the doctor squeezes the superficial masseter muscles from the anterior to the posterior margins in

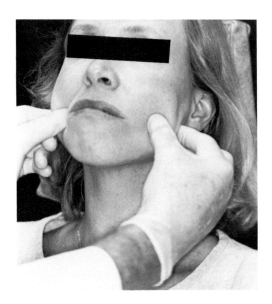

*Fig. 7–12.* Palpating the superficial masseter muscle.

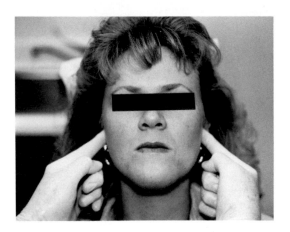

*Fig. 7–13.* Palpating the masseteric aponeurosis and deep masseter fibers.

the lower third of the muscle, asking the patient to compare the two sides (Fig. 7–12). Next, the index fingers are pressed against the face overlying the base of the coronoid processes just beneath the zygomatic arches, while asking the patient to report any difference (Fig. 7–13). These palpations test for tenderness of the superficial masseteric aponeurosis and the deep masseter muscle fibers.

If either of these locations is tender, the entire masseter is palpated progressively, be-

ginning just beneath the zygomatic arch by pressing each finger, in sequence, against the muscle in a rolling motion (Fig. 7–14). A trigger point in the muscle will roll back and forth between two palpating fingers. The fingers are lowered approximately 8 mm and are pressed again, in sequence, to locate any firm muscles or trigger points lower in the muscle. The entire masseter muscle can be rapidly scanned in four or five sequences of palpation. Trigger points are treated by vapocool-

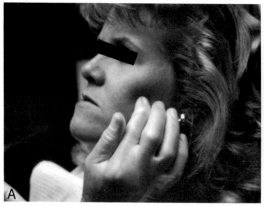
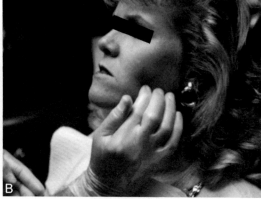

*Fig. 7–14.* A. Palpating across the upper masseter muscle in a rolling motion to detect a firm trigger point that will deflect under a palpating finger. This progessive palpation is repeated, lowering about 8 mm inferiorly with each scan, until the entire muscle is palpated. B. Fourth scan across the masseter muscle.

ant spray-stretch, injection with local anesthetic without constrictor, or transcutaneous nerve stimulation therapy.

## Temporalis Muscles

The index fingers are next pressed against the lateral rim of the orbit at the lateral canthus of the eye and rotated back into the anterior margin of the temporalis muscle. The patient is asked to report any difference between the two sides (Fig. 7–15). The index fingers are then pressed into the horizontal fibers of the temporalis muscles just above and behind the pinna of the ear. Again, the patient should report any differences noted (Fig. 7–16). If either or both of these two points on the temporalis muscle are tender, the clinician brings the fingers forward across the muscle every 8 mm to test for trigger points.

## Pterion Pain

If the palpating finger presses on pterion beneath the upper anterior temporalis muscle, the patient will report pain (Fig. 7–17). At pterion, four corners of bone meet: frontal, parietal, tip of greater wing of sphenoid, and temporal squama. The middle meningeal artery runs just beneath pterion. In almost all individuals, these four bones move enough

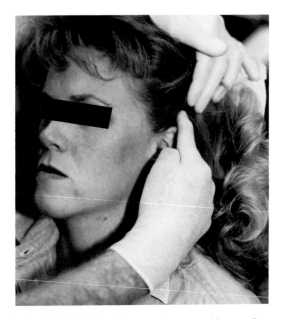

*Fig. 7–16.* Palpating the posterior temporalis muscle.

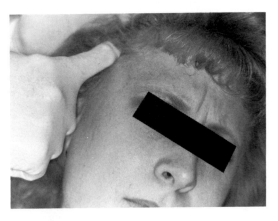

*Fig. 7–17.* Four corners of bone meet at pterion. Almost all patients report pain with palpation of the temporalis muscle over this point.

to stimulate free nerve endings in the dura along the middle meningeal artery, with a normal painful response.

## Sternocleidomastoid Muscles

The insertion of the sternocleidomastoid (SCM) muscles are palpated by squeezing just beneath the mastoid processes, the patient reporting any difference in sensation (Fig. 7–18). If either SCM is tender, the muscle is palpated by squeezing in the middle of the muscle (Fig. 7–19). Patients with tender SCM muscles often complain of vertigo. The ves-

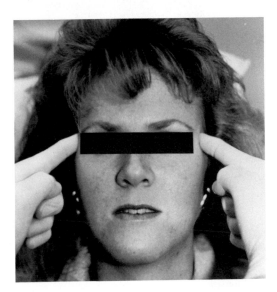

*Fig. 7–15.* Palpating the anterior temporalis muscle.

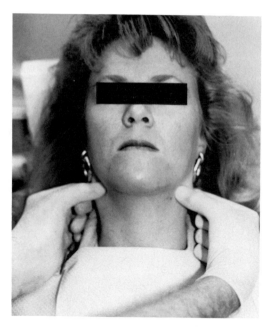

*Fig. 7–18.* Palpating the insertion of the sternocleidomastoid muscles beneath the mastoid processes.

tibular system and proprioceptive system of the SCM muscles interact in the righting reflex, which enables mammals to upright themselves when falling through space so as to land on their feet. Apparently, when the SCM muscles are in spasm, the vestibular system, which interacts physiologically, also malfunctions producing vertigo.

### Splenius Capitis Muscles

The index fingers are pressed against the posterior mastoid processes until they slide downward into a concavity on each side (Fig. 7–20). The fingers are located over the splenius capitis and are pressed inward to test for tenderness. The patient again reports any difference in pain.

### Trapezius Muscles

The index fingers are moved more posteriorly around a margin of muscle so they are about 1½ inches apart (Fig. 7–21); at this position, they are located over the insertion of the trapezius. The fingers are pressed into the

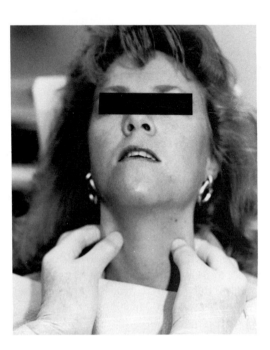

*Fig. 7–19.* Palpating the middle sternocleidomastoid muscle.

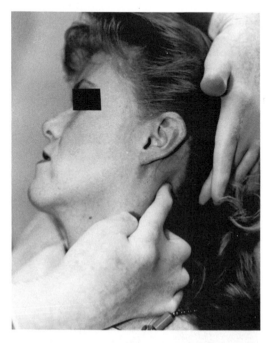

*Fig. 7–20.* Palpating the splenius capitis muscle in the concavity just behind and below the mastoid process. This point is usually painful in post-whiplash patients.

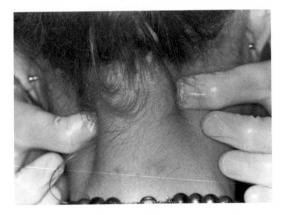

*Fig. 7–21.* Palpating the insertions of the trapezius muscles.

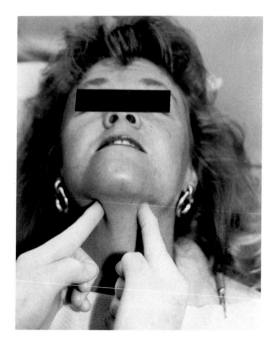

*Fig. 7–23.* Palpating the anterior bellies of the digastric and mylohyoid muscles.

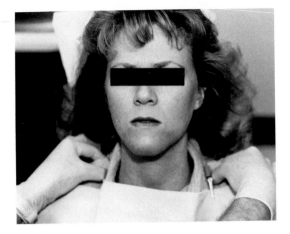

*Fig. 7–22.* Palpating the anterior margins of the trapezius muscles.

muscle and the patient reports the comparison of sensation.

After grasping the anterior margins of the trapezius muscles in the lateral base of the neck, light squeezing pressure is applied (Fig. 7–22). The patient reports any difference in sensation.

## Mylohyoid and Anterior Belly of the Digastric Muscles

After asking the patient to protrude the mandible and elevate the chin by looking up to the ceiling, the clinician presses the index fingers into the floor of the mouth halfway between the midline and the inferior border of the mandible on each side (Fig. 7–23). The patient reports any difference in sensation

from anterior bellies of the digastric and mylohyoid muscles.

## Posterior Belly of the Digastric Muscles

The index fingers are placed on the angles of the mandible with the patient still looking upward, and the fingers are rolled under the angle and pushed upward and backward to palpate the posterior belly of the digastric muscle (Fig. 7–24). This palpation also presses on several branches of the carotid artery; therefore, pain at this location may be vascular rather than muscular in origin.

## Medial Pterygoid Muscles

The medial pterygoid muscles are examined next, by palpating the painless side first. The patient is asked to note the sensation and to then compare it to the sensation elicited on the painful side, which is immediately palpated.

The right medial pterygoid is palpated by placing the right index finger on the patient's right maxillary tuberosity, and asking the patient to note the sensation as the finger is moved posteriorly off the tuberosity into the

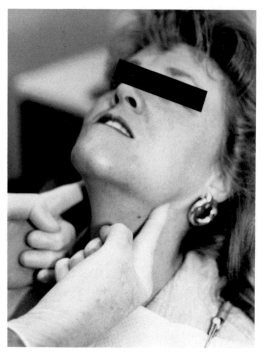

**Fig. 7–24.** Palpating the posterior belly of the digastric muscles and several branches of the external carotid arteries.

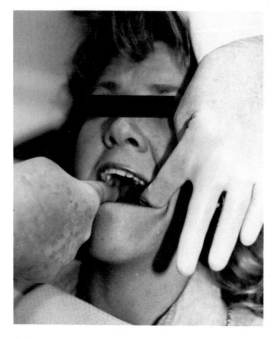

**Fig. 7–25.** Palpating the patient's right medial pterygoid muscle. The left corner of the mouth is being retracted to better visualize the palpating finger.

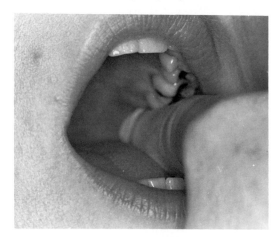

**Fig. 7–26.** Palpating the left medial pterygoid muscle.

anterior margin of the medial pterygoid muscle (Fig. 7–25).

Care is taken to avoid pressing on the hamulus as the finger is moved posteriorly from the tuberosity, because this bony spine is painful. If the hamulus is palpated and the patient flinches, the clinician should go back to the hamulus and press gently on it, telling the patient, "Not this point, but the sensation back here in this sling," as the finger slides back on the medial pterygoid muscle. If the patient does not gag, the clinician can move the finger up and down to palpate more of the muscle and the styloid process if it is elongated.

The left medial pterygoid is palpated with the clinician's left index finger starting with the maxillary tuberosity and sliding back onto the muscle as described for the right side (Fig. 7–26). The medial pterygoids are often tender on the side opposite the direction of the slide from retruded contact to intercuspal position in patients receiving prochlorperazine (Compazine),[40] in patients with degenerative arthritis in the ipsilateral TM joint,[72] and in pa-

tients with a masticator space infection on the ipsilateral side.

### Lateral Pterygoid Muscles

Because part of the medial pterygoid is lateral to the lateral pterygoid muscle at its origin on the lower lateral pterygoid plate, the medial pterygoid covers the lateral pterygoid in all areas that are palpable.[73]

The lateral pterygoid is not accessible to

palpation alone since the medial pterygoid intervenes at all palpation locations. A provocation test instead of palpation is used to evaluate the lateral pterygoid by placing the thumb on the mandibular symphysis and instructing the patient to protrude against the thumb pressure.[74] The lateral pterygoid inferior bellies are tensed to protrude and, if they are in spasm, pain will be elicited in the deep preauricular area (Fig. 7–27).

The lateral pterygoid is usually painful along with the ipsilateral medial pterygoid, because they function in harmony to position the mandible in the horizontal plane. In patients with pain associated with malocclusion, the pterygoids are usually tender to palpation when the acquired bite requires excessive contraction of the pterygoids to position the mandible in the eccentric registration.

## Provoked Myalgias

Painful pterygoids are found in patients with degenerative arthritic involvement of the ipsilateral TM joint, patients receiving prochlorperazine therapy, individuals with ipsilateral masticator space infection, as well as persons in whom traumatic occlusion requires excessive function of the pterygoids.

If the anterior and posterior digastric bellies as well as the posterior temporalis are painful, the upper anterior teeth are examined for overcontoured and abraded lingual surfaces of full crowns. The lower anterior incisal edges also are often abraded to fit the upper lingual surfaces precisely. An example of a muscular disability originating in the dental arch is a patient who reports that artificial crowns on maxillary anterior teeth have never been comfortable. In addition, the patient has a history of temporal and occipital headaches. This condition developed because the patient learned to hold the mandible in retrusion during final closure to avoid striking the overcontoured lingual surface of the upper teeth. The digastric and posterior temporalis muscles contracting simultaneously retrude the mandible, so they become tender to palpation with excessive function. If the patient is unable to avoid occluding against the upper anterior teeth, the incisors may tip labially, with visible diastemata as the teeth flair anteriorly in the dental arch.

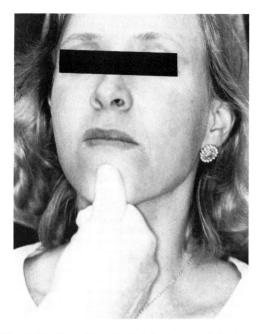

*Fig. 7–27.* Provoking the inferior heads of the lateral pterygoid muscles.

## References

1. Stacey M.J.: Free nerve endings in skeletal muscle of the cat. J Anat, *105*:231, 1969
2. Tabary J.C., et al: Physiological and structural changes in the cat's soleus muscle due to immobilization at different lengths by plaster casts. J Physiol (Lond.), *224*:231, 1972
3. Williams P.E. and Goldspink G.: The effect of immobilization on the longitudinal growth of striated muscle fibers. J Anat, *116*:45, 1973
4. Rugh J.D. and Drago C.J.: Vertical dimension: A study of clinical rest position and jaw muscle activity. J Prosthet Dent, *45*:670, 1981
5. Manns A., et al: Influence of the vertical dimension in the treatment of myofascial pain-dysfunction syndrome. J Prosthet Dent, *50*:700, 1983
6. Travell J.G. and Simons D.S.: Myofascial Pain and Dysfunction: The Trigger Point Manual. Baltimore, Williams and Wilkins, 1983
7. Awad E.A.: Interstitial myofibrositis: Hypothesis of the mechanism. Arch Phys Med Rehabil, *54*:449, 1973
8. Park S.R. and Rodbard S.: Effects of load and duration of tension on pain induced by muscular contraction. Am J Physiol, *203*:735, 1962
9. Mahan P.E., et al: Superior and inferior bellies of the lateral pterygoid muscle EMG activity at basic jaw positions. J Prosthet Dent, *50*:710, 1983
10. Gibbs C.H., et al: EMG activity of the human superior lateral pterygoid in relation to other jaw muscles. J Prosthet Dent, *51*:691, 1984
11. Asmussen E.: Positive and negative work. Acta Physiol Scand, *28*:364, 1952

12. Bigland-Ritchie B. and Woods J.J.: Integrated electromyogram and oxygen uptake during positive and negative work. J Physiol (Lond.), 260:267, 1976
13. Miles T.S. and Wilkinson T.M.: Limitation of jaw movement by antagonist muscle stiffness during unloading of human jaw closing muscles. Exp Brain Res, 46:305, 1982
14. Mills K.R., et al: Muscle pain. In Textbook of Pain. Edited by P.D. Wall and R. Melzack. New York, Churchill Livingstone, 1984
15. McArdle B.: Myopathy due to a defect in muscle glycogen breakdown. Clin Sci, 10:23, 1951
16. Morgan-Hughes J.A.: Painful disorders of muscle. Br J Hosp Med, 22:360, 1979
17. DeVere R. and Bradley W.G.: Polymyositis: Its presentation, morbidity and mortality. Brain, 98:637, 1975
18. Riddach J. and Morgan-Hughes J.A.: Prognosis in adult polymyositis. J Neurol Sci, 26:71, 1975
19. DuBois E.L.: Lupus Erythematosus. 2nd Ed, Los Angeles, Southern California Press, 1974
20. Golding D.N.: Polyarteritis presenting as leg pains. Br Med J, 1:277, 1970
21. Ettlinger R.E., et al: Polymyalgia rheumatica and giant cell arteritis. Annu Rev Med, 29:15, 1978
22. Perkoff G.T., et al: Reversible acute muscular syndrome in chronic alcoholism. N Engl J Med, 274:1277, 1966
23. Lane R.J.M. and Mastaglia F.L.: Drug-induced myopathies in man. Lancet, II:562, 1978
24. Tarui S., et al: Phosphofructokinase deficiency in skeletal muscle. A new type of glycogenosis. Biochem Biophys Res Commun, 19:517, 1965
25. Morgan-Hughes J.A., et al: A mitochrondrial myopathy characterized by a deficiency of reducible cytochrome B. Brain, 100:617, 1979
26. Coonan T.J., et al: Ankylosis of the temporomandibular joint after temporal craniotomy: A cause of difficult intubation. Can Anaesth Soc J, 32:158, 1985
27. Volkman R.: Die ischaemischen muskellahmungen und kontrakturen. Zentralbl Chir, 8:801, 1881
28. Smythe H.A. and Moldofsky H.: Two contributions to understanding of the "fibrositis" syndrome. Bull Rheum Dis, 28:928, 1977–1978
29. Yunus M., et al: Primary fibromyalgia (fibrositis): Clinical study of 50 patients with matched normal controls. Semin Arthritis Rheum, 11:151, 1981
30. Epstein W.V. and Henke C.J.: The nature of U.S. rheumatology practice, 1977. Arthritis Rheum, 24:1177, 1981
31. Waxman J. and Zatzkis S.M.: Fibromyalgia and menopause, examination of the relationship. Postgrad Med, 80:165, 1986
32. Wolfe F. and Catey M.A.: Prevalence of primary and secondary fibrositis. J Rheumatol, 10:965, 1963
33. Carette S., et al: Evaluation of amitriptyline in primary fibrositis, a double-blind, placebo-controlled study. Arthritis Rheum, 29:655, 1986
34. Benoit P.W. and Belt W.D.: Destruction and regeneration of skeletal muscle after treatment with a local anesthetic, bupivacaine (Marcaine). J Anat, 107:547, 1970
35. Dolwick M.F., et al: Degenerative changes in masseter muscle following injection of lidocaine: A histochemical study. J Dent Res, 56:1395, 1977
36. Benoit P.W.: Microscarring in skeletal muscle after repeated exposure to lidocaine with epinephrine. J Oral Maxillofac Surg, 36:530, 1978
37. Zener J.C. and Harrison D.C.: Serum enzyme values following intramuscular administration of lidocaine. Arch Intern Med, 134:48, 1974
38. Benoit P.W. and Belt W.D.: Some effects of local anesthetic agents on skeletal muscle. Exp Neurol, 34:264, 1972
39. Frost F.A., et al: Control, double-blind comparison of mepivacaine injection versus saline injection for myofascial pain. Lancet, I:499, 1980
40. Kraak J.G.: A drug-initiated dislocation of the temporomandibular joint: Report of a case. J Am Dent Assoc, 74:1247, 1967
41. Abelson C.B.: Phenothiazine-induced neck-face syndrome: Report of case. J Oral Maxillofac Surg, 26:649, 1968
42. Chiles J.A.: Extrapyramidal reactions in adolescents treated with high-potency antipsychotics. Am J Psychiatry, 135:239, 1978
43. Menuck M.: Laryngeal-pharyngeal dystonia and haloperidol. Am J Psychiatry, 138:394, 1981
44. Klawans H.L.: The pharmacology of tardive dyskinesias. Am J Psychiatry, 130:82, 1973
45. Klawans H.L., et al: Toward an understanding of the pathophysiology of Huntington's chorea. Contin Neurol, 33:297, 1981
46. Weiner W.J. and Klawans H.L.: Lingual-facial-buccal movements in the elderly. I. Pathophysiology and treatment. J Am Geriatr Soc, 21:314, 1973
47. Tolosa E.S.: Clinical features of Meige's disease (idiopathic orofacial dystonia): A report of 17 cases. Arch Neurol, 38:147, 1981
48. Buxton P.H.: Pathology of muscle. Br J Anaesth, 52:139, 1980
49. Ringquist M.: Histochemical fiber types and fiber sizes in human masticatory muscles. Scand J Dent Res, 79:366, 1971
50. Ringquist M.: Histochemical enzyme profiles of fibers in human masseter muscles with special regard to fibers with intermediate myofibrillar ATPase reaction. J Neurol Sci, 19:133, 1973
51. Ringquist M.: A histochemical study of temporal muscle fibers in denture wearers and subjects with natural dentition. Scand J Dent Res, 82:28, 1974
52. Steinhauser E.W., et al: Correction of severe openbite associated with muscular disease. Report of a case. Oral Surg Oral Med Oral Pathol, 39:509, 1975
53. Bottomley W.K. and Terezhalmy G.T.: Management of patients with myasthenia gravis who require maxillary dentures. J Prosthet Dent, 38:609, 1977
54. Bland J.H. and Frymoyer J.W.: Rheumatic syndromes of myxedema. N Engl J Med, 282:1171, 1970
55. Beumer J., et al: Radiation therapy of the oral cavity: Sequelae and management. Part I. Head Neck Surg, 1:301, 1979
56. Stone J., et al: Trismus after injection of local anesthetic. Oral Surg Oral Med Oral Pathol, 48:29, 1979
57. Bullock K.N.: Salivary duct calculi presenting as trismus in a child. Br Med J, 280:1357, 1980
58. Waite P.D. and Alling C.C. III: Management of oral and maxillofacial infectious disease. In Clark's Clinical Dentistry, Vol. 1. Philadelphia, J.B. Lippincott, 1987
59. Marback J.J.: Hysterical trismus: A study of six cases. N.Y. State Dent J, 32:413, 1966
60. Lagundoye S.B.: Radiologic examination of trismus as a complication of cancrum oris. Oral Surg Oral Med Oral Pathol, 39:812, 1975
61. Smith M.J., et al: Tetanus: Review of the literature and report of a case. Oral Surg Oral Med Oral Pathol, 41:451, 1975

62. Furman R.E. and Barchi R.L.: Pathophysiology of myotonia and periodic paralysis. *In* Diseases of the Nervous System: Clinical Neurobiology. Edited by A.K. Asbury, G.M. McKhann, and W.I. McDonald. Philadelphia, Ardmore Medical Books, 1986

63. Brown G.L. and Harvey A.M.: Congenital myotonia in the goat. Brain, *64*:341, 1939

64. Becker P.E.: Myopathies. *In* Humangenetik. Vol. 31. Edited by P. Becker. Stuttgart, Thieme, 1964

65. Roses A.D., et al: Myotonic muscular dystrophy. *In* Diseases of Muscle, Part 2; Handbook of Clinical Neurology. Vol. 41. New York, Elsevier North Holland, 1979

66. Bucher N.L.: Effects of 2,4-dichlorophenoxyacetic acid on experimental animals. Proc Soc Exp Biol Med, *63*:204, 1946

67. Winer N., et al: Induced myotonia in man and goat. J Lab Clin Med, *66*:758, 1965

68. Blatt I.M.: Parotid-masseter hypertrophy-traumatic occlusion syndrome. Laryngoscope, *79*:624, 1969

69. Wade W.M. Jr.: Idiopathic masseter muscle hypertrophy: Report of cases. J Oral Maxillofac Surg, *29*:196, 1971

70. Friedman M.H.: Tenomyositis of the masseter muscle: Report of cases. J Am Dent Assoc, *110*:201, 1985

71. Hellinger M.J.: Myositis ossificans of the muscles of mastication. Oral Surg Oral Med Oral Pathol, *19*:581, 1965

72. Kreutziger K.L. and Mahan P.E.: Temporomandibular degenerative joint disease, Part II. Diagnostic procedure and comprehensive management. Oral Surg Oral Med Oral Pathol, *40*:297, 1975

73. Johnstone D.R. and Templeton M.: The feasibility of palpating the lateral pterygoid muscle. J Prosthet Dent, *43*:318, 1980

74. Thomas C.A. and Okeson J.P.: Evaluation of lateral pterygoid muscle symptoms using a common palpation technique and a method of functional manipulation. J Craniomandib Pract, *5*:125, 1987

# 8

# *Facial Skeletal Deformities*

Facial pain patients often have orthognathic skeletal deformities that may be primary factors in the etiology of their musculoskeletal problems, but the facial skeletal deformities may not have been recognized in previous history and physical evaluations.

Facial pain patients with a clinically apparent facial skeletal deformity should be examined for orthognathic surgical relations using appropriate methods, including cephalometric analyses and study casts, as indicated. If the findings are not within normal limits, then prudent planning would include consideration for surgical intervention to improve the skeletal and soft tissue deformities. This improvement results in correction of the positions of the dentition and other intraoral structures, the primary and secondary muscles of mastication, and the temporomandibular (TM) joints.

The location of occlusal surfaces of teeth and the general position of teeth depend on the alveolar processes. Deformities of these processes that prevent teeth from having normal occlusal contacts frequently are the result of facial skeletal deformities. An example is evident in a patient with a retrognathic mandible. The anterior dentition may have no normal occlusal contacts. Overeruption occurs, with the mandibular teeth moving toward the anterior hard palate and causing the accompanying alveolar process to become hyperplastic and deformed. Similarly, the maxillary teeth may overerupt inferiorly, causing the accompanying alveolar process to become hyperplastic and the teeth to become malpositioned posteriorly owing to lip and tongue pressures (Fig. 8–1).

In this chapter, we review correction of facial skeletal orthognathic deformities, facial pain patients with facial skeletal orthognathic deformities, as well as orthognathic surgery and how it may assist these patients. Craniofacial deformity syndromes are not discussed.

## Patients with Facial Skeletal Orthognathic Deformities

When considering patients presenting for correction of orthognathic deformities, although the signs and symptoms of mastica-

tory pain and dysfunction were slightly more common in female than in male patients, Edwards and colleagues noted that the prevalence of masticatory pain and dysfunction in 57 class II patients and 34 class III patients was about the same as in the general population.[1]

Laskin and associates, in a survey of oral and maxillofacial surgery training programs, found that fewer than 20% of the patients undergoing orthognathic surgical procedures had preoperative symptoms of TM joint abnormalities and related dysfunctions.[2] Results of this retrospective study included a wide range, with symptoms noted in 75% of orthognathic surgery patients in two programs and no patients with symptoms in five programs. Laskin and co-workers did not investigate the prevalence of significant facial skeletal orthognathic deformities in patients with TM joint-related facial pain.

Patients expect and appreciate the positive aspects of orthognathic surgical procedures, such as improved masticatory capability, preservation of teeth, and enhanced appearance.[3] Another interesting benefit noted by Gunther and colleagues is increased nasopharyngeal airway capacity after LeFort I maxillary intrusion procedures.[4]

If the patient is properly prepared as to expectations of surgical correction of skeletal deformities and is appropriately supported by friends and family members, a high degree of acceptance and reinforcement of the surgical results are likely.

## Patients with Facial Pain

As noted previously, most orthognathic surgical patients with facial skeletal deformities and consequent dental occlusal abnormalities have no more complaints regarding the TM joint or the supporting myofascial structures than the general population. On the other hand, most facial pain patients in the musculoskeletal category, which includes the TM joint, have facial skeletal deformities. Weinberg noted that 57% of his TM joint surgical patients " . . . had class II malocclusion, characterized by deep overbite, . . . "[5]

In facial pain patients with facial skeletal deformities, a summation of factors puts the

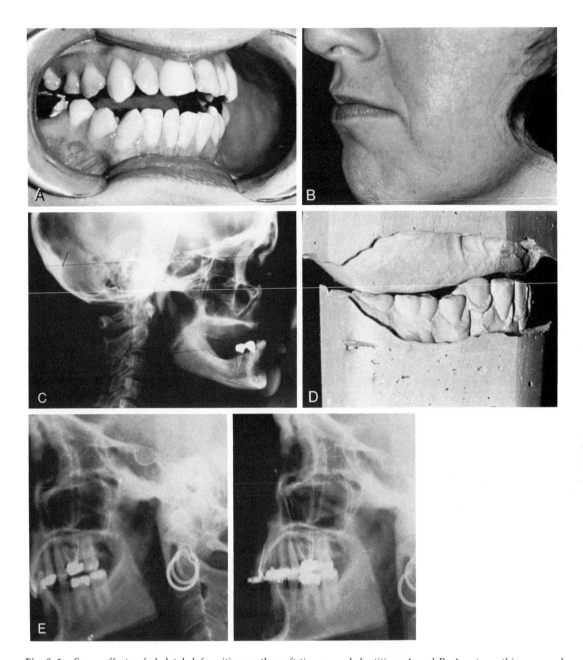

***Fig. 8–1.*** Some effects of skeletal deformities on the soft tissues and dentition. A and B. Apertognathism caused strain in obtaining lip closure. Patient's chief complaint was related to pain in the muscles of mastication. C and D. Loss of maxillary dentition and mandibular posterior dentition in a patient who had a mandibular prognathism, resulting in ever-increasing overclosure of the mandible and lack of stability of a series of maxillary dentures caused by absorption of the anterior maxilla. Patient's chief complaint was unilateral painful TM joint meniscus subluxation (click). E. Super-eruption and palatal tipping of the anterior maxillary teeth (left) was treated with presurgical orthodontia (right) prior to orthognathic surgery. Patient's chief complaint was intermittent and recurring bilateral meniscus dislocations.

TM joint and the associated musculature and ligaments at risk. A steep occlusal plane, mandibular retrognathism, and/or maxillary prognathism change the locus of vectors of the muscles of mastication and may overload the TM joint.[6] Another factor is gender, female patients having less connective tissue stability of the joints as compared to their male counterparts.[7] Other factors include malocclusal relations when the mandible moves from the centric position to a closed position; an open bite deformity with an anterior tongue thrust, either a congenital problem or an acquired habit, that stabilizes the skeleton in an apertognathism; and a psychologically motivated tendency to carry a retrognathic mandible in a forward position for esthetics (we had a patient who called this her "Sunday position!") (Fig. 8–2).

## Compromised Treatment

Compromised treatment may be planned and performed for patients whose basic problems are orthognathic deformities. These procedures include treatment of the malocclusion produced by a facial skeletal deformity by moving teeth within the limits of the alveolar

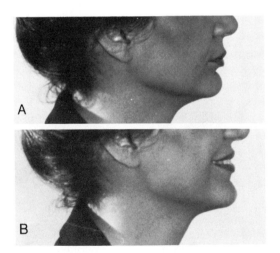

*Fig. 8–2.* A 35-year-old patient with a long habit of carrying her retrognathic mandible in a forward position for esthetics. Her chief complaints were painful TM joints, menisci subluxation (click) at 20 mm opening, occasional dislocations (closed lock) of the menisci, and generalized pain in the major and accessory muscles of mastication. A. Teeth in centric relations; B. mandible in the habitual forward position. The successful treatment plan included orthognathic surgery.

processes; by producing temporary or permanent alterations of the occlusion; and by the performance of masking facade operations to lengthen the mandible by placing an alloplastic device in the symphyseal area (Fig. 8–3).

## Disabling TM Joint Maladies and Orthognathic Deformities

If a patient has a disabling intracapsular malady that requires a surgical solution and a facial skeletal deformity that was probably a factor in the etiology of the TM joint problem, we believe the orthognathic deformity should be corrected first. After a period of repair and adaptation of the new skeletal relationships, the TM joint malady is then assessed and treated in its new anatomic and functional relations to the corrected facial skeleton. The performance of the orthognathic surgical procedure may eliminate the need for an open surgical procedure involving the TM joint.

When performing the orthognathic surgical procedure for patients with a TM joint malady, the surgeon should consider the use of transosseous wires and intermaxillary fixation instead of rigid transosseous fixation at the osteotomy sites. This approach permits more latitude for the condyles and menisci to accommodate to their new relationships as well as a period of rest for the TM joints during the 6 to 8 weeks of postoperative immobilization.

## Restructuring and Adaptation of Maxillofacial Tissues

The delicacy of the balance within the TM joint capsule has been demonstrated time and again by intracapsular reactions to deflective contacts, the use of occlusal borne splints, placement of coronal prostheses, and occlusal equilibrations. Also, psychopathologic maladies may produce intracapsular reactions secondary to muscular stresses. The intracapsular TM joint relationships are changed by all surgical procedures that alter the osseous form and/or the muscular attachments of the mandible or maxilla. The new muscular functioning vectors and stresses influence both

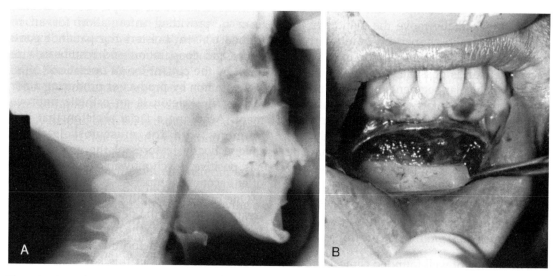

*Fig. 8–3.* Lateral cephalometric radiograph of a silicone rubber chin implant being forced into the supporting bone by the mentalis muscle, A. The patient had musculoskeletal facial pain. The treatment consisted of removal of the implant, B, and orthognathic surgery which relieved the muscular pain.

the intracapsular relationships and the eventual form of the bone.

For example, sagittal osteotomy of the rami may be performed to permit movement of the body of the mandible to a proper anatomic relationship with the maxilla. When performing this procedure, the main bodies of the lateral pterygoid, the masseter, and temporalis muscles may remain virtually untouched. Postoperatively, however, the proximal and distal segments of the rami are in different positions relative to their positioning preoperatively. These new osseous relationships of the proximal segments result from the new horizontal dimension at the osteotomy site of the anterior segment, it having been advanced or retruded (depending on the operation), and the type fixation employed between the proximal and distal segments. Thus, the location of the osseous base for attachment of all the major and accessory muscles of mastication is altered. Dechow and Carlson expressed this concept as follows: "Maxillofacial surgery restructures the craniofacial skeleton and associated soft tissues . . . (and) . . . may also have a direct effect on masticatory function. This effect is mediated . . . directly by the surgical procedures . . . (and also more subtly) . . . through postsurgical adaptation of the temporomandibu-lar joints, skeletal structures, periodontium and neuromusculature."[8]

### Acquired Facial Deformities

Orthognathic surgical procedures, when indicated, may correct facial skeletal deformities acquired from injuries, such as malunited fractures, and from diseases, such as rheumatoid arthritis and acromegaly. As an example of the application of these techniques, consider the patient with acromegaly in whom the disease process was arrested by surgical management or irradiation of the pituitary gland and/or with the prescription of pharmacotherapeutic agents, but the facial skeletal deformities persist. Myofascial pain, secondary to unusual muscular and ligamentous vectors and to psychologic factors, as well as painful intracapsular TM joint dysfunction, may be noted by acromegalic patients. A logical approach to this patient, in whom acromegaly is controlled, is orthognathic surgical correction, including possible glossoplasties, supported by pre- and postoperative occlusal and/or orthodontic care.[9]

## Orthognathic Surgery

Orthognathic surgical procedures are performed to correct facial skeletal deformities.

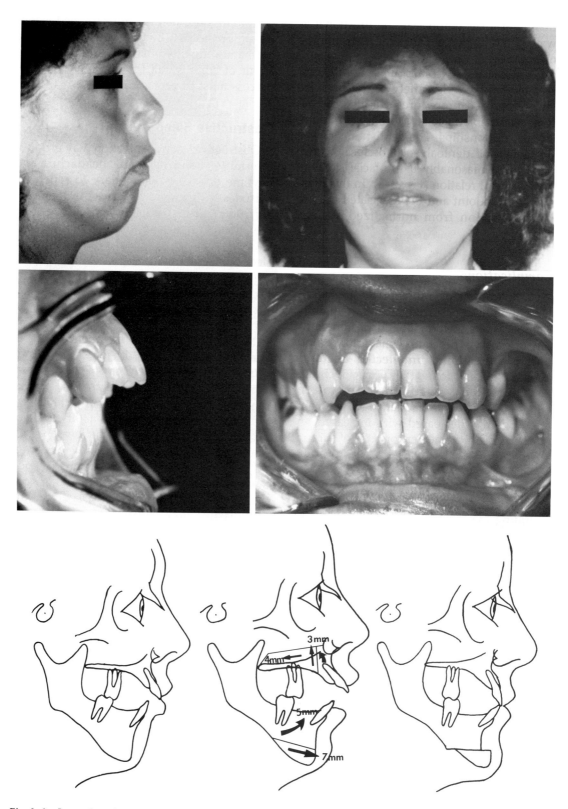

*Fig. 8–6.* Legend on facing page.

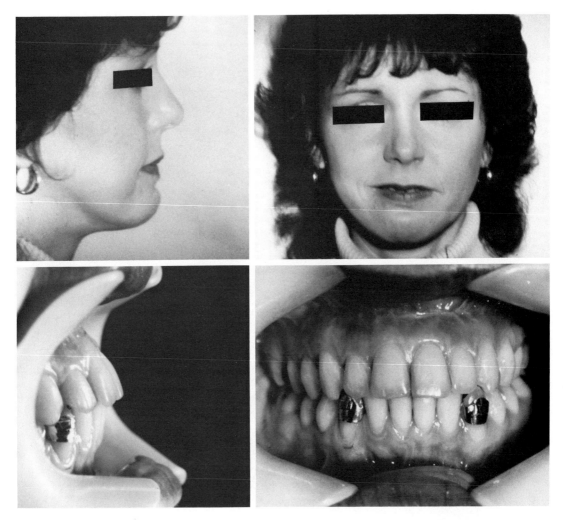

*Fig. 8–6.* Examples of orthognathic surgical procedures to relieve myofascial and TM joint pain and dysfunction. A 30-year-old, well-adjusted married woman had bilateral moderate TM joint pains. Evaluations revealed class II malocclusion, irregularity of the maxillary occlusal plane, lateral deviation of the left mandibular ramus, lip seal incompetence, bilaterally small rami,[1-5] and moderately severe degenerative joint disease. Following 6 months of orthodontic preparation, the patient underwent an anterior maxillary and segmental 3-mm intrusion and 4-mm retrusion, osteotomy with mandibular autorotation, and an anterior horizontal advancing sliding osteotomy of the mandibular base.[6,7] Postoperatively, the patient has been free of pain with stable occlusion for 5 years.[8-10,14]

nasal reconstructive surgery may be indicated. Kuo and colleagues described etiologies of sleep apnea and, where indicated, surgical solutions.[29] Riley and associates described the logical combination of evaluations and surgical treatments.[30] Waite and associates' study confirmed that combining maxillomandibular advancements with other procedures, especially uvulopalatopharyngoplasty, gave the highest success rate for treating obstructive sleep apnea syndrome.[31]

## Diagnosis

A diagnosis of sleep apnea may be made with the medical and personal histories. Detailed confirmation of the diagnosis involves studies of sleep and awake states with polysomnographic instrumentation that records vital signs and activities of the heart, brain, eyes, musculoskeletal system, cardiovascular system, and respiratory activities including abdominal and chest movements, airflow, and oximetric analysis of the exchanged air.

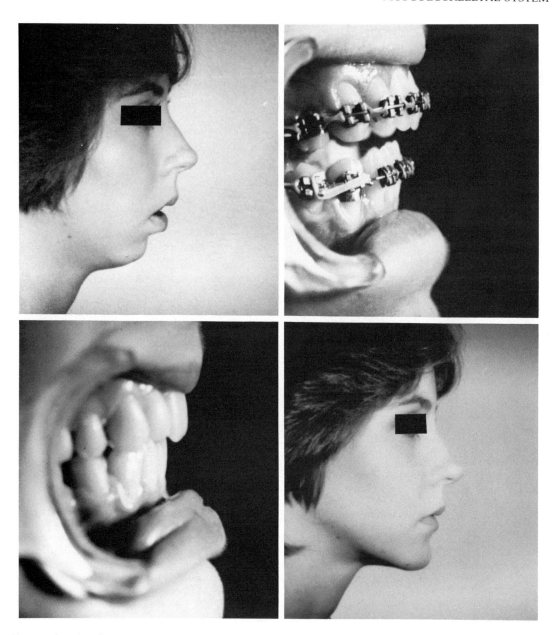

*Fig. 8–6 (continued).* Examples of orthognathic surgical procedures to relieve myofascial and TM joint pain and dysfunction. A 19-year-old female college student was unable to chew her food and had left-sided TM joint pain. The preoperative evaluations revealed a class II malocclusion with anterior open bite, increased lower facial height caused by vertical maxillary excess, mandibular retrognathia, and left TM joint degenerative arthritis.[1,2] She had a retained thumb habit and tongue thrust with associated speech problems; the patient spoke very little and avoided eye contact. The patient received 1 year of orthodontic presurgical preparation. The skeletal surgery consisted of a 4-mm LeFort I maxillary intrusion osteotomy, bilateral sagittal rami osteotomies with advancement, and anterior horizontal advancing sliding osteotomy of the anterior base of the mandible. For over 5 years postoperatively, she has been pain free and without recurrence of her open bite.[3,4]

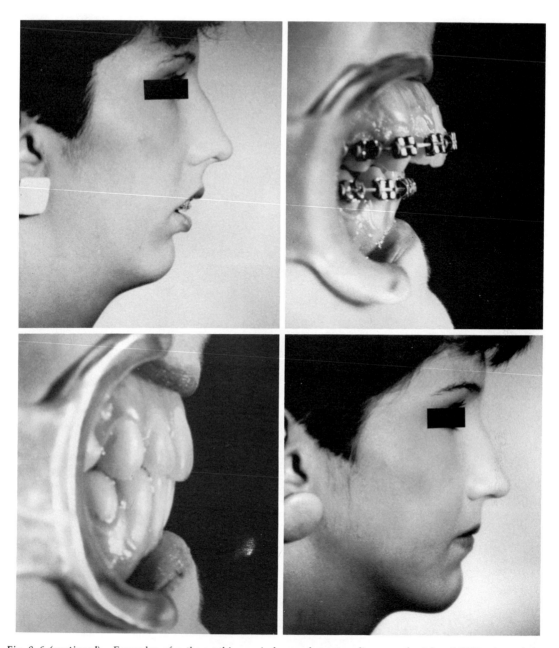

*Fig. 8–6 (continued).* Examples of orthognathic surgical procedures to relieve myofascial and TMJ pain and dysfunction. A 14-year-old girl was referred with a complaint of being "unable to bite and chew correctly" and left TM joint pain. Evaluations revealed a severe class II malocclusion with a large amount of excessive gingiva showing in her high smile, lip closure incompetence, and facial muscle strain.[1,2] After 1 year of presurgical orthodontic therapy, the patient underwent a LeFort I maxillary osteotomy, with 4 mm intrusion and 3 mm advancement and bilateral sagittal split rami osteotomies with 2 cm advancement. She was stable at 5 years postoperatively without change in occlusion and with resolution of her left TM joint pain.[3,4]

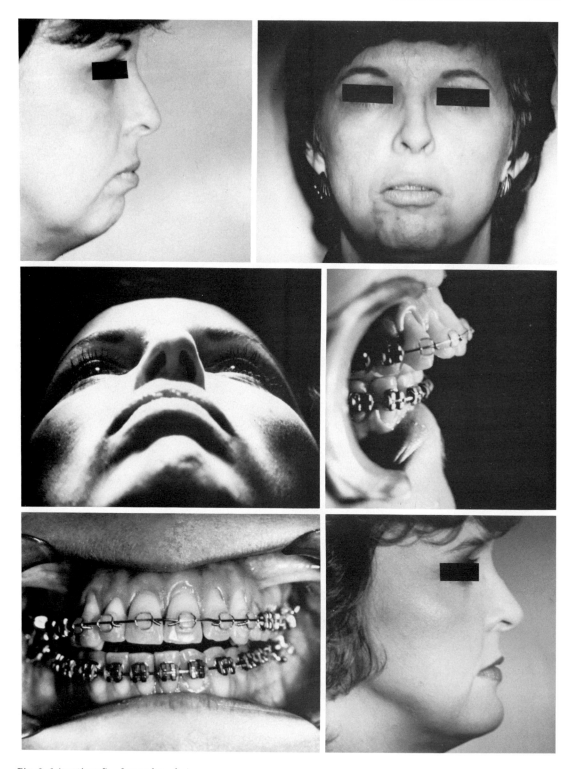

*Fig. 8–6 (continued).*   Legend on facing page.

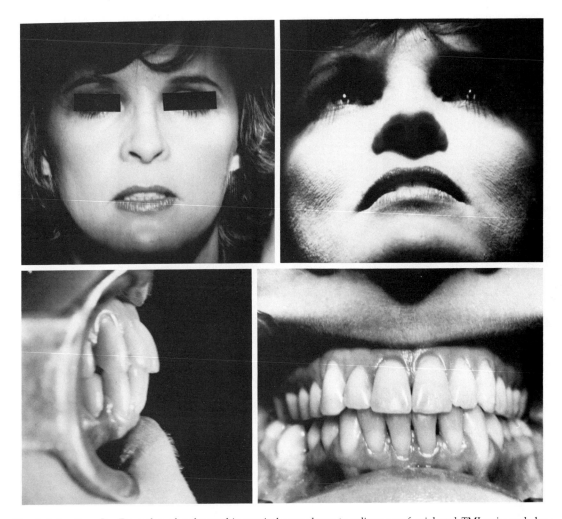

*Fig. 8–6 (continued).* Examples of orthognathic surgical procedures to relieve myofascial and TMJ pain and dysfunction. A 37-year-old married woman had paroxysmal bilateral TM joint pain and a tired feeling "in the jaws" as a result of constant mandibular protrusive posturing. Evaluations revealed a class II malocclusion, procumbent maxillary incisors, excessive gingiva showing with high smile, lip closure incompetence, and extreme facial muscle pain. Other indications were maxillary and mandibular retrusion, moderate vertical maxillary excess, maxillary incisor protrusion, bilateral mild degenerative joint disease with anterior spur formation indicative of excessive external pterygoid pull and protrusive posturing.[1-5] Following 1 year of presurgical orthodontic preparation, the patient underwent a LeFort I maxillary osteotomy with 4 mm intrusion and 2 mm advancement. An augmentation nasolabial graft of hydroxylapatite was placed for additional fullness. Mandibular bilateral sagittal rami osteotomies with advancement and an advancing horizontal sliding osteotomy of the anterior mandibular base with hydroxylapatite graft were performed. Postoperatively, the patient's occlusion was stable at 4 years with resolution of muscle and TM joint pain.[6-10] (Appreciation is extended to the *Journal of the Alabama Dental Association* for permission to use the case reports in Fig. 6 which originally appeared as part of an article by Brindley, H.P., Alling, C.C., and Cale L.T.: Orthognathic surgery, combined maxillary and mandibular procedures. J Al Dent Assoc *70:*37, 1986.)

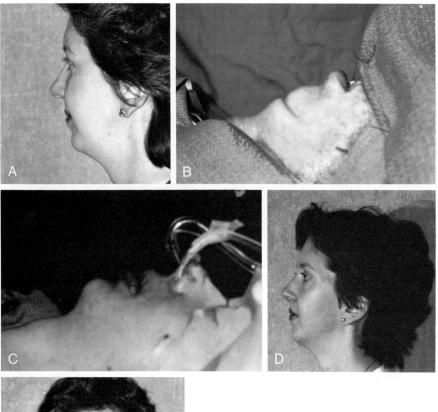

*Fig. 8–7.* Sleep hypopnea patient. A 35-year-old woman with a history of sleep hypopnea. A. Preoperative profile disclosed an obvious mandibular retrognathism and probable maxillary retrognathism. The SNA was 74°, the ANB, 7°; the pharyngeal airway space, 6 mm; the hyoid bone, 15 mm below the cephalometric mandibular plane. B. and C. Immediate pre- and postoperative views. The patient received advancement of the mandible, maxilla, base of the mandible, with rigid fixation of all osteotomy sites. D. and E. One year postoperative facial views. The patient had no recurrence of the signs and symptoms of hypopnea.

The detailed analysis includes audio recordings of breathing and snoring episodes.

In patients with a history of sleep deprivation and related symptoms, deformities of the facial skeleton may be the etiology or be a contributing problem producing obstructive sleep apnea or hypopnea. As measured on lateral cephalometric radiographic films, the following are indicative of possible obstruction of the upper airway due to a deficient forward support of the pharyngeal soft tissues: a pharyngeal airway space of less than 6 mm, a SNB (sella-nasion-supramentale) angle less than 76 degrees, ANB (subspinale-nasion-supramentale) angle greater than 5 de-

grees, and a placement of the hyoid bone more than 15 mm below the cephalometric mandibular plane.

## Orthognathic Surgical Correction

The basic surgical procedure, mandibular advancement utilizing bilateral sagittal osteotomies of the rami, is supplemented with a horizontal sliding osteotomy of the anterior base of the mandible to advance the attachments of the genial and diagastric muscles and to assist in closure competence of the lips. The procedure is based on the midfacial skeleton being in a normal position as a guide for advancing the mandible; this normal position of the midfacial skeleton is either present as a preoperative finding in the patient or is produced by concurrent orthognathic surgical procedures.

For a patient with obstructive sleep apnea, the normally positioned maxilla may be advanced one standard deviation from the normal to permit even greater advancement of the mandible and the stomatognathic system.

## References

1. Edwards S.M., et al: Prevalence of masticatory pain and dysfunction in skeletal II and III patients. Study Guide for AAO-AAOMS 1983 Clinical Conference on Surgical-Orthodontic Challenges. American Association of Orthodontists and American Association of Oral and Maxillofacial Surgeons, St. Louis, 1983
2. Laskin D.M., Ryan W.A., and Greene C.S.: Incidence of temporomandibular symptoms in patients with major skeletal malocclusions. A survey of oral and maxillofacial surgery training programs. Oral Surg Oral Med Oral Pathol, 61:537, 1986
3. Nagamine T., Kobayshi T., Hanada K, and Nakajima T.: Satisfaction of patients following surgical-orthodontic correction of skeletal class III malocclusions. J Oral Maxillofac Surg, 44:944, 1986
4. Gunther T.A., et al: Effect of LeFort I maxillary impaction on nasal airway resistance. Study Guide for AAO-AAOMS 1983 Clinical Conference on Surgical-Orthodontic Challenges. American Association of Orthodontists and American Association of Oral and Maxillofacial Surgeons, St. Louis, 1983
5. Weinberg S.: Eminectomy and meniscorrhaphy for internal derangements of the temporomandibular joint. Oral Surg Oral Med Oral Pathol, 57:241, 1984
6. Storey A.T.: Joint and tooth articulation disorders of jaw in movements. In Oral-Facial Sensory and Motor Functions. Edited by Y. Kawamura and R. Dubner. Chicago, Quintessence Publishing, 1981
7. Waite P.D.: Evaluation of 49 mitral valve prolapse patients for maxillofacial deformities and temporomandibular joint dysfunction. Oral Surg Oral Med Oral Pathol, 63:496, 1986
8. DeChow P.C. and Carlson D.S.: Occlusal force after mandibular advancement in adult rhesus monkeys. J Oral Maxillofac Surg, 44:887, 1986
9. Hampton R.E.: Acromegaly and resulting myofascial pain and temporomandibular joint dysfunction: Review of the literature and report of case. J Am Dent Assoc, 114:625, 1987
10. Hullihen S.P.: Case of elongation of the lower jaw. Am J Dent Sci, 9:157, 1849
11. Blair V.P.: Operations on the jaw-bone and face. Surg Gynecol Obstet, 4:67, 1907
12. Kazanjian V.H.: Surgical correction of deformities of the jaws and its relation to orthodontia. Am J Orthod, 22:259, 1936
13. Caldwell J.B. and Letterman G.S.: Vertical osteotomy in the mandibular rami for correction of prognathism. J Oral Maxillofac Surg, 12:185, 1954
14. Hinds E.C.: Surgical correction of mandibular deformities. Am J Orthod, 43:160, 1957
15. Robinson M.: Prognathism corrected by open vertical condylotomy. J South Calif Dent Assoc, 24:22, 1956
16. Goldstein A.: Appraisal of results of surgical correction of class III malocclusions. Angle Orthod, 17:59, 1947
17. Dingman R.O. and Alling C.C.: Open reduction and internal wire fixation of maxillofacial fractures. J Oral Maxillofac Surg, 12:140, 1956
18. Obwegeser H.: The surgical correction of mandibular prognathism and retrognathia with consideration of genioplasty, Part I. Oral Surg Oral Med Oral Pathol, 10:677, 1957
19. Trauner R.: The surgical correction of mandibular prognathism and retrognathia with consideration of genioplasty, Part II. Oral Surg Oral Med Oral Pathol, 10:787, 899, 1957
20. Köle H.: Surgical operations of the alveolar ridge to correct occlusal abnormalities. Oral Surg Oral Med Oral Pathol, 12:515, 1959
21. Bell W.H., Fonseca R.J., Kennedy J.W., and Levy B.M.: Bone healing and revascularization after total maxillary osteotomy. J Oral Maxillofac Surg, 33:253, 1975
22. Bell W.H.: LeFort I osteotomy for correction of maxillary deformities. J Oral Maxillofac Surg, 33:412, 1975
23. Bell W.H., et al: Surgical Correction of Dentofacial Deformities. Vols. I and II. Philadelphia, W.B. Saunders, 1980
24. Epker B.N. and Wolford L.M.: Dentofacial Deformities Surgical-Orthodontic Correction. St. Louis, C.V. Mosby, 1980
25. Jacobson A.: Orthognathic diagnosis using the proportionate template. J Oral Maxillofac Surg, 38:820, 1980
26. Jacobson A. and Kilpatrick M.: Proportionate templates for orthodontic diagnosis in children. J Clin Orthod, 17:180, 1983
27. Morris J.H.: Personal communication, 1988
28. Aragon S.B., Van Sickels J.E., Dolwick M.F., and Flanary C.M.: The effects of orthognathic surgery on mandibular range of motion. J Oral Maxillofac Surg, 43:939, 1986
29. Kuo P.C., et al: The effect of mandibular osteotomy in three patients with hypersomnia sleep apnea. Oral Surg Oral Med Oral Pathol, 48:385, 1979
30. Riley R.W., et al: Current surgical concepts for treating obstructive sleep apnea syndrome. J Oral Maxillofac Surg, 45:149, 1987
31. Waite P.D., et al: Maxillomandibular advancement surgery in 23 patients with obstructive sleep apnea syndrome. J Oral Maxillofac Surg, 47:1256, 1989

# 9

## Occlusion and Occlusal Pathofunction

For purposes of this chapter, we define occlusal function as the manner in which the opposing teeth contact, interdigitate, and move against each other. The functional range is defined as all contact positions of the teeth from buccal cusp to buccal cusp contact on the right to those on the left, forward to incisal edge against incisal edge contact in protrusive, and back to retruded contact (RC) from intercuspal position (IP). When the lower teeth are moved to the right, left, or forward beyond the functional range, the position is called crossover. Pathofunction is defined as any function that produces pathology if continued beyond some critical time limit. Occlusal pathofunction both in the functional range and in crossover may affect teeth, periodontium, muscles, and the temporomandibular (TM) joints in producing pain and/or pathologic change.

To diagnose pain arising from occlusal pathofunction, the clinician must understand the characteristics of healthy and stable occlusal function. The studies of Posselt, in which he described the movement space of the mandible, provide a basis for understanding occlusal function.[1] Posselt assumed that harmony between the movements of the arches of teeth and those of the two TM joints is required to maintain a stable and healthy stomatognathic system, because these structures are analogous to the three legs of an upside-down stool. Two posterior legs represent the condyles in the fossae and the anterior leg represents the occlusion of the arch of teeth. Anytime one leg is altered in shape or length, the other two change their relationship to their supporting surface, but the stool stabilizes and reseats against the supports. Because the two arches of teeth provide such a large, complex foot of the anterior leg of the stool, if either or both of the posterior legs (the TM joints) change their supporting position, points of great stress may develop in one localized area of the anterior leg (the dentition). Such reciprocal interaction occurs between any pair of the three legs. As long as harmony exists between the two joints and the occlusion of the teeth, points of stress or heavy forces on one pair of teeth do not develop. Such harmony produces a stable re-

lationship and the teeth remain in place in the dental arch in a healthy condition.

## Movement Space of the Mandible

Posselt characterized the movement space of the mandible by recording the border movements of the mandible at many increments of mouth opening from occlusal contact of the teeth to maximum opening. These movements were recorded as intraoral needle point tracings of the extreme movement of the mandible to the right, forward, to the left, then back in retrusive, and across to the starting point on the right. The tracings were oriented one above the other to produce a solid that represents the movement space of the mandible.

Examination of a midsagittal section through the Posselt movement space (Fig. 9–1) describes many functional characteristics of occlusion and jaw movement. Posselt seated the condyles superiorly in the fossa so the posterior legs of the stool positioned the mandible. He found that the lower teeth could be rotated up and down about 20 mm

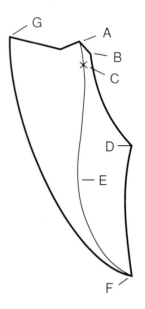

**Fig. 9–1.** Posselt movement space. A midsagittal section through the mandibular movement space. A—intercuspal position (IP); B—retruded contact (RC); C—rest position; D—deflection point at which condyle begins to translate out of the fossa on opening; E—free opening-closing path; F—maximum opening; G—maximum occluded protrusion.

with the condyles remaining up in the fossae. The mandible was essentially rotating on an arc about an axis running through or near the medial poles of the condyles seated in the fossae. This arc of closure is called the *centric relation closure arc*, and its axis of rotation is called the *terminal hinge axis*.

When the mouth is opened to the deflection point at the bottom of the centric relation closure arc, the condyles can no longer remain seated in the glenoid fossae, but translate down and forward. The posterior border movement below the deflection point represents a combination of translation and rotation of the condyles until maximum opening is reached. This movement has a constantly changing center of rotation.

The maximum protruded closure arc extends from maximum opening to maximum occluded protrusion. In many cases, the condyles are located forward and anterior to the eminence during this closure.

The irregular path from maximum occluded protrusion to IP represents the gliding of cuspal inclines of the teeth over one another. IP represents the point of maximum intercuspation of the teeth. Posselt found that 88% of several hundred subjects first contacted in an RC position when closing in the centric relation closure arc. From this initial contact, they deflected up and forward to maximum intercuspation of the teeth. This distance had a horizontal component of 1.25 mm and a vertical component of 0.9 mm relative to the sella nasion line. In recent studies, authors reported slides from RC or centric relation to IP or central occlusion in 57 to 100% of subjects studied.[2-8] These studies involved different types of subjects and different methods of measurement, which should account, in part, for the wide range in the data.

The distal inclines of buccal cusps of lower posterior teeth occlude against the mesial inclines of lingual cusps of upper posterior teeth in the slide from RC to IP. Because the lower teeth are moving forward in an arc during the final increment of jaw elevation, interfering tooth substance that deflects the mandible forward is greatly minimized. Slight removal of enamel from these inclines eliminates what had seemed a long, pronounced slide from RC to IP.

Interferences in the slide from RC to IP are sometimes associated with TM joint pain in patients with psychic tension.[9] The RC position is rarely used in normal masticatory function,[10,11] but this fact does not seem to prevent this interference from playing a role in facial pain in some patients. When 12 subjects with a dual bite (2.5 to 5 mm between the retruded and intercuspal positions) were compared to 12 control subjects with physiologic occlusion, investigators noted that the dual bite subjects used the retruded mandibular position during chewing.[12] Findings of studies involving electromyography of mandibular muscles show that occlusal interferences result in asynchronous contraction patterns in the muscles and increased muscle activity at rest during function.[9,13-15] In some patients, interferences or prematurities in the slide from RC to IP must be eliminated completely before synchronous muscle contraction patterns are re-established.[9]

## Examination of Occlusal Function

Seven occlusal abnormalities can be identified in a matter of a few minutes to help determine if occlusal dysfunction plays a role in a facial pain problem (Table 9–1).

### Interceptive Occlusal Contacts

To examine for interceptive occlusal contacts in the centric relation closure arc, the clinician can use a bimanual manipulation method of seating the condyles superiorly in the fossae (Fig. 9–2).[16] The patient is instructed to relax the mandibular muscles, and the condyles are seated superiorly in the fossa by the last three fingers positioned at the angle of the mandible, elevating superiorly to-

**TABLE 9–1.** *Occlusal Abnormalities Diagnosed by Mandible Manipulation*

1. Interceptive occlusal contacts
2. Lateral deviation in slide from retruded contact to intercuspal position
3. Lateral guidance on posterior teeth
4. Retrusive ("distalizing") lateral guidance
5. Balancing interference
6. Protrusive guidance on posterior teeth
7. Excessive or inadequate occlusal vertical dimension

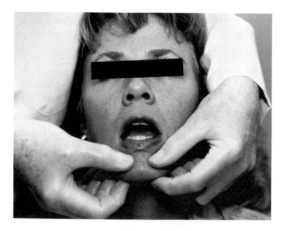

*Fig. 9–2.* Patient with mandible positioned in centric relation by bimanual manipulation. The clinician elevates the posterior mandible with the last 3 fingers positioned on the inferior border of the mandible, beginning at the angle. The force directed superiorly must be equal on the two sides. The thumbs are positioned on the symphysis and force is exerted downward tending to rotate the mandible so the condyles are seated upward and anterior-ward against the roof of the fossa and posterior incline of the articular eminence. The patient relaxes the mandibular muscles and the clinician rotates the mandible up and down in the centric relation closure arc.

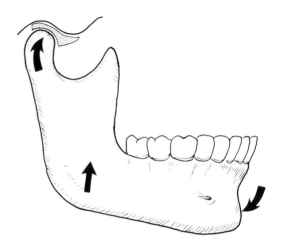

*Fig. 9–3.* Seating of the condyle by bimanual manipulation. Force applied by the thumbs is directed as shown by the arrow at the symphysis of the mandible. Force applied by the last 3 fingers is directed superiorly as shown by the arrow at the angle of the mandible. The resultant force at the condyle seats the condyle superiorly canted forward against the posterior incline of the articular eminence as shown by the arrow in the condyle.

ward the fossae. The thumbs push downward on the symphysis as the condyles are seated superiorly and the mandible is rotated around the condyles seated in the fossae (Fig. 9–3). As the mandibular teeth approach the maxillary teeth, the closing movement is slowed and the teeth are lightly tapped into occlusion several times. The patient is asked to note where the teeth are touching: right or left side, front or back of the mouth. With this procedure, the typical patient can localize the interceptive contact for the clinician.

An alternative method of accomplishing the same examination is illustrated in Figure 9–4. The patient is seated in the chair. The left hand is inverted so the thumb can be pressed upward at the angle of the patient's right mandible with the clinician standing right-front of the patient. The index and third finger of the left hand hold the lips apart exposing the anterior teeth so they can be easily observed (see Fig. 9–4). The right hand is positioned with the index finger pressing superiorly on the angle of the mandible to balance the thumb pressure on the opposite side. The right thumb grasps the lower lip and mentalis muscle without pressing the finger-

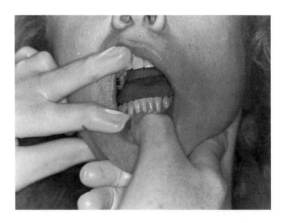

*Fig. 9–4.* Alternative method of manipulating the mandible into centric relation. The dentist stands right front of the patient. The patient is seated upright in the dental chair. The left thumb is positioned under the patient's right mandibular angle on the inferior border. The right index finger is positioned under the left angle of the patient's mandible. These two fingers push superiorly on the posterior mandible with the same force on each side. The dentist's right thumb grasps the patient's lower lip and his last three fingers are curled around the chin. Force is directed inferiorly by the thumb so the resultant force seats the condyle superiorly and anteriorly in the fossa. The index and third finger of the dentist's left hand retracts the lips so all the anterior teeth can be observed during manipulation.

nail into the labial gingiva. The remaining three fingers of the right hand curve under the chin to help provide a firm grasp of the mandibular symphysis. The condyles are elevated superiorly several times as the patient is instructed to relax and let the clinician rotate the mandible up and down freely. When the patient relaxes the mandibular muscles, the clinician torques downward on the symphysis with the right thumb and rotates the mandible up and down with the condyles seated in the fossae superiorly. The teeth are then lightly tapped into occlusion. The patient is asked to tell where the teeth are touching. This process represents closure in centric relation. No distracting devices, such as articulating ribbon or ribbon holders are needed. The patient with physiologic occlusion will report that teeth are touching simultaneously on the two sides and the contacts will include a number of teeth on each side. When only one pair of teeth are touching in centric relation, the next procedure is to determine how the interfering teeth deflect the mandible in the slide from RC to IP.

## Lateral Deviation in Slide from Retruded Contact to Intercuspal Position

To evaluate the slide, the clinician grasps the mandible by either of the two methods used to find the interference and closes the mouth to lightly contact the interfering teeth. After observing the upper and lower midlines of the central incisors, the clinician instructs the patient to bite or close tightly (Fig. 9–5). The length and direction of the slide is observed and related to the proportion of the lower incisors overlapped by the upper incisors at each end of the slide. If the slide has a lateral component and is erratic and irregular, the posterior two legs of the mandibular stool (condyles in the fossae) are being displaced by the lateral shifting of the mandible. This condition is often associated with the symptoms of myofascial pain, and such symptoms are usually eliminated by the use of an occlusal splint, which is constructed to eliminate the lateral deviation in the slide.

When patients with a lateral deviation in the slide open and close normally, they do

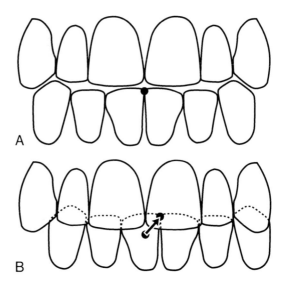

*Fig. 9–5.* Drawing demonstrating a lateral deviation in the slide from RC to IP. A. The relationship of anterior teeth when the teeth first contact on elevation of the mandible in the centric relation closure arc (RC). B. The relationship of anterior teeth when the patient bites down closing into intercuspal position (IP). Arrow shows the direction and magnitude of the slide from RC to IP at the incisors.

not close on the interfering contact and slide into their lateral position. They close directly into the lateral position or their acquired bite.

When pain is related to this occlusal interference, both pterygoid muscles on the side opposite the direction of the slide are typically painful to palpation. This tenderness occurs because these muscles must contract more continuously during closure to position the mandible laterally to the opposite side, allowing the teeth to seat in their acquired bite. It does not matter which side has the premature contact. The important factor is the direction of the slide.

## Lateral Guidance on Posterior Teeth

To evaluate lateral guidance, the patient closes the teeth lightly, and the clinician places the left index finger on the labial surface of the right maxillary canine. The right thumb pushes against the lateral chin on the patient's left side so the mandible is guided into a straight right lateral bite (Fig. 9–6). The index finger is used to stop the lateral excursion as the canine labial surfaces become flush. The patient is instructed to hold that

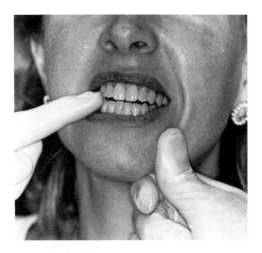

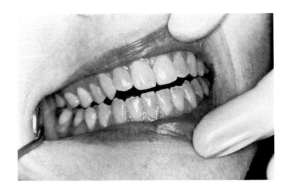

*Fig. 9–8.* When the patient's mandible has been positioned straight laterally the dentist can observe contact on the molars and lack of contact of the canines.

*Fig. 9–6.* Method of manipulating the patient's mandible into a straight lateral bite. The index finger will stop the mandibular canine as it moves edge to edge with the maxillary canine. The thumb of the opposite hand is used to push the patient's mandible straight laterally.

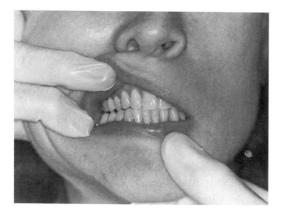

*Fig. 9–7.* The patient has been positioned straight laterally and instructed to hold that position. The lips and cheeks are retracted so tooth contacts and relative positions can be observed.

position and the lips and cheek are deflected laterally so the right posterior teeth can be observed (Fig. 9–7). Only the two canines are in contact in most patients under 30 years of age.[17] In older patients, the canines are likely abraded enough to allow the posterior teeth to contact buccal cusp to buccal cusp. If the canines are not in contact and the molars are guiding the mandible by occluding on the buccal cusps, the patient has, in effect, an anterior opened bite in lateral or a working side interference (Fig. 9–8).

Findings of a study involving 50 young adults and 50 children showed lateral guid-

ance is provided by the first permanent molars in 11-year-old children and it moves forward to the canines in the 23-year-old young adults.[18] The canines are not fully erupted in the 11-year-old child, but they provide lateral guidance when they reach their position in the arch. Lateral guidance at the anterior of the mandible provides a longer lever arm from the joints to the tooth contact than to the mathematic center of the elevator muscles. The canine periodontal ligament mechanoreceptors inhibit the jaw elevating muscles,[19,20] and this mechanical advantage helps to protect the canines and their periodontium from excessive muscle force in the lateral contacting positions.

Because lateral guidance moves anteriorly during normal development of occlusal function, providing a mechanical advantage for canine lateral guidance, we consider lateral guidance by the posterior teeth only an abnormality or pathofunction.

## Retrusive Lateral Guidance

When patients with steep cuspal inclines on the canines are positioned in straight right lateral, the distal incline of the lower canine should guide against the mesial incline of the upper canine, creating a protrusive component to the lateral guidance (Fig. 9–9). If the patient is less than a full cusp class II at the canines, the mesial incline of the lower canine guides against the distal incline of the upper canine so the lateral guidance has a retrusive component (Fig. 9–10). This retrusive com-

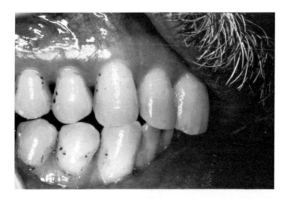

**Fig. 9–9.** This patient has been manipulated straight laterally and the dentist can observe the contact between the distal incline of the mandibular canine and mesial incline of the maxillary canine while there is space between the mesial incline of the mandibular first premolar and distal incline of the maxillary canine. There is a protrusive component to this type of lateral guidance.

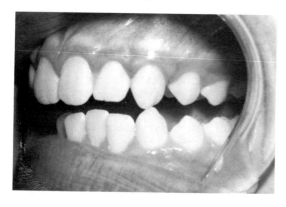

**Fig. 9–10.** This patient has been manipulated straight laterally and the dentist can observe the contact between the mesial incline of the mandibular canine and the distal incline of the maxillary canine. There is a space between the distal incline of the mandibular canine and the mesial incline of the maxillary first premolar. This tooth guidance produces a lateral retrusive or distalizing guidance.

ponent tends to displace the lateral pole of the ipsilateral condyle distally into the retrodiskal tissues during lateral movement. The authors have noted lateral retrusive guidance in patients with an early, reciprocal click in the ipsilateral TM joint, and the lateral one third of the posterior band of the disk is obliquely displaced anterior to the lateral pole of the condyle when the teeth are in occlusion. This problem is described in Chapter 10. This condition is also seen in some class II, division 2 patients in whom the deep anterior bite retrudes the mandible during lateral movement.

The function of incising food on the anterior teeth establishes the length of the anterior teeth and abrades and shapes their incisal edges. When patients wear segmental appliances covering the posterior teeth only, and the anterior teeth cannot contact in protrusion because of acrylic or metal between the posterior occlusal surfaces, the anterior teeth usually elongate. When this elongation produces a retrusive lateral guidance at the canines, the patient often develops anterior displacement of the lateral aspect of the posterior band of the disk. Long-term, repetitive retrusion of the lateral pole of the condyle appears to cause anterior displacement of the ipsilateral disk.

## Balancing Interference

When the patient is positioned in straight right lateral, and none of the teeth on the right side are in contact, the patient has a balancing interference on the left side (Fig. 9–11). To confirm this diagnosis, the patient is instructed to attempt to close the right canines together and rub them against each other. After such an attempt, the clinician touches the left cheek in the molar region and asks the patient if teeth are contacting on that side. The patient will report a balancing side contact. No articulating ribbon or efforts to work floss forward from the third molars are needed to detect a contact on the balancing side.

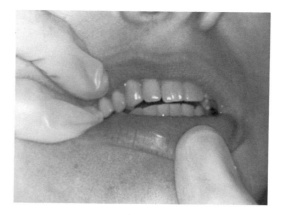

**Fig. 9–11.** This patient has been manipulated into a straight lateral position. Since none of the right teeth are in contact, a balancing or cross arch contact exists in the molar region of the left side.

A balancing interference is the second most significant trigger for bruxing after the discrepancy between CR and IP.[21] Balancing interferences often develop in patients with missing mandibular first molars and mesial drifting of second and third molars. The distobuccal cusps of these tipped molars clash with a lingual cusp of the opposing upper molar when the mandible moves to the opposite side.

### Protrusive Guidance on Posterior Teeth

With the patient's mouth closed in IP, cheeks are retracted laterally to observe any crossbite relationships of posterior teeth (Fig. 9–12). Any findings are noted in the patient's record. The clinician then places the thumb against the labial surface of the upper central incisors to stabilize the edge-to-edge contact position, and instructs the patient to hold the anterior teeth in contact and push the lower jaw straight forward, pushing against the upper teeth (Fig. 9–13). The cheek is retracted laterally as the patient makes the protrusive excursion to observe if the posterior teeth disclude as the anterior teeth guide the mandible in straight protrusion. The patient is asked to retrude (pull the lower jaw back) and the opposite cheek is retracted laterally to observe

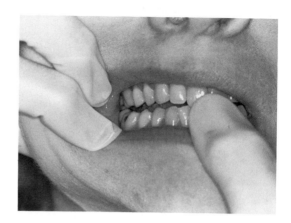

**Fig. 9–13.** This patient has moved into straight protrusive until stopped at incisal edge to edge by the dentist's thumb. The cheek is retracted to observe the manner in which the posterior teeth disclude as the mandible moves forward. If posterior tooth contacts interfere in protrusive excursion, the dentist will be able to detect them.

that side as the patient repeats the protrusive excursion.

Patients with protrusive guidance on the posterior teeth may have facial pain and bilateral temple and occipital headaches. Many patients who have their anterior guidance removed for restorative reasons become nocturnal bruxers and develop sore muscles and other symptoms of bruxism.[22]

Protrusive guidance on the anterior teeth is the more physiologic protrusive pattern, but patients with advanced rheumatoid arthritis, who have anterior opened bite and fibrosis with condylar erosion, are able to function without anterior guidance when the disease goes into remission. They usually have minimum protrusive excursive range because of the fibrosis in the joints. This exception is fortuitous, because restoration of anterior guidance in these patients is difficult for both esthetic and functional reasons, and surgical intervention is often required to correct their anterior opened bite.

### Excessive or Inadequate Occlusal Vertical Dimension

To evaluate the interocclusal distance (free way space) and to estimate occlusal vertical dimension, the patient opens the mouth in a relaxed manner and slowly closes until the lips just touch lightly and stops. This maneu-

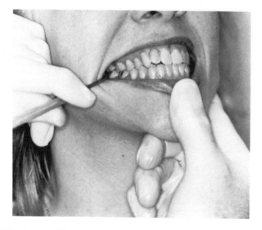

**Fig. 9–12.** This patient has closed into IP; the cheek is retracted to check for teeth in crossbite. Note that the right upper first premolar is in crossbite.

ver typically positions the mandible in rest position. The clinician then quickly opens the lips, noting the position of the lower incisors relative to the upper incisors, and instructs the patient to close or bite down into IP. The amount of superior movement of the lower incisors during this closure is estimated. It can be measured with a ruler placed between marks on the nose tip and chin before and after the closure from rest position to IP (Fig. 9–14).

In patients with angles class I; class II, division 1; and class III jaw relationships, the interocclusal distance should be 1.0 to 3.0 mm at the anterior teeth.[23] In patients with class II, division 2 jaw relationship, the interocclusal distance measures 3.5 to 8 mm.[24] If the interocclusal distance is too small, the occlusal vertical dimension is too great by the same amount. If the interocclusal distance is too great, the occlusal vertical dimension is too small by the excess increment.

Patients with new complete dentures in which the occlusal vertical dimension is excessive often develop denture-sore mouth and tired or sore muscles of mastication, a clear indication of a dimension that is not correct.

## Types of Occlusal Function

A simple examination of the occlusion enables the clinician to classify the type of oc-

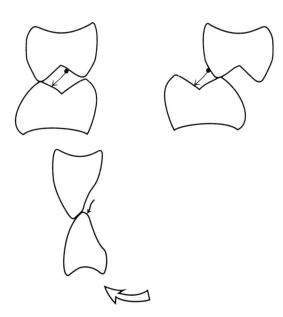

*Fig. 9–15.* Balanced occlusal function. Second molar relationships bilaterally and right canine relationship in balanced occlusal function. Note the right canine and molar facial cusps are in contact and the left second molars are contacting palatal cusp of upper against buccal cusp of lower in right lateral position of the mandible.

clusal function in most patients as balanced occlusal function, group function, or cuspid protected occlusal function. The type of occlusal function in a given patient may not be bilateral; e.g., a patient may have cuspid protected occlusion on one side and group function occlusion on the other. All three types assume bilateral contact of posterior teeth in IP.

### Balanced Occlusal Function

When the mandible is moved laterally from IP, one or more buccal cusp to buccal cusp contacts are noted on the working side and one or more contacts are noted on the balancing side (Fig. 9–15). The balancing side contacts are usually between the lingual cusps of upper molars and the distobuccal cusps of lower molars. This type of occlusion is considered ideal in complete dentures, because the bilateral contact helps to keep the lower denture base seated against the lower ridge during lateral biting.

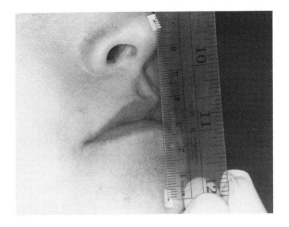

*Fig. 9–14.* The distance between dots on the nose tip and chin is measured with the mandible in rest position and then with the teeth closed in IP. The difference between these measurements represents the interocclusal distance (free-way space).

## Group Function

When the canines and one or more posterior teeth contact on the working side in lateral excursion and no tooth contact occurs on the balancing side, the function is classified group function. Many older patients acquire this type of function when they abrade the canines enough to bring the posterior buccal cusps into contact on the working side in lateral excursion (Fig. 9–16).

## Cuspid Protected Occlusal Function

In this type of occlusion, even centric stops are noted around the arch in IP, but lateral movement of the mandible immediately discludes the posterior teeth, with the lower canine contacting the lingual surface of the upper canine. No contacts are evident on the balancing side (Fig. 9–17).

D'Amico highlighted the significance of cuspid protected occlusal function when he noted that ancient California Indian skulls showed abraded canines and incisors with functional side occlusion, whereas the mod-

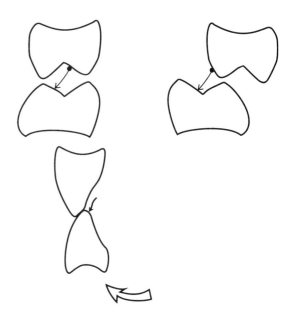

*Fig. 9–17.* Cuspid protected occlusal function. Drawing of second molar relationships bilaterally and right canine relationship in cuspid protected occlusal function. Note the right canine teeth are in contact in right lateral position but the molars are not contacting on either side. The steepness of the right canine guidance and condylar path down the left articular eminence direct the posterior mandible inferiorly so all teeth except the guiding canines are discluded.

ern California Indian (eating a less abrasive diet) has cuspid protected occlusion.[25] Cuspid protected occlusion tends to put heavy forces on the canines in eccentric occlusal positions. The periodontal ligaments of the teeth, especially the anterior teeth, are richly innervated with mechanoreceptors, the primary cell bodies of which lie in the mesencephalic nucleus of the trigeminal nerve.[26] These receptors are directionally oriented around the tooth roots so that slight displacement of the canine inhibits the motor output to the jaw-elevating muscles and stimulates the anterior belly of the digastric muscle. These periodontal ligament receptors and their neurons constitute the sensory side of a jaw-opening reflex. The intractable bruxer seems able to override or inhibit this "protective" jaw opening reflex.

### Incidence

In several studies, investigators determined the incidence of different types of occlusal function in man.[17,18,27] The subjects in

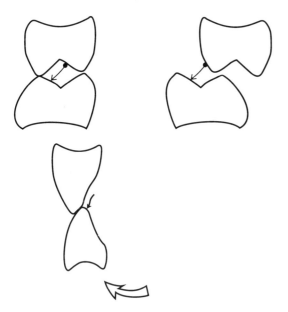

*Fig. 9–16.* Group function. Second molar relationships bilaterally and right canine relationship in group function. Note the right canine and molar facial cusps are in contact and the left second molars are not contacting in right lateral position. The balancing path of the left condyle against the articular eminence directed the left posterior mandible inferiorly so steeply that the left second molars were discluded.

one study by Weinberg had at least 28 natural teeth and ranged from 17 to 69 years of age.[27] The incidence of types of occlusal function was reported to be 19% cuspid protected occlusion, 65% group function, and 16% balanced occlusion, with no indication of unilaterality or bilaterality. In another study involving 1200 men between 17 and 25 years of age, 73% of the subjects had cuspid protected occlusion on at least one side.[17]

The great difference in incidence of cuspid protection reported in these two studies could be related to the difference in the age of the subjects. The older patients in the study by Weinberg[27] had abraded their canines so that posterior teeth made contact in lateral excursions.

In another study, 50 young adults (average age of 23 years) and 50 children (average age of 11 years) were examined by using a static method of classifying occlusal function.[18] In these subjects, lateral movement was exactly 3 mm, as indicated by a marking device fixed to the labial surface of the incisors. Quick set alginate was placed on the occlusal surfaces of the lower teeth and the subjects held the lateral position until the alginate had set. Any perforation in the alginate registrations was considered a tooth contact. If unilateral and bilateral functions are combined, the children had single tooth contact on the working side 42% of the time, and contact usually involved the first permanent molar. The adults had single tooth contact on the working side 58% of the time, usually on the canines. Greater than 84% of both the children and adults had balancing side contacts. The balancing contacts were on the first molars in children and on the second molars in the adults. No other studies have demonstrated this high an incidence of balanced occlusal function. This finding can be interpreted to show that balancing side contact can be achieved when a static lateral position is maintained, even though it may not occur during mastication.

If these few studies are sufficient to represent the population at large, the dentist can expect to find more group function in older patients and more cuspid protected occlusion in younger patients who have not abraded their canines excessively. A small percentage of patients will have balanced occlusal func-

tion of their natural teeth. All three of these types of occlusal function are noted in patients with no evidence of malocclusion.

## Clinical Application of Occlusal Function Data

A dentist should take a few minutes to classify the occlusal function of a patient before beginning restorative therapy. This analysis facilitates treatment planning as well as the restorative procedure. If a patient with a cuspid protected occlusion needs a crown on an upper canine, the dentist must decide whether to restore cuspid protected occlusion and make a conservative lingual reduction on the canine or to consider elective endodontics on the canine and reduce the lingual surface enough to provide a less steep lateral guidance in group function.

If a patient with badly abraded canines and group occlusal function needs extensive restorative dental work, the clinician may consider restoring cuspid protected function. Many factors such as periodontal health, tooth mobility, number of teeth remaining, jaw relationship, and noxious occlusal habits warrant consideration when determining whether or not to restore cuspid protected occlusal function or group function.

If a patient has cuspid protected occlusal function, an adjustment of posterior teeth, such as carving a fresh amalgam restoration, is critical only at the centric stops. After the central fossae and marginal ridges are adjusted, no posterior interferences in right and left lateral positions are likely. If the patient has group function, the posterior adjustment is critical over a larger area of the occlusal surfaces of the teeth.

If posterior occlusal surfaces are to be restored in a patient with balanced occlusal function, the dentist must pay particular attention to mesiolingual inclines of lower buccal cusps and distobuccal inclines of upper lingual cusps.

## Crossover Pathofunction

The dentist should examine occlusal function beyond the functional range, because occlusal contact beyond this point can become the position of noxious clenching and bruxing in some patients. The crossover usually results in a contact of the anterior teeth when the mandible is elevated into occlusion. Thus, thin incisal edges provide the only occlusal contacts to which bruxing forces are applied. In other cases, the posterior teeth may also contact and show abrasive facets.

A diagnostic sign of crossover bruxing is notching in the incisal edges of opposing anterior teeth. The notches or abraded facets are typically polished to a shiny surface with sharp edges. This habit often develops after some dental pathologic process or discomfort in the posterior teeth on one side prompts the patient to brace the mandible to the opposite side (Fig. 9–18).

Crossover bruxing can be diagnosed by using a provocation test of positioning the teeth in the crossover position with the notches fitting together precisely. The patient clenches or bites in this position and reports the resulting sensation. In the crossover bruxing patient, this maneuver elicits the pain that is the chief complaint. These patients invariably deny that they ever clench in the crossover position. This denial is pathognomonic, because it indicates the patient is unaware of the habit of abrading the teeth and eliciting pain. The site of pain is usually located in the TM joint contralateral to the side of the crossover, and involves the mandibular muscles on that side. The condyle on the contralateral side may show evidence of flattening on the anterior aspect where it has been positioned

against the articular eminence in the braced, crossover position for long periods. The affected condyle may also be hypermobile from the many years of stretching of the capsule and ligaments in the translated position. Family members often confirm that the patient is habitually postured in the noxious crossover position.

Making these patients aware of the crossover bruxing habit and teaching them to avoid it is therapeutic in many patients. The use of a repeat timer to accomplish this training is described in detail in the section concerning bruxism in this chapter. Occlusal splint therapy, which prevents occlusion in the crossover position by filling in the abraded facets, prevents the habit from recurring. Also, electromyographic biofeedback and muscle relaxation therapy are often effective in alleviating this noxious habit.

## Mandibular Dimensional Stability

Investigators have demonstrated that mandibular arch width decreases when the lower jaw is protruded, depressed, or moved laterally.[28-31] An average convergence was 0.07 to 0.40 mm at the first or second molar region on wide opening of the jaws. The decrease in arch width was greater at maximum protrusion, averaging 0.09 to 0.50 mm, and was least in lateral movement, averaging 0.1 mm.

When long-span fixed bridges are seated on the lower arch, stimulation of the periodontal ligament mechanoreceptors of the abutment

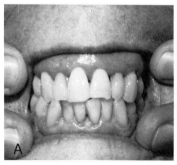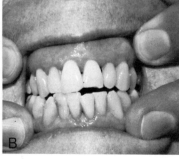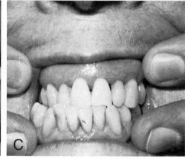

**Fig. 9–18.** Crossover bruxing facets. This patient has been bruxing in right lateral protrusive crossover for approximately 17 years and has suffered a dull pain in the left preauricular region. A. Teeth in IP only reveal notching in upper central incisors. B. Teeth in edge to edge protrusive show right incisors guiding the movement and facets in the lower left incisors are revealed. C. When the patient closes in right lateral protrusive, note that the tooth facets fit together perfectly.

teeth resulting from jaw function is abnormal. When the lingual wall of the lower first molar alveolus moves lingually as a patient opens the mouth, the receptors in the periodontal ligament are stimulated as though a lateral force from lingual to buccal was applied to the molar. This decrease in arch width not only abnormally stimulates periodontal ligament mechanoreceptors, but also applies torque to bridge abutment teeth and breaks the cement seal of the crowns in their retainers. These patients often seek help for a vague feeling of confinement of lower teeth or a sensation of a foreign body lodged in the lingual periodontium.

To diagnose this problem, the patient puts the mandible in a relaxed, rest position, and a provocation test is applied by pushing inward on both angles of the mandible (Fig. 9–19). The patient is asked if the chief complaint sensation occurs. The treatment for this problem is to replace the long-span bridge with one with flexible connectors at the distal of each canine.

The authors had a patient who incurred a mandibular symphysis fracture secondary to flexing of the mandible by muscular activity. The patient was a 59-year-old man who had undergone horizontal advancement of the anterior inferior border of the mandible, an advancing sliding genioplasty. The patient had been edentulous in the mandibular incisor area for the preceding three decades, and the alveolar process of the anterior mandible had undergone the usual physiologic resorption. After the genioplasty, the remaining unoperated bone of the anterior mandible was the thinned superior margin of the alveolar process. Six weeks after the operation, during a yawn, the mandible fractured in the midline (Fig. 9–20). Bone repair followed stabilization of the mandible with a rigid lingual splint; a bone graft was not necessary.

## Bruxism

Bruxism is defined as nonfunctional clenching, grinding, or gnashing of the teeth. Clenching of the teeth has been called centric bruxism; in this text, we use the term clenching. Grinding and gnashing of the teeth has been called eccentric bruxism; we use the term bruxing. Clenching involves mostly the masseter and temporalis muscles, whereas bruxism also involves the medial and lateral pterygoid muscles.

Bruxing is a common oral-motor behavior; the reported incidence varies between 15 and 88% of adult subjects studied.[32] It is believed that all humans engage in bruxism at some stage of their life. This parafunctional habit may result in headache, muscle pain, muscle hypertrophy, sore teeth, tooth abrasion, pulpal exposure, mobile teeth, periodontal injury, mandibular muscle fatigue, and TM joint changes. Bruxing and clenching may occur predominantly during the day (diurnal bruxism or clenching), predominantly at night (nocturnal bruxism or clenching), or during both periods. Most people brux about 10 seconds per hour on the average during sleep.[33]

### Diurnal and Nocturnal Bruxism

Findings of several studies indicate that diurnal and nocturnal bruxing are two distinct problems with different etiologies.[34-38] Nocturnal bruxing seems to be a stress-related behavior during sleep, whereas diurnal bruxing is often a learned behavior. A careful and complete history helps to identify subtle factors that lead to diurnal bruxing and clenching. Such factors as holding a telephone between the chin and shoulder, playing a violin

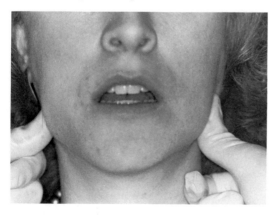

*Fig. 9–19.* Provocation test for mandibular flexibility causing noxious discomfort in a patient with a long span bridge on the lower arch. The patient opens slightly and the dentist pushes medially on the angles of the mandible, on and off, to test for the chief complaint when the mandible converges.

turnal bruxing is often associated with tension or muscle contraction headache. This headache may include the preauricular region along the origin of the masseter muscles and the occipital region along the insertion of the trapezius. In one study of 62 patients with bruxism and headache,[57] 87% of the headaches were controlled effectively by wearing a posterior discluding (Hawley-type) bite plate at night. In 7 cases, the patients were treated with a placebo splint for 1 to 2 months, and none of them had relief of the headaches. The placebo splints were then altered to provide anterior support only, and 5 of the 7 patients became completely free of headaches, 1 was improved, and 1 was unchanged.

Bruxism can occur periodically, so the presence of wear facets on the teeth is not proof that the patient is bruxing at the time of examination.[58] The facets appear shiny and well polished when the bruxing is active and they appear dull after the bruxing has stopped. Muscle tenderness subsides when bruxing ceases, so masseter tenderness is an excellent indicator of ongoing bruxism. The massive hypertrophy of the masseter muscle that often occurs with bruxism disappears within 1 or 2 weeks after cessation of the noxious habit.[59]

## Stages of Sleep

Several different methods of staging sleep based on systematic changes in electroencephalographic recordings have been identified.[60,61] All of these methods include two different types of sleep. Paradoxical sleep is called REM (rapid eye movement) sleep, and even though it seems to be a light stage of sleep, it is difficult to arouse a person during this stage. REM sleep has only one stage. Non-REM sleep ranges from light to very deep sleep, and is usually divided into three or four different stages.

### Non-REM Sleep

During wakefulness, the electroencephalogram typically shows an alpha activity of 8 to 12 cycles per second (cps), with a minimum amplitude of 40 microvolts ($\mu$V) peak to peak. Stage 1 sleep shows less than 50% alpha activity, with bursts of activity at 12 to 14 cps for about 2 seconds (sleep spindles). This stage of sleep is very light. Stage 2 is also a light stage and is characterized by slower theta waves at 4 to 7 cps, with sharp spontaneous rises followed by a slow descent (K complexes). Sleep spindles may also be seen in stage 2. Stage 3 shows 20 to 50% slow delta waves at 0.5 to 3 cps at an amplitude of at least 40 $\mu$V. Stage 4 shows more than 50% delta waves at an amplitude higher than 40 $\mu$V and constitutes a deep stage of sleep. Stages 3 and 4 non-REM sleep are usually called, simply, delta stage sleep.

### REM Sleep

The REM stage of sleep shows the alpha and theta pattern of stage 1 non-REM sleep with the addition of eye movement potentials in the tracings. Subjects typically dream during REM sleep. Again, trying to arouse a person during REM sleep is difficult.

### Typical Pattern of Sleep Stages and Bruxism

A pleasantly fatigued person lying down to sleep rapidly falls into a deep delta stage, passing through stages 1 and 2 non-REM sleep. After 50 to 100 minutes in delta, the subject moves into a lighter stage of sleep, either stage 2 non-REM or REM sleep. This light stage usually lasts 5 to 20 minutes. If the person goes into stage 2 non-REM, the skeletal muscles typically become active and the subject rolls over in bed or flails the arms or legs. Most nocturnal bruxing occurs in stage 2, but it may not be associated with pain.[62] Subjects that brux during REM sleep are likely to have pain when they awake.[63]

At the end of this period of light sleep, the subject drops back into delta stage for another 50 to 100 minutes. The subject cycles through the stages in this fashion throughout 7 or 8 hours of sleep. The ratio of delta to REM sleep is critical to normal sensitivity and balance between different parts of the central nervous system. Prolonged wakefulness leads to progressive central nervous system malfunction, such as irritability and sometimes psychosis. Medications such as L-dopa, phenothiazines, and amphetamines decrease REM sleep.[44,64,65]

Bruxism has been identified during all stages of sleep, even though it is seen more frequently in stage 2 non-REM. Subjects who brux during delta stage sleep grind with massive force and have been observed to chew up a hard acrylic splint in 3 weeks. They are especially resistant to treatment.

## Diagnosis

To diagnose diurnal and nocturnal bruxism, many of the following signs and symptoms must be present.

1. Abrasive facets on the occlusal and incisal surfaces of the teeth in excess of that expected for the patient's age and diet.
2. The patient awakens with sore teeth and tired mandibular muscles.
3. The patient awakens frequently with a headache and/or a lateral face ache.
4. The patient experiences numbness or paresthesia of the cheek.
5. Noxious occlusion may be present.
6. The patient is enduring great anxiety and emotional stress.
7. Habitual, unusual posturing of the neck that involves occlusal contact of the teeth may be present.
8. A provocation test of biting down with abrasive facets fitted together elicits the pain that is the chief complaint.
9. The patient awakens with the teeth tightly clenched.
10. The patient finds the teeth tightly clenched during the daytime when concentrating on a difficult task or when in a stressful situation.
11. The patient's spouse or roommate reports that the patient grinds the teeth at night.
12. The mandibular elevator muscles, especially the masseters, are hypertrophied, bulge outward, and harden when the patient clenches the teeth together.

## Treatment

The clinician should attempt to determine whether the bruxing or clenching habit is diurnal, nocturnal, or both. The history and examination, as just described, usually provide adequate information to make this determination.

### Diurnal Bruxism

If diurnal bruxism is present and the patient is under great stress, an explanation of the relationship of anxiety and emotional stress to bruxing often helps the patient to reduce the noxious habit. The repeat timer procedure for eliminating a daytime clenching habit is then described and demonstrated for the patient. The clinician should have a repeat timer available for the demonstration and possibly keep a supply on hand to give to the patient (Fig. 9–21). The authors set the timer to 1 minute instead of 15 minutes for the demonstration and it signals at the correct time in the discussion to teach the procedure.

A patient who appears extremely anxious or stressed is informed that behavior modification therapy helps patients respond more appropriately to events in their lives. The authors use the analogy of a coach who can observe behavior and, being an expert, the clinician can teach a patient to correct an inappropriate response to stimuli just as a golf instructor can watch a golfer, detect a flaw in a golf swing, and teach the pupil how to correct it. Without this coaching, the golfer continues to practice the flawed swing and never improves his score. Occasionally, a diurnal bruxist benefits from splint therapy, but this approach is not the first unless the patient has both diurnal and nocturnal bruxing.

### Nocturnal Bruxing

If nocturnal bruxism is diagnosed by history and examination, occlusal splint therapy verifies the diagnosis, protects the teeth from further abrasion, and often eliminates or greatly reduces the bruxing.[66,67] The diagnosis is verified by inspecting the splint and noting the amount of abrasion on the splint. If a bruxist destroys a splint in 3 weeks or cannot wear it because of tooth soreness, the patient is probably a delta stage bruxer. This patient usually responds to 10 to 50 mg of desipramine (Norpramin) at bedtime. Desipramine is contraindicated in patients taking monoamine oxidase inhibitors or with cardiovascular disease, glaucoma, urinary retention, thyroid disease, or seizure disorder.

To treat nocturnal bruxing, the authors usually construct a maxillary, full arch splint with simultaneous contact of buccal cusps of lower posterior teeth and incisal edges of anterior teeth. A mandibular splint may be indicated by such factors as patient preference, esthetics, speech, mobility of anterior teeth, and prosthetic devices.

Assuming that a maxillary splint is constructed, the articulator is opened 1 mm at the second molars and an anterior lingual table is added to the splint to produce a posterior discluding splint. Only the six lower anterior teeth contact the anterior table of the splint on closure. The patient wears the splint for 3 weeks only at night. The patient is told that the teeth will move, producing a malocclusion if the splint is worn 24 hours per day. If the symptoms are controlled and the splint is not badly abraded in 3 weeks, the anterior table is ground off using articulating ribbon until the mandibular posterior teeth buccal cusps contact the flat occlusal table of the splint. A gentle anterior guidance is created where the lingual table had prevented posterior contact before this adjustment.

At a 3-week follow-up examination, the amount of abrasion of the splint is evaluated again. If the abrasion is minimal and the patient remains comfortable, the patient is instructed to leave the splint out every other night and gradually discontinue wearing the splint. If the patient remains comfortable after discontinuing use of the splint, we recommend keeping the splint in a self-sealing plastic bag in the refrigerator for use if the bruxing recurs.

While the bruxist is testing the splint for relief of pain, the clinician continues to teach the patient the role of stress and anxiety in nocturnal bruxing. If the splint therapy is not effective, the patient may be referred for behavior modification or doxepine (Sinequan, 25 mg at bedtime) and baclofen (Lioresal, 5 mg tid) are prescribed. This combination of muscle relaxant and psychotropic medication usually reduces or eliminates nocturnal bruxing when used in combination with a splint.

When bruxism occurs in patients after operations involving the TM joint, diagnosis and treatment of the problem are critical to the outcome of the procedure. If such a patient begins bruxing within 10 to 14 days postoperatively, the effect on the healing joint is as detrimental as an orthopedic patient running a 100-yard dash 10 days after knee surgery.

In a recent pilot study using an intrasubject replication experimental design,[68] we found that night time use of an occlusal and placebo splint reduced the frequency of masseter EMG activity but did not affect the duration or amplitude of the activity. In another study using an EMG-activated alarm, two staff clinical psychologists at our facial pain center studied 10 nocturnal bruxers, recording bruxing episodes for 28 nights.[69] They found that EMG-triggered alarms reduced bruxing rates and did not adversely affect self-reports of sleepiness, vigor, or fatigue. They recounted some evidence that reduced bruxing rates were maintained after the alarm was discontinued. A great need exists for more research designed to identify better methods of treating and eliminating bruxing and clenching habits.

### Bruxism in Children

The incidence of bruxism in children varies from 5 to 81% of the children studied.[70,71] One infant with newly erupted lower central incisors lacerated the upper anterior gum pad before the upper central incisors erupted.[72] A moderate amount of occlusal wear is consistently observed on the primary teeth. Because the enamel is thin on primary teeth, extensive occlusal abrasion occurs in children who brux. Production of secondary dentin may not keep pace with abrasion in the child bruxer, so pulpal exposure and dental abscess may occur.[73]

Systemic factors that may cause bruxism in children include calcium and vitamin deficiencies, intestinal infestation with pinworms, food allergy, recurrent urologic dysfunction, hyperthyroidism, hyperkinesia, and pubertal growth spurt.[48]

Occlusal interferences and deflective occlusal contacts may trigger bruxism in children. Incisor crossbite, class II malocclusion, and buccal crossbite of posterior teeth are listed as the most common types of occlusal interference.[74] Anterior guidance on posterior teeth rather than the anterior teeth has also been correlated with bruxism in children.

Headaches in school children are often correlated with bruxism and dental abrasion. The authors treated an 8-year-old boy who had suffered incapacitating headaches for 4 years. Radiographic and neurologic examination had not revealed the cause of the headaches. A maxillary, full arch splint built in centric relation with moderate anterior guidance relieved his headaches as long as he wore the splint. Over 13 months, we constructed three splints to allow for tooth eruption and maxillary growth. After this 13-month period of treatment, the headaches subsided.

## Pinworm Infestation

One of the causes of forceful nocturnal bruxing, especially in children, is pinworm (*Enterobius vermicularis*) infestation. The symptoms of pinworm infestation are perianal, perineal, and vaginal irritation; local pruritis and discomfort; disturbed sleep; debilitation; and nocturnal bruxism. Children infested with pinworms convert from sound, quiet sleepers to violent bruxers, making enough noise to waken their parents and siblings in separate bedrooms. The condition is diagnosed by applying an adhesive tape swab to the perianus in the early morning hours before the child awakens. The swab is then examined for pinworm eggs.

Misconceptions about pinworm infestation are numerous. Man is the only host of the pinworm. It does not attach to the intestine, has no tissue-migrating stage, and causes no blood changes. This information is reassuring to a concerned parent. Dogs and cats can only help to spread the disease among humans by carrying the eggs from an infected child on their fur. Kindergarten and play schools are fertile sources for passage of the pinworm.

The gravid female pinworm contains as many as 11,000 eggs, and she migrates to the perianal region in the early morning hours where the eggs are expelled. The eggs remain infectious from 3 hours to 2 days. Pinworm infestation affects 18 million people in North America. The incidence is higher in whites than in blacks. The infestation is cured with pyrantel pamoate (Antiminth oral suspension, 11 mg/kg orally as a single dose and a repeat dose 2 weeks later). The maximum dosage is 1 gram. Transient elevations in SGOT occur infrequently, so caution is indicated in patients with liver disease.

## Hereditary Factors

In a study of twins, monozygotic twins had a significantly higher frequency of identical dental bruxing facet patterns than did dizygotic twins.[75] Environmental factors such as imitation of the parent's habits by the child may play a role in the etiology of bruxing, as evidenced by a high incidence of bruxing in children and their parents.[76]

## Allergy

Itching, sneezing, and coughing during the night in allergic children may be relieved by clenching and grinding. In one study, investigators reported that the incidence of bruxing in allergic children is 60% whereas the incidence in nonallergic children is 20%.[47] Marks postulated that allergic edema of the mucosa in the auditory tubes may lead to nocturnal bruxism.[47] The mucosal swelling closes the auditory tube orifice at torus tubarius, which reduces the pressure in the middle ear by absorption of the trapped gases into the water of the vascular bed of the cavity lining. The dilator tubae and tensor veli palatini are attached to the fibrous anterior wall of the auditory tube. When they contract, their tension pulls the tube open. During sleep, these muscles scarcely function, but with decreased pressure stimulus in the middle ear, the patient bruxes to secrete saliva and swallows to open the auditory tube when the tensor veli palatini and dilator tubae contract. In these patients, bruxism has been eliminated or reduced significantly with appropriate treatment of allergies.

## Psychologic Factors

Anxiety from stresses at school or in the home can lead to nocturnal bruxing in children just as in adults. Children under great pressure to excel in competitive sports clench their teeth on the playing field. An effective measure is to hold a conference with the parents to discuss possible pressure placed on the child. Relaxation exercises and biofeedback may be as effective in children as in adults.

# References

1. Posselt U.: Studies in the mobility of the human mandible. Acta Odontol Scand, 10 (Suppl. 10), 1952
2. Beyron H.: Occlusal relationship and mastication in Australian aborigines. Acta Odontol Scand, 22:597, 1964
3. Kydd W.L. and Sander A.: A study of posterior mandibular movements from intercuspal occlusal position. J Dent Res, 49:419, 1961
4. Hodge L.C. and Mahan P.E.: A study of mandibular movement from centric occlusion to maximum intercuspation. J Prosthet Dent, 18:19, 1967
5. Graham M.M., et al: A study of occlusal relationship and the incidence of myofascial pain. J Prosthet Dent, 47:549, 1982
6. Solberg W.K., et al: Prevalence of mandibular dysfunction in young adults. J Am Dent Assoc, 98:25, 1979
7. Rieder C.E.: The prevalence and magnitude of mandibular displacement in a survey population. J Prosthet Dent, 35:299, 1976
8. Maruyama T., et al: Analysis of the mandibular relationship of TMJ-dysfunction patients using the mandibular kinesiograph. J Oral Rehabil, 9:217, 1982
9. Ramfjord S.P.: Bruxism, a clinical and electromyographic study. J Am Dent Assoc, 62:21, 1961
10. Graf H. and Zander H.A.: Tooth contact patterns in mastication. J Prosthet Dent, 13:1055, 1963
11. Pameijer J.H.N., et al: Intraoral occlusal telemetry. III. Tooth contacts in chewing, swallowing and bruxism. J Periodontol, 40:253, 1969
12. Ingervall B. and Egermark-Eriksson I.: Function of temporal and masseter muscles in individuals with dual bite. Angle Orthod, 49:131, 1979
13. Moyers R.E.: Temporomandibular muscle contraction patterns in angle class III, division I malocclusions: An electromyographic analysis. Am J Orthod, 35:837, 1949
14. Jarabak J.R.: An electromyographic analysis of muscular and temporomandibular joint disturbances due to imbalances in occlusion. Angle Orthod, 26:170, 1956
15. Perry H.T. and Harris S.C.: Role of the neuromuscular system in functional activity of the mandible. J Am Dent Assoc, 48:665, 1954
16. Dawson P.E.: Evaluation, Diagnosis and Treatment of Occlusal Problems. St. Louis, C.V. Mosby, 1974
17. Scaife R.R. and Holt J.E.: Natural occurrence of cuspid guidance. J Prosthet Dent, 22:225, 1969
18. Ingervall B.: Tooth contacts on the functional and nonfunctional side in children and young adults. Arch Oral Biol, 17:191, 1972
19. Jerge C.R.: The neurologic mechanism underlying cyclic jaw movements. J Prosthet Dent, 14:667, 1964
20. Sessle B.J. and Schmitt A.: Effects of controlled tooth stimulation on jaw muscle activity in man. Arch Oral Biol, 17:1587, 1972
21. Ramfjord S.P. and Ash M.M.: Occlusion. 2nd Ed. Philadelphia, W.B. Saunders, 1971
22. Shyrock E.: Personal communication, Sept. 1973
23. Tallgren A.: Positional changes of complete dentures. A 7-year longitudinal study. Acta Odontol Scand, 27:539, 1969
24. Ingervall B.: Relation between contact, intercuspal, and rest positions of mandible in children with Angle class II, division 2 malocclusion. Odontol Rev, 19:1, 1968
25. D'Amico A.: Canine teeth: Normal functional relation of the natural teeth of man. J Southern Calif Dent Assoc, 26:6, 1958
26. Jerge C.R.: Organization and function of the trigeminal mesencephalic nucleus. J Neurophysiol, 26:379, 1963
27. Weinberg L.A.: A cinematic study of centric and eccentric occlusions. J Prosthet Dent, 14:290, 1964
28. McDowell J.A. and Regli C.P.: A quantitative analysis of the decrease in width of the mandibular arch during forced movements of the mandible. J Dent Res, 40:1183, 1961
29. Osborne J. and Tomlin H.R.: Medial convergence of the mandible. Br Dent J, 117:112, 1964
30. Regli C.P. and Kelly E.K.: The phenomenon of decreased mandibular arch width in opening movements. J Prosthet Dent, 17:49, 1967
31. Burch J.G.: Patterns of change in human mandibular arch width during jaw excursions. Arch Oral Biol, 17:623, 1972
32. Scharer P.: Bruxism. Front Oral Physiol, 1:293, 1974
33. Powell R.N.: Tooth contact during sleep: Association with other events. J Dent Res, 44:959, 1965
34. Rugh J.D. and Solberg W.K.: Electromyographic studies of bruxist behavior before and during treatment. J Calif State Dent Assoc, 3:56, 1975
35. Funch D.P. and Gale E.N.: Factors associated with nocturnal bruxism and its treatment. J Behav Med, 31:385, 1980
36. Ingle J.I.: Occupational bruxism and its relation to periodontal disease. J Periodontol, 23:7, 1952
37. Robinson J.E., et al: Nocturnal teeth-grinding: A reassessment for dentistry. J Am Dent Assoc, 78:1308, 1969
38. Rugh J.D. and Ohrback R.: Occlusal parafunction. In A Textbook of Occlusion. Edited by N.D. Mohl, G.A. Zarb, G.E. Carlsson, and J.D. Rugh. Chicago, Quintessence Publishing, 1988
39. Rieder C.E.: Possible premature degenerative temporomandibular joint disease in violinists. J Prosthet Dent, 35:662, 1976
40. Friction J.: Personal communication, March, 1989
41. Vernallis F.F.: Teeth-grinding: Some relationships to anxiety, hostility and hyperactivity. J Clin Psychol, 11:389, 1955
42. Randow K., et al: The effect of an occlusal interference on the masticatory system. An experimental investigation. Odont Rev, 27:245, 1976
43. Thaller J.I.: The use of the Cornell Index to determine the correlation between bruxism and the anxiety state: A preliminary report. J Periodontol, 31:138, 1960
44. Ashcroft G.W., et al: Recognition of amphetamine addicts. Br Med J, 1:57, 1965
45. Lindqvist B. and Heijbel J.: Bruxism in children with brain damage. Acta Odontol Scand, 32:313, 1974
46. Satoh T. and Harada Y.: Electrophysiological study on tooth grinding during sleep. Electroencephalogr Clin Neurophysiol, 35:267, 1973
47. Marks M.B.: Bruxism in allergic children. Am J Orthod, 77:48, 1980
48. Ahmad R.: Bruxism in children. J Periodont, 10:105, 1986
49. Christensen L.V.: Facial pain and internal pressure of masseter muscle in experimental bruxism in man. Arch Oral Biol, 16:1021, 1971
50. Clark T.D. Jr.: A neurophysiologic study of bruxism in the rhesus monkey. Meeting of the American Dental Association, Las Vegas, 1970
51. Ramfjord S. and Ash M.M.: Bruxism and related oc-

clusal habits: Epidemiology, etiology and significance. *In* Occlusion. 3rd Ed. Philadelphia, W.B. Saunders, 1983

52. Krogh-Poulsen W.: The significance of occlusion in temporomandibular function and dysfunction. *In* Temporomandibular Joint Problems: Biologic Diagnosis and Treatment. Edited by W.K. Solberg and G.T. Clark. Chicago, Quintessence Publishing, 1980

53. Lundeen H.C. and Gibbs C.H.: Advances in Occlusion. Edited by J. Wright. Boston, PSG Inc, 1982

54. Murphy T.R.: The relationship between attritional facets and occlusal plane in aboriginal Australians. Arch Oral Biol, *9*:269, 1964

55. Mongini F.: Dental abrasion as a factor in remodeling of the mandibular condyle. Acta Anat (Basel), *92*:292, 1975

56. Ingle J.I.: Alveolar osteoporosis and pulpal death associated with compulsive bruxism. Oral Surg Oral Med Oral Pathol, *13*:1371, 1960

57. Berlin R. and Dessner L.: Bruxism and chronic headache. Lancet, *2*:289, 1960

58. Graf H.: Bruxism. Dent Clin North Am, *31*:659, 1969

59. Ahlgren J., et al: Bruxism and hypertrophy of the masseter muscle. A clinical, morphological and functional investigation. Pract Oto-laryngol, *31*:22, 1969

60. Dement W.C. and Kleitman N.: Cyclic variations in EEG during sleep and their relation to eye movements, body motility and dreaming. Electroencephalogr Clin Neurophysiol, *9*:673, 1957

61. Webb W.B., ed.: Research: An Introduction. *In* Biological Rhythms, Sleep and Performance. New York, John Wiley and Sons, 1982

62. Reding G.R., et al: Nocturnal teeth-grinding: All night psychophysiologic studies. J Dent Res, *47*:786, 1968

63. Rugh J.D. and Ware J.C.: Polysomnographic comparison of nocturnal bruxists with and without facial pain. J Dent Res (Special Issue), *65*:180, 1986

64. Magee K.R.: Bruxism related to levodopa therapy. JAMA, *214*:147, 1970

65. Kamen S.: Tardive dyskinesia: A significant syndrome for geriatric dentistry. Oral Surg Oral Med Oral Pathol, *39*:52, 1975

66. Solberg W.K. and Rugh J.D.: Nocturnal electromyographic evaluation of bruxism patients undergoing short-term splint therapy. J Oral Rehabil, *2*:215, 1975

67. Sheikholeslam A., et al: A clinical and electromyographic study of the long-term effects of an occlusal splint on the temporal and masseter muscles in patients with functional disorders and nocturnal bruxism. J Oral Rehabil, *13*:137, 1986

68. Cassisi J.E., et al: Occlusal splint effects on nocturnal bruxing: An emerging paradigm and some early results. J Craniomandib Pract, *5*:64, 1987

69. Cassisi J.E. and McGlynn F.D.: Effects of EMG-activated alarms on nocturnal bruxism. Behav Res Ther, *19*:133, 1988

70. Leof M.: Clamping and grinding habits: Their relation to periodontal disease. J Am Dent Assoc, *31*:184, 1944

71. Reding G.R., et al: Incidence of bruxism. J Dent Res, *45*:1198, 1966

72. Arnold M.: Bruxism and the occlusion. Dent Clin North Am, *25*:395, 1981

73. Schneider P.E.: Oral habits: Consideration in management. Pediatr Clin North Am, *29*:523, 1982

74. Egermark-Eriksson I. and Ingervall B.: Anomalies of occlusion pre-disposing to occlusal interference in children. Angle Orthod, *52*:293, 1982

75. Lindqvist B.: Bruxism in twins. Acta Odontol Scand, *32*:177, 1974

76. Kuch E.V., et al: Bruxing and non-bruxing children: A comparison of their personality traits. Pediatr Dent, *1*:182, 1979

## Anatomy

Most of the synovial, diarthrodial, or freely moveable joints of the body develop in a primary cartilaginous matrix. They have articular surfaces of hyaline cartilage that articulate directly against each other with an incomplete cartilaginous meniscus intervening. The temporomandibular (TM) joint is an exception in that it does not form in a primary cartilaginous matrix. The condylar process of the mandible forms by endochondral ossification of a secondary cartilage. The glenoid fossa and articular eminence form in the temporal bone by intramembranous ossification. Meckel's cartilage, the primary cartilage of the first branchial arch, forms the malleus and incus bones, the anterior malleolar ligament (Pinto's ligament), and the sphenomandibular ligament. It does not contribute to the formation of the TM joint, but the relationship of its structures to the joint are discussed later in this chapter.

The articular surfaces of the glenoid fossa, articular eminence, and condyle consist essentially of collagen. Small areas of cartilage cells are seen on the crest of the articular eminence, but on the condyle, the secondary cartilage is completely covered by collagen. For the purposes of this book, we define meniscus as all the tissues located between the condyle and the articular eminence, glenoid fossa, and tympanic plate of the temporal bone, and the disk is the avascular part of the meniscus that lies above and anterior to the condyle.

This disk consists of collagen that is organized in sheets of anterior-posteriorly oriented fibers on the superior and inferior surfaces, whereas the thicker, peripheral areas show fibers oriented in all three directions in space.[1] Chondroid cells have been identified in menisci from subjects 30 years of age and older, but no parallel rows of chondrocytes in a cartilaginous matrix as seen in hyaline cartilage are evident.[2] In the TM joint of 60- to 80-year-old patients, lacunae are visible in the thicker portions of the disk with a chondroid cell nucleus in the center. The anterior edge of the disk (in a sagittal section) is shaped like a foot (pes meniscus). The central portion of the disk is thinner and the posterior margin lo-

cated just superior to the condyle is called the posterior band. The pliable disk is thus able to provide stabilization of the condyle against the articular eminence, even though the embrasure between the two bones varies greatly as the condyle translates from a concave fossa to a convex eminence. A stiff, cartilaginous meniscus could not serve such a function. The volume of the flexible disk is adequate to fill the potential spaces during all functional positions of the condyle when these spaces are not filled with contrast media, medicine, or fluids used during arthroscopic procedures.

Synovial tissues that line the periphery of the superior cavity appear as villi in sagittal sections of the joint (Fig. 10–1). The villi are actually folds of synovial membrane that extend from the medial to the lateral region of the joint. These folds allow the condyle-disk assembly to translate as far as 15 mm anteriorly by unfolding with movement of the condyle. The synovial tissues of the inferior cavity are also folded into villi. This synovial membrane allows the meniscus to rotate posteriorly as the condyle translates forward. Lymphatic capillaries are located in the synovial villi and provide lymph fluid for the creation of the small amount of synovial fluid necessary to lubricate the articular surfaces of the joint. When a needle is inserted into the superior and inferior cavities of the healthy TM joint, synovial fluid cannot be aspirated. The passive fill volume of the superior cavity, however, averages 1.2 ml and that of the inferior cavity averages 0.9 ml.[3] Studies in 11 patients with hypermobility of the TM joint revealed a 60% increase in the superior cavity passive fill volume (1.9 ml) and 20% increase in the inferior cavity (1.1 ml).

The posterior attachments of the disk are complicated. This region of the meniscus, the bilaminar zone, contains two strata of fibers with loose, areolar connective tissue, blood vessels, and nerves filling the space between the layers (Fig. 10–1). The superior stratum is rich in elastin and is loosely attached to the tympanic plate and tragal cartilages. Elastin is the only connective tissue of the body that has a true modulus of elasticity. Because the meniscus in the healthy TM joint is tightly attached to the medial and lateral pole of the

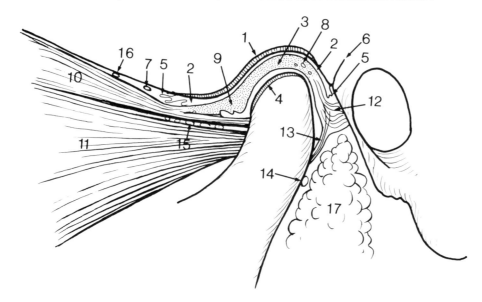

*Fig. 10–1.* Parasagittal cut through middle of the human temporomandibular joint angled 25° medially toward the anterior. 1. Articular surface of glenoid fossa; 2. Superior cavity; 3. Disk (avascular); 4. Articular surface of condyle; 5. Synovial membranes; 6. Squamo-tympanic suture; 7. Masseteric nerve; 8. Vascular knee of meniscus; 9. Pes meniscus; 10. Superior head of lateral pterygoid; 11. Inferior head of lateral pterygoid; 12. Superior stratum of bilaminar zone of meniscus; 13. Inferior stratum of bilaminar zone of meniscus; 14. Auriculotemporal nerve; 15. Blood vessels; 16. Posterior deep temporal nerve; 17. Parotid gland.

condyle (see Fig. 10–2), its attachment to bone posteriorly must be loose and elastic to allow the disk to translate forward with the condyle.[4] The inferior stratum of the bilaminar zone is not stretched as the condyle translates forward, because the meniscus rotates posteriorly, relieving tension in this stratum (see subsequent discussion).

Pressure changes in the bilaminar zone of the TM joint meniscus become negative when the condyle translates forward and positive when it moves back into the fossa.[5] The maximum pressure measured was +16 mm Hg with rapid retrusion of the condyle in an angle class III subject, but the usual range was ± 1 mm Hg. These pressures are not remarkably high considering that the pressure in the lung alveoli varies from −1 to +3 mm Hg during normal breathing. This passive pressure gradient is actually applied across the cardiovascular system so blood is aspirated into the capillaries and venous sinuses that abound in this zone when the mouth is opened and the condyle translates forward. Magnetic resonance imaging of the TM joint reveals a high signal in the retrodiskal zone, indicating water in this area in the mouth open view. This influx of blood moves the synovial membranes into the embrasures between the condyle and temporal bone during function. This synovial membrane function allows a near constant volume for the joint cavities as the mouth opens and closes. The volume of synovial fluid cannot change as rapidly as the condyles move during talking and eating, so the synovial membranes must move rapidly into the embrasures supported by the blood that moves into the retrodiskal zone in response to the pressure gradient during mouth opening. In patients with TM joint internal derangement, the abused synovial membranes may be caught momentarily or pinched in the embrasure during condylar translation, producing a soft clicking sound, which accounts for some of the aberrant sounds heard in dysfunctioning joints.

Behind the superior aspect of the condyle and anterior to the bilaminar zone, the meniscus is vascular. Tissue in this region, called the vascular knee (genu vasculosa),[6] extends throughout the bilaminar zone and may contain glomus cell arteriovenous shunts. Actually, blood vessels completely encircle the avascular central area of the meniscus.[7] Blood is shunted back and forth with jaw function to compensate for the volume of the condyle as it leaves the glenoid fossa and translates to the region of the crest of the eminence. The zone between the bellies of the lateral pterygoid, just anterior to the foot of the disk, is also vascular. These blood vessels supply the two bellies of the lateral pterygoid muscle as well as the anterior joint structures. At birth, the entire meniscus and the superior surface of the condyle are vascularized. The central region of the meniscus, the disk area, becomes avascular soon after birth. The fetal condyle is penetrated by vascular canals, with their blood vessels anastomosing over the articular surface.[8] These vessels normally disappear by age 3 years. Results of studies in monkeys revealed that perforations in the avascular disk do not heal and lead to degenerative arthritic changes, whereas those at the disk periphery involving a vascular zone sometimes fill in and heal completely.[9]

The medial one half of the anterior aspect of the TM joint has no capsule. The superior head or belly of the lateral pterygoid muscle sends a small percentage of its fibers into the foot of the disk at the medial corner. Most of the lateral pterygoid fibers continue under the foot of the disk to attach into the condylar neck (pterygoid fovea). Lateral to the attachment of the muscle into the disk, the connective tissue forms a capsule-like structure with the appearance of loose, areolar connective tissue. This lack of anterior capsule at its medial or deep side is the anatomic Achilles heel of the TM joint. Hypertranslation of the condyle is not prevented by a sturdy anterior capsule, so injury to the synovial tissues and areolar connective tissue can occur with excessive translation. This anatomic feature is probably related to the reported high incidence of TM joint pain and dysfunction after whiplash injury.[10] With rapid extension of the neck in a whiplash, the supra- and infrahyoid muscles cannot lengthen rapidly enough; they hold back on the mandibular symphysis, whipping the condyles forward excessively. The posterior deep temporal and masseteric nerves are located on the temporal bone just anterior to the articular eminence, near the path of hypertranslation of the condyles, and they could also be injured. The lateral one half of the condyle is thrust into the posterior margin of the temporalis and these fibers can be

bruised and stretched. Hypertranslation of the condyle during medical and dental procedures may lead to pain that is usually transient.

The capsule on the medial and lateral wall of the joint comprises well-organized collagen fibers, but the fibers are not under tension. This laxity in the fiber arrangements does not firmly support the joint, but allows the medial and lateral poles of the condyles to translate forward without tearing the capsule.

Unlike the capsular attachments, the disk is tightly attached to the lateral and medial poles of the condyle in the healthy TM joint. No meniscus-condyle discoordination with joint clicking or popping occurs unless these attachments are loosened or torn (Fig. 10–2).

Excising the TM joint capsule over the lateral pole of the condyle allows access to the superior cavity of the joint. With the usual lateral surgical approach to the TM joint, the disk must be released from its tight attachment at the lateral pole to allow entry into the inferior cavity. It follows that the disk should not be sutured to the capsule during closing,

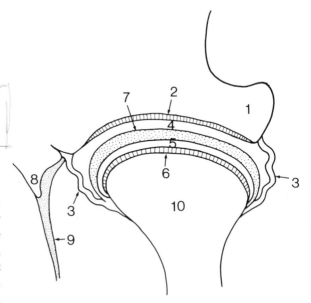

*Fig. 10–2.* Coronal cut through the human temporomandibular joint along the long axis of the condyle. 1. Posterior root of zygomatic arch; 2. Articular surface of glenoid fossa; 3. TM joint capsule; 4. Superior joint cavity (potential space); 5. Inferior joint cavity (potential space); 6. Articular surface of the condyle; 7. Disk; 8. Spinous process of sphenoid bone; 9. Sphenomandibular ligament; 10. Condyle.

because this attachment would fix the lateral aspect of the disk to the lateral lip of the glenoid fossa. In this instance, the disk could not translate with the condyle, as seen in normal joint function. The posterior wall of the joint lacks a well-organized capsule. The loose, vascular tissue in this zone constitutes a meshwork of connective tissue fibers, including collagen, reticulin, and elastin. When the anatomist bluntly dissects supraperiosteally in a superior direction along the posterior surface of the ramus to the level of the tragal cartilages and tympanic plate, the dissection creates a connective tissue sheet that has been misconstrued as a well-organized capsule. As shown in Figures 10–3 to 10–8, retrodiskal tissue is not organized in this fashion.

Several structures actually pass through the medial side of the TM joint. In the medial wall of the glenoid fossa, where the squamotympanic, petrotympanic, and squamopetrosal sutures meet, the anterior tympanic artery and vein, the chorda tympani nerve, and the anterior malleolar ligament enter the superior cavity. The anterior malleolar ligament (Pinto's ligament) is attached to the anterior process of the malleus superiorly.[11] It passes through the petrotympanic fissure and medial capsule, then continues as the sphenomandibular ligament inferiorly to attach to the lingula of the mandible.[12] In a study of 52 TM joints, 3 anterior malleolar ligaments were large diameter ligaments that could be mobilized in the petrotympanic fissure.[13] Most of the sphenomandibular ligaments had a broad band extending into the fissure and a smaller band attaching to the spinous process of the sphenoid bone.

Both open and arthroscopic TM joint surgical procedures have been associated with tearing of the posterior-superior quadrant of the tympanic membrane and loss of hearing. This trauma can result from tension on the anterior malleolar ligament via the sphenomandibular ligament as the mandible is depressed inferiorly by instrumentation (Fig. 10–9). In a recent arthroscopic examination of the TM joint, the patient became deaf on the side of the examination. The stapes plate was torn out of the oval window and the tympanic membrane was torn in the posterior-superior quadrant, but no penetration into the middle ear was found. Tapes of the procedure showed significant inferior deflection of the condyle by pressure of the irrigating fluid and leverage by the scope against the condyle. The logical explanation for these findings is that this patient had a large anterior malleolar ligament that was mobilized by inferior displacement of the mandible. Tension on the malleus tore the tympanic membrane and pulled the stapes plate out of the oval window.

The collateral ligament of the joint, the temporomandibular ligament, extends from the lateral and inferior surface of the zygomatic arch to the lateral neck of the condylar process and into the lateral capsule and disk in some cases. The posterior and inferior direction of this ligament allows it to function like a pendulum during translation of the condyle, so it resists excessive posterior-inferior condylar

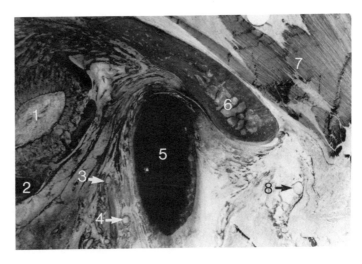

*Fig. 10–3.* Sagittal cut through 45-year-old male TM joint at lateral pole of condyle. 1. External auditory meatus; 2. Tragal cartilage; 3. Frontal branch of cranial nerve VII; 4. Zygomatic branch of cranial nerve VII; 5. Condyle; 6. Posterior root of zygomatic arch; 7. Temporalis muscle; 8. Masseteric nerve. (Figures 10–3 to 10–8 courtesy of Drs. Richard Marguelles, J.P. Young, P. Carpentier, and M. Meunissier, Paris, France.)

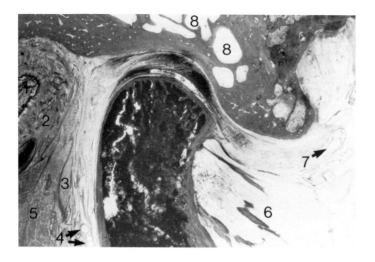

*Fig. 10–4.* Sagittal cut at junction of lateral and medial thirds of condyle of cadaver shown in Fig. 10–3. 1. External auditory meatus; 2. Tragal cartilage; 3. Auriculotemporal nerve; 4. Three upper branches of cranial nerve VII; 5. Parotid gland; 6. Inferior head of lateral pterygoid muscle; 7. Masseteric nerve; 8. Mastoid air cells.

*Fig. 10–5.* Sagittal cut through middle of condyle of cadaver shown in Fig. 10–3. 1. Parotid gland; 2. Posterior band of disk; 3. Mastoid air cell; 4. Foot of disk; 5. Superior head of lateral pterygoid muscle; 6. Anterior extent of superior cavity; 7. Masseteric nerve; 8. Inferior head of lateral pterygoid muscle.

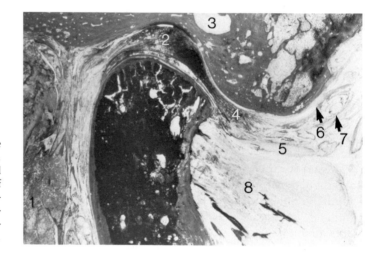

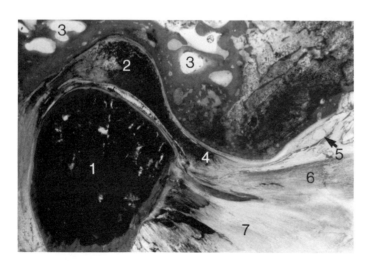

*Fig. 10–6.* Sagittal cut through junction of middle and medial thirds of condyle of cadaver shown in Fig. 10–3. 1. Condyle; 2. Posterior band of disk; 3. Mastoid air cell; 4. Foot of disk; 5. Masseteric nerve; 6. Superior head of lateral pterygoid muscle; 7. Inferior head of lateral pterygoid muscle.

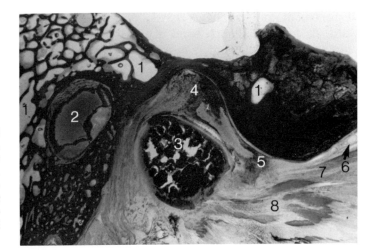

*Fig. 10–7.* Sagittal cut through medial pole of condyle of cadaver shown in Fig. 10–3. 1. Mastoid air cells; 2. Tympanic membrane; 3. Medial pole of condyle; 4. Posterior band of disk showing chondroid cells; 5. Foot of disk; 6. Masseteric nerve; 7. Superior head of lateral pterygoid muscle; 8. Inferior head of lateral pterygoid muscle.

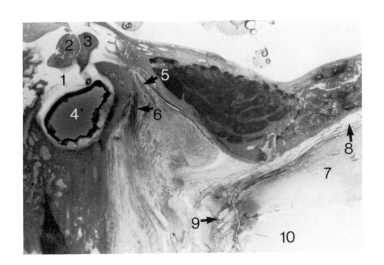

*Fig. 10–8.* Sagittal cut through medial capsule of the TMJ of cadaver shown in Fig. 10–3. 1. Middle ear cavity; 2. Incus; 3. Malleus; 4. Tympanic membrane; 5. Anterior malleolar (Pinto's) ligament in petrotympanic fissure; 6. Discomalleolar ligament; 7. Superior head of lateral pterygoid muscle; 8. Masseteric nerve; 9. Auriculotemporal nerve; 10. Inferior head of lateral pterygoid muscle.

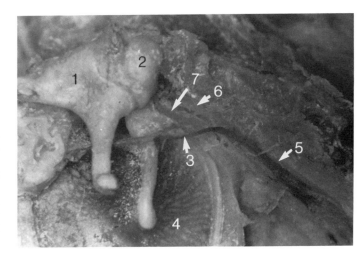

*Fig. 10–9.* View of medial side of tympanic membrane from within the middle ear cavity. 1. Incus; 2. Malleus; 3. Chorda tympani nerve; 4. Tympanic membrane; 5. Petrotympanic fissure; 6. Anterior malleolar ligament; 7. Discomalleolar ligament. (Courtesy of Dr. Barry Loughner, University of Florida Facial Pain Center.)

displacement and still allows translation forward. A deep, horizontal band of the temporomandibular ligament may extend from the crest of the articular tubercle to the lateral pole of the condyle.[14]

The sphenomandibular and stylomandibular ligaments span the TM joint. The sphenomandibular ligament extends from the spine of the sphenoid bone to the lingula on the mandibular foramen in the medial surface of the ramus. This ligament represents a remnant of Meckel's cartilage and is a well-formed structure. The stylomandibular ligament extends from the styloid process to the posterior border of the ramus above the angle. This ligament is broad and appears to represent a confluence of fascial planes.

The medial, posterior, and lateral walls of the TM joint capsule and the lateral one half of the anterior wall are innervated by a large branch of the auriculotemporal nerve as it crosses posterior to the neck of the condylar process.[15] Blocking this nerve just posterior to the condylar neck anesthetizes the TM joint. The posterior deep temporal and masseteric nerves supply the anterior region of the joint, but many of their fibers are larger than the C and A delta fibers that subserve pain. They probably, therefore, subserve proprioception more than nociception.

Findings of studies in both monkey and man demonstrated that the two heads of the lateral pterygoid muscle function antagonistically.[16,17] The large inferior head contracts on mouth opening and the superior head contracts on closing. The inferior head extends from the pterygoid fovea in the neck of the condylar process, inferiorly and medially to the lateral surface of the lateral pterygoid plate (Fig. 10–10). When it contracts, it translates the condyle down onto the articular eminence and pulls medially.

The superior head inserts into the anterior-medial margin of the disk and to the pterygoid fovea (condylar neck). Its origin is at the orbital lip of the greater wing of the sphenoid bone. When it contracts or is in the active state, the condyle-disk assembly is typically moving posteriorly, up into the fossa. The condyle and disk, therefore, are held against the posterior incline of the articular eminence during closing of the mouth by the eccentric work of the superior head. The small percentage of fibers attaching to the medial corner of the disk tend to rotate the disk back to the anterior articular surface of the condyle during mouth closing (Fig. 10–11). Thus, the eccentric work of the superior head maintains contact of TM joint articular surfaces during mouth closure and brings the disk back onto the anterior aspect of the articular surface of the condyle as it moves back and up into the fossa. This repositioning of the disk is necessary because the elastic superior stratum of the bilaminar zone exerts passive, elastic tension on the disk during opening and rotates the disk backward on the condyle. Because this tension is passive and is maintained (in diminishing amount) during closure, the disk tends to stay on the posterior of the condyle at intercuspal position unless the superior head pulls anteriorly on the disk during closure.

The thinnest and most compact part of the disk is in its central zone and is positioned between the posterior incline of the articular eminence and the anterior-superior surface of the condyle when the mouth is closed in intercuspal position. The dense zone usually extends over the medial pole of the condyle at the medial aspect of the joint and supports stress in the intercuspal position. This relationship between condyle, disk, and articular eminence at intercuspal position, routinely observed in cadavers when the joint is healthy, is the relationship the surgeon attempts to restore in patients with an anteriorly displaced disk.

## Joint Sounds

The normal TM joint moves silently within the usual opening and closing pathways. More than 50% of normal joints, however, produce a click-like sound at maximal opening.[18] However, sounds at maximal opening may be a click of disk displacement or a dull thud-like sound of deflection of condyle-disk assembly up and anterior to the eminence at maximum opening, and should not be confused with the normal sound.

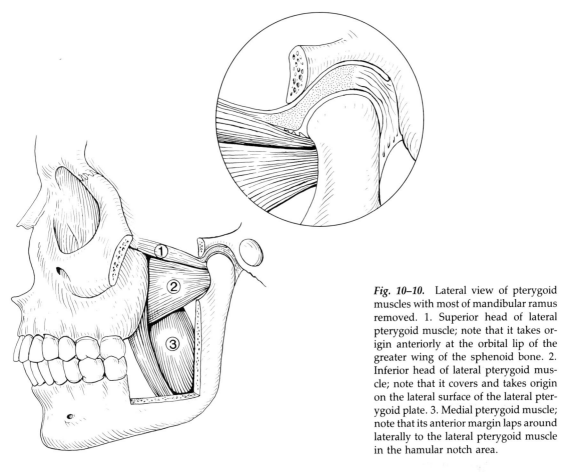

*Fig. 10–10.* Lateral view of pterygoid muscles with most of mandibular ramus removed. 1. Superior head of lateral pterygoid muscle; note that it takes origin anteriorly at the orbital lip of the greater wing of the sphenoid bone. 2. Inferior head of lateral pterygoid muscle; note that it covers and takes origin on the lateral surface of the lateral pterygoid plate. 3. Medial pterygoid muscle; note that its anterior margin laps around laterally to the lateral pterygoid muscle in the hamular notch area.

## Noncrepitus Joint Sounds

### Single, Painless Early Click on Opening

Several types of painless joint sounds occur only during opening, i.e., no reciprocal clicking (a click or popping sound made during opening and another, usually softer sound made during closing). One sound is a single, painless click heard early in the opening movement. This click is not loud, but it is usually sharp or staccato. It likely occurs because of a temporary fixation of the disk to the posterior incline of the articular eminence as the condyle begins to translate down the eminence. As soon as the compromised attachments at the medial and/or lateral poles of the condyle become taut, the fixation is released and the disk pops forward into place on the condyle with a clicking sound (Fig. 10–12). The clinical sign of this click, during dynamic palpation with the index finger, is feeling the anteriorward, rapid deflection of

tissue catching up with the condyle as it begins to translate forward.

The mechanism of the temporary fixation of the disk is unknown. It may result from roughing of the disk and articular eminence surfaces with interlocking of the irregular surfaces, or from changes in viscosity of synovial fluid. In the knee, with a period of rest, the osmolality of the synovial fluid measures 404 mOsmol/L.[19] After exercise, the osmolality decreases to approximately that of blood serum (305 mOsmol/L). The temporary fixation may also involve the forces of physical adhesion that occur when a thin layer of liquid is pressed between two surfaces so that hydrogen bonding and van der Waals forces become effective. These forces are exerted over short distances, so as soon as the disk is pulled away slightly from the articular surface of the eminence, the disk is released to pop forward.

The patient who exhibits this type of click is usually a young person who reports symp-

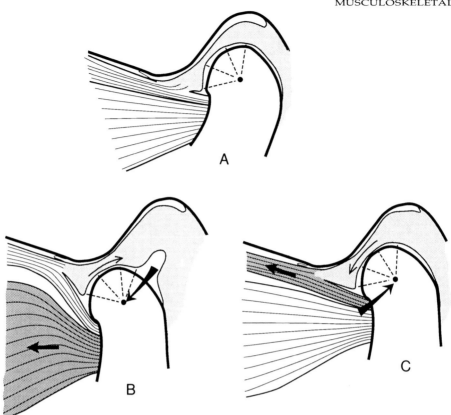

*Fig. 10–11.* Relationship between disk, articular eminence and condyle during opening and closing the mouth. A. Condyle in fossa with mouth closed and both heads of lateral pterygoid muscle relaxed. B. During mouth opening, the inferior head of the lateral pterygoid muscle is contracting (shaded), pulling the condyle down the eminence. Since the superior head is not contracting, the disk rotates backward on the condyle. C. During mouth closing, the superior head is contracting (in the active state) while it lengthens, since the condyle is translating back-up into the fossa. This eccentric contraction serves to rotate the disk forward on the condyle during mouth closure to its normal position in the fossa.

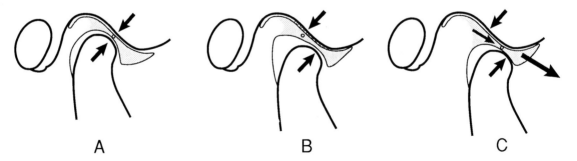

*Fig. 10–12.* Single, painless, early click on opening. A. Position of condyle and disk in the fossa with mouth closed. The dot represents the thinnest part of the disk and the arrows mark the spot on the condyle and articular eminence that oppose the dot when condyle is seated in the fossa. B. Early in opening, the disk remains fixed and the condyle translates until lateral and medial attachments of disk to condyle become taut. C. At the instant of the click, the disk is released from the articular eminence and rapidly deflects forward.

toms of nocturnal clenching or is undergoing orthodontic therapy. A universal, full arch splint or an anterior deprogrammer or Sved type splint (worn only at night) often reduces nocturnal clenching and stops this type of opening click. A lateral pterygoid isometric exercise performed 30 times per set, 4 sets per day for 4 weeks also usually stops this type of click (Fig. 10–13).

This exercise is performed by having the patient close the teeth in intercuspal position and place the palm of the hand on the chin, pushing upward and backward, forcing the teeth together. The patient then opens the teeth a few millimeters against the force of the hand. The patient attempts to hold this open position, but then increases the hand force pushing the mouth closed. This routine is repeated 30 times at a rate of 1 second opening and 1 second closing so it only takes 1 minute. The clicking may stop during the second week, but the patient should continue for the full 4-week regimen. If the patient has an interceptive occlusal contact in the centric relation closure arc or a lateral deviation in

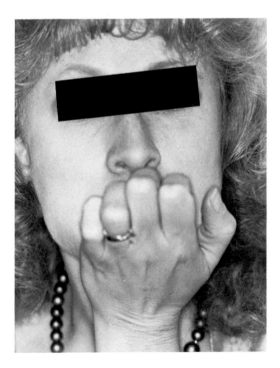

**Fig. 10–13.** Lateral pterygoid isometric exercise. The patient demonstrates correct method of applying force to elevate mandible while making opening effort and to force it closed while trying to hold open.

the slide from retruded contact to maximum intercuspation, the patient should wear a full arch occlusal splint while performing this exercise.

### Single, Painless Late Click on Opening

A second type of painless click on opening occurs at three fourths or two thirds of the opening excursion. The clinical sign noted with dynamic palpation (described in Chapter 2) is that tissue deflects back against the palpating index finger at the instant of the click. This click is also soft but staccato, and it is easy to palpate because the space behind the condyle for the palpating finger is greater when it occurs. The mechanism of this click involves a temporary fixation of the disk to the condyle as it begins to translate. The loose and elastic superior stratum of the bilaminar zone is therefore stretched excessively, because the disk is positioned further forward than normal for the amount of opening. The laxity in this disk attachment allows the condyle disk assembly to translate farther before the tension is sufficient to release the disk (Fig. 10–14). Light pressure behind the condylar lateral pole as it translates downward may prevent this click. It typically returns as soon as the palpating finger is removed.

The mechanism of the temporary fixation in this click is also unknown; roughening of the articulating surfaces, increased viscosity of synovial fluid, and physical adhesion can be postulated. These patients are typically the same group that demonstrate the first type of click. These patients also usually respond to the lateral pterygoid isometric exercise or wearing the full arch splint or anterior, deprogrammer-type splint that tend to reduce nocturnal bruxing and clenching.

### Painless Thud-Like Sound at Crest of Articular Eminence (Eminence Click)

A third type of joint sound is not a click, but rather is a dull "thunk" sound that occurs with rapid deflection of the condyles upward, anterior to the crest of the eminence (Fig. 10–15). This sound does not manifest until age 12 or 13 years at the earliest, when the articular eminence is fully formed. It may not occur in patients who develop a bulbous eminence with a steep anterior incline until years

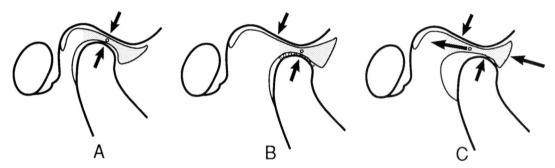

**Fig. 10–14.** Single painless late click on opening. A. Condyle in fossa with mouth closed; B. During opening the disk remains fixed to the condyle translating excessively down eminence; C. At the instant of the click the disk releases from the condyle and rapidly deflects back toward the fossa.

later, when they have extraction of lower third molars, endodontic treatment of molars, tonsillectomy, endotracheal intubation for general anesthesia, wide yawning, whiplash injury, or parkinsonian-like spasm of lateral pterygoid muscles as a drug side effect. At the instant of this sound, the entire mandible rapidly moves as the condyles deflect upward anterior to the eminence. If the patient has a tapered arch form and, therefore, a tapered face, the condyles bulge outward in two swellings just below the zygomatic arch in the preauricular region of the face. The authors have seen two patients who thought they had cancer because of these swellings.

This condition can be diagnosed by watching the bulge of the translating condyle in the face move down the eminence and then "jump" upward. Objective data are obtained by taking lateral transcranial radiographs of the patient with the mouth closed and then opened maximally. The condyle in the maximally opened position is anterior and superior to the crest of the eminence. More objective data are obtained from axiographic tracings of the condyles during the maximum opening and closing movement (Fig. 10–16).

The condyles trace a path superiorly anterior to the eminence and may be as high anteriorly to the eminence as they are in the fossa.

This condition is typically bilateral, but one condyle always moves higher than the other as it "jumps" forward. The sounds usually occur simultaneously in the two joints during opening, but one side occurs first on closing. The mandible quickly swings to the side that deflects back into the fossa first, then swings back to the midline when the second condyle deflects back into the fossa, creating one sound on opening and one sound per side on closing. This patient often reports that his mouth has locked open in the past or it feels like it is going to lock open.

The treatment for this condition is to stop opening wide. The patient is instructed to avoid biting thick sandwiches or apples, to learn to stifle yawns, and, anytime the sounds occur to stop, note what he just did to cause the sound, and avoid that action in the future. This subluxation beyond the eminence is not painful because the condyle and disk move together as they deflect anterior to the eminence; the superior stratum of the bilaminar zone is stretched excessively and rotates the

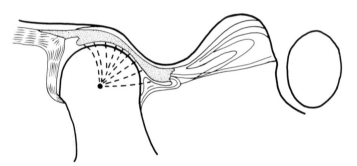

**Fig. 10–15.** The position of the condyle and disk after the opening "thud," which is painless and occurs at the crest of the eminence (eminence click). The superior stratum of the bilaminar zone is stretched excessively. The disk is still attached to the lateral pole of the condyle. This patient developed an anterior incline to the articular eminence at age 12 to 13.

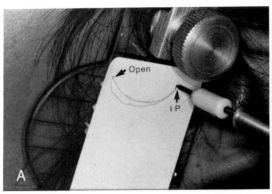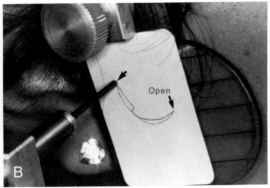

*Fig. 10–16.* Left and right axiographic tracings of a patient with a painless eminence click. A. Tracing of left condyle in which the upper tracing was recorded on opening and the lower tracing was recorded on closing. Note that the condyle was as high at maximum opening as it was in the fossa. The movement of the stylus was rapid from the lowest point in the opening pathway to the maximum open position. As the patient began to close, wedging of the disk deflected the stylus inferiorly initially. At the lowest point in the tracing (at the notch) the opposite condyle deflected rapidly around the eminence and up into the fossa. Movement was also rapid from the notch to the final position in the fossa (IP). B. Tracing of right condyle in which the opening path begins as a lower tracing, then crosses the closing trace about midway down the eminence. Note that the right condyle does not deflect as high as the left condyle when it moves anterior to the eminence. With closing, the disk does not wedge as much as the left did. At the lowest point in the closing pathway, the condyle moves rapidly back up into the fossa. Note the deflection upward in the closing tracing when the left condyle deflected rapidly around the eminence. The right condyle was already moving rapidly up the posterior eminence when the left condyle deflected around the crest of the eminence. This patient's mandible deflected to the right and then back to the midline during closing.

disk backward on the condyle farther than it normally rotates. The compressive forces in this joint position are exerted superiorly and posteriorward against the anterior slope of the eminence. The disk is still positioned in the zone of maximum compressive force because it is rotated excessively into the zone. The superior stratum is loose and elastic and the disk is avascular and not innervated, and so no pain occurs. Many patients can learn to prevent this subluxation and manage the problem after it has been explained to them. Those who cannot stop the problem often develop a painful condition that requires extensive surgical intervention to correct.

### Painful, Thud-Like Sound at Crest of Articular Eminence (Eminence Click)

When the painless subluxation of the third sound cannot by controlled by the patient, continued excessive stretching of the superior stratum of the bilaminar zone leads to injury and repair. With repair of elastic connective tissues, the elastin is replaced by collagen (scar formation). Collagen does not stretch like elastin, so more and more force is exerted on the normally tight lateral and medial attachments of the disk to the condyle. If this "tug of war" loosens the attachments to the condylar poles sufficiently, the collagenized superior stratum displaces the disk posteriorly as the condyle deflects upward, anterior to the eminence (Fig. 10–17). Because a small percentage of muscle fibers from the superior head of the lateral pterygoid are attached to the disk, deflection of the disk posterior to the condyle tears muscle fibers into the superior head and pulls them into the compressive zone of the joint, causing excruciating pain. These patients will no longer open enough to produce the subluxation because of the pain. They speak through their teeth with little mandibular movement and cannot masticate solid food. This condition cannot be diagnosed unless the patient opens maximally to demonstrate the subluxation, but accomplishing such movement is too painful. An auriculotemporal nerve anesthetic block normally relieves pain from the TM joint, but not in patients with this condition. The patient reports only 70 to 80% reduction in pain from the auriculotemporal nerve block. The pain can be relieved by a second infiltration of anesthetic (without vasoconstrictor) just

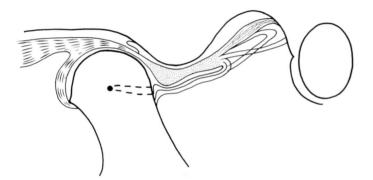

*Fig. 10–17.* Painful thud-like sound at the crest of the eminence (eminence click); the position of the condyle and disk after the painful opening "thud." The superior stratum of the bilaminar zone is scarred and will stretch less than it did in the healthy state. Consequently, the disk attachments to the medial and lateral poles are stretched or torn. As the condyle deflects upward, anterior to the eminence, it tears into the insertion of the superior head of the lateral pterygoid muscle applying pressure against the fibers attached to the disk.

anterior to the articular eminence into the superior head of the lateral pterygoid. After the two injections, the patient can open to produce the subluxation and the diagnosis can be made. A significant increase in pain is often noted when the local anesthesia wears off. Posterior displacement of the disk with anterior-superiorly displaced condyles such as described here was also reported by authors of arthrographic and magnetic resonance imaging studies of the TM joint.[20,21]

This fourth type of condition usually requires an operation to relieve the pain and pathofunction. Several surgical procedures for this condition have been reported. Because these joints are internally deranged, the disk must be repositioned on the condyle. In addition, the anatomic abnormality allowing deflection of the condyle upward and anterior to the articular eminence must be corrected. An eminectomy has been advocated to eliminate or reduce the upward deflection of the condyle. Postsurgical scarring of the joint capsule helps to prevent the condylar deflection. Approximately 2.6% of a group of more than 1000 dental patients had radiographic evidence of mastoid air cells pneumatizing the articular eminences.[22] The authors have observed a higher percentage of patients with the third and fourth type clicks who have pneumatized eminences. The clinician planning to operate on the articular eminence should be aware of the presence of these air cells. Partial myotomy of the inferior belly of the lateral pterygoid muscle weakens the muscles so they cannot pull the condyle forward beyond the eminence. Metal cribs placed at the anterior slope of the eminence in the superior cavity cause the condyle to

translate onto the crib and not deflect superiorly. Down-fracturing of the zygomatic arch, locking it under the stub of the posterior root of the arch, provides a bony stop to limit translation of the condyle. This method shortens the length of the posterior fibers of the masseter muscle. These fibers may adjust to their decreased length by a decrease in the number of sarcomeres. Sclerosing solution injected on the lateral capsule of the joint leads to scarring and prevention of translation of the condyle far enough to deflect anterior to the eminence.

### Defect in Form Click

A fifth type of noncrepitus joint sound occurs in joints with defects in form (Fig. 10–18). These articular surface abnormalities are seen in cadavers and appear to be developmental. They have rounded, smooth margins and surfaces and are normal in color. No evidence of inflammation or degeneration at the defect is noted. A concavity in the articular surface is associated with an elevation in the disk that fits into it. The clinical sign of a defect in form is that the opening click occurs at the same place as the closing click. Any hysteresis or lag of disk movement behind condylar movement is minimal. These clicks are soft and difficult to palpate. At the palpating finger, the clinician feels a vibration with minimal movement of tissues under the skin. These clicks can be verified by laminographic arthrography, if necessary. Because the clicks are usually painless, radiography is seldom performed. Instead, the patient is instructed to use care with mandibular function, to avoid chewing gum, and to use the masticatory system only when necessary.

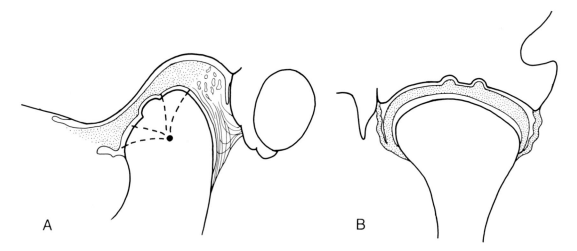

*Fig. 10–18.* Defect in form clicks. A. Protuberance on condyle located within concavity in inferior surface of disk. During opening as disk rotates around medial and lateral attachment, protuberance snaps out of concavity. During closing the protuberance snaps back into the concavity. B. Grooves of concavities in posterior incline of articular eminence. An elevation in the disk conforms to the bony defect in form. During translation anteriorly in opening or anteriorly and medially during lateral movement (balancing movement), the disk elevations snap out of the bony defect. On closing, they snap back into the defects at the same location as on opening.

Most patients manage this type of clicking when the condition has been explained to them.

### Oblique, Anteriorly Displaced Posterior Band of the Disk Click

When the posterior band of the disk is anteriorly displaced at the lateral pole and the medial aspect of the disk is still in place, the condyle sits in a groove or concavity in the posterior band (Fig. 10–19). When this condition exists, the retrodiskal tissue behind the lateral pole is usually scarred and little or no pain is associated with function. When the condyle translates forward in opening or balancing side movement, the anteriorly displaced mass of the posterior band deflects outward and backward around the condylar lateral pole. This deflection typically occurs early on opening and late on closing and is palpated easily when the index finger is positioned over the lateral pole. The posterior band movement is detected like a push button jumping outward and immediately back inward above the translating condyle. Another clinical sign is an immediate click with contralateral (balancing) movement after seating the condyles in the fossa in intercuspal position but no ipsilateral click occurs after seating the condyles in intercuspal position. Be-

cause the condyles rotate in the posterior band groove and produce no movement out of the groove with ipsilateral movement, no deflection of tissue or clicking are noted.

The authors have observed that this sixth type of click often occurs on the side of retrusive lateral guidance when the condition is unilateral. In a study of eight subjects in which we traced the movement of the condylar lateral poles with a computerized jaw tracking (Gibbs-Messerman) instrument, we found that retrusive lateral guidance does indeed "move" the condylar lateral poles distally on the ipsilateral side.[23] A slight pressure wave produced by the distal movement of the condylar lateral pole might, with time and repetition, displace the lateral aspect of the posterior band forward, anterior to the condyle. When entering this joint, a surgeon's first impression is that the disk is anteriorly displaced when only the lateral one third or one half of the posterior band is displaced.

This condition is often treated successfully with use of a full arch, lower universal splint with flat anterior guidance and simultaneous posterior stops for each upper lingual cusp (Fig. 10–20). The elimination of retrusive lateral guidance by wearing the splint usually stops the clicking in 1 to 3 months; permanent elimination with restorative dentistry or or-

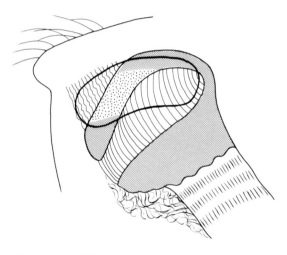

*Fig. 10–19.* Oblique, anteriorly displaced posterior band: a horizontal view of the clicking joint when the condyle is in the fossa and the mouth is closed. The left side depicts the side of the face and tragus turning into the anterior wall of the external auditory meatus at the top. The condyle is shaped like a kidney bean with the lateral pole to the left and the medial pole to the right. The posterior band of the disk runs obliquely across the condyle. The stippled zone represents a groove in the posterior band into which the lateral half of the condyle seats. The wavy lines above the lateral pole of the condyle represent the stretched and scarred retrodiskal tissue sitting above the condylar lateral pole. The zone with slightly curved, parallel lines represents the thin part of the disk, or the pocket in the disk that normally houses the condyle. The more darkly stippled zone below the condyle represents the foot of the disk. The superior head of the lateral pterygoid projects medially below the foot with loose capsular tissue attached to the foot lateral to the muscle. The triangular shaded zone of the posterior band just below the lateral pole of the condyle deflects rapidly around the condylar lateral pole early in the opening movement.

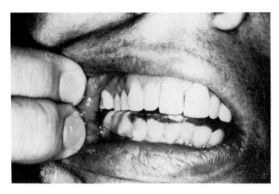

*Fig. 10–20.* Lower universal splint providing flat anterior guidance for upper central incisors and canines and occlusal stops for lingual cusps of upper posterior teeth on a flat posterior table. Christensen's phenomenon opens the posterior contacts in all excursions as the central incisors and canines glide on the flat anterior table. This patient is positioned in a straight right lateral excursion to demonstrate the flat lateral guidance.

thodontics is then required. Without this step, the click returns when use of the splint is discontinued.

### Painful Anteriorly Displaced Disk

When the disk is positioned anterior to the condyle with the mouth closed and the retrodiskal tissue above the condyle is vascularized and innervated, the patient usually experiences constant pain that exacerbates with function (Fig. 10–21). This condition occurs after hypertranslating trauma as well as retrusive trauma to the mandible. Many patients do not recall any trauma that could have released the disk from its attachment to the posterior condylar neck and the lateral and

medial poles of the condyle. Clinical evidence indicates that bruxing with retrusive occlusal contacts may be related to loosening of the attachments of the disk to the condyle, leading to disk displacement in some patients, but this relationship has not been scientifically proven.

When the disk is anteriorly positioned with the mouth closed, a click-like sound usually occurs during opening of the mouth and a softer click is noted during closure of the mouth (reciprocal clicking). The opening click is usually noted at a point one fourth to one half the excursion of the opening movement and the closing click occurs only a few millimeters from closure. The opening click occurs when the condyle rapidly translates forward, snapping into the "pocket" on the inferior surface of the disk. The closing click occurs as the condyle snaps posteriorward over the posterior band of the disk, seemingly when the redundant retrodiskal tissue packs up behind the disk, stopping its posteriorward movement. The condyle continues to translate posteriorward snapping across the posterior band of the disk. The condyle is therefore located under the disk after the opening click and holds this position until the closing click, when the disk snaps back again anterior to the condyle. When the joint is palpated dynamically, tissue deflects back against the palpating finger at the instant of the opening

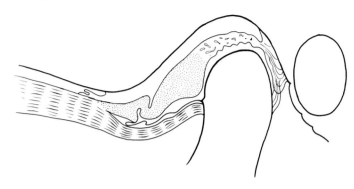

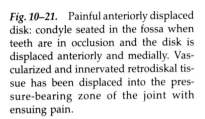

*Fig. 10–21.* Painful anteriorly displaced disk: condyle seated in the fossa when teeth are in occlusion and the disk is displaced anteriorly and medially. Vascularized and innervated retrodiskal tissue has been displaced into the pressure-bearing zone of the joint with ensuing pain.

click and deflects forward with the closing click. Frequently, pain resulting from elevating the condyle superiorly ceases after the opening click when the disk slips back onto the condyle. The inflamed, vascularized, innervated retrodiskal tissue becomes painful when the pressure of the condyle is applied, but no pain is noted when the collagenous, noninnervated disk absorbs the pressure of the condyle.

Internal derangement of the TM joint may be treated by several means. Anterior repositioning splints (ARS) hold the condyles forward under the disk, preventing the closing click. These splints are effective when the painful reciprocal clicking is acute, resulting from a recent trauma to the mandible. In longstanding, chronic cases, such therapy is not effective in recapturing and holding the disk. Another approach involves the use of a universal, nondirective splint for a few months to allow the "freed-up" mandible to reposition the disk, if possible. In a few patients, reciprocally clicking joints spontaneously stop the clicking.

*Painless Anteriorly Displaced Disk*

In some patients, the TM joints click on opening and click on closing without pain. This condition is related to an anteriorly displaced disk, but the retrodiskal tissue is a noninnervated scar composed mostly of collagen (Fig. 10–22). Because this extension pad is not innervated, it is not painful when forces from the condyle are applied. In essence, this patient has a double pocket in the disk. When the mouth opens, the condyle translates forward until the extension pad of scar becomes taut. Then, the condyle snaps under the posterior band of the disk into the inferior surface

of the disk proper. With closing, the condyle carries the disk back up into the fossa until the extension pad of scar blocks any further posterior movement of the disk. The condyle then snaps across the posterior band and back onto the extension pad.

These clicks may be loud or soft. If the embrasure between the condyle and articular eminence is wide, the posterior band is thick and the clicking sound is loud as the condyle rapidly deflects across the thicker barrier. The rapid acceleration and deceleration of condylar movement occurs with more force, producing vibrations of greater amplitude that are detected by the ear as louder sound. When the embrasure between the condyle and articular eminence is narrow, the posterior band of the disk is narrow and the clicking sound is softer.

It is unlikely that this painless reciprocal clicking can be reversed with ARS therapy. The retrodiskal scarring creates a constant volume tissue replacing a rich vascular bed whose volume can decrease and expand with condylar movement. The constant volume blocks the posterior movement of the disk during mouth closure and the condyle deflects behind the disk. The scarred tissue cannot be converted back into vascular tissue to recreate normal disk-condyle function. When the patient can tolerate the clicking and has no pain and only minimal headache, no treatment is indicated. If this patient requires extensive dental restoration, the dentition should be restored using the registration produced by the condyle positioned behind the disk. The fact that the teeth are restored with the condyle off the disk should be explained to the patient. If the teeth were restored with the condyle under the disk, malocclusion

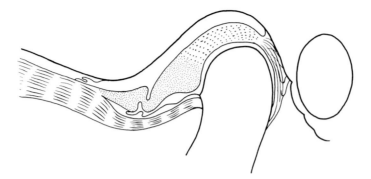

*Fig. 10–22.* Painless anteriorly displaced disk: condyle seated in the fossa when teeth are in occlusion and the disk is displaced anteriorly and medially. Retrodiskal tissue that has been displaced into the pressure-bearing zone of the joint has been converted into scar and is not innervated.

would exist each time the condyle deflects off the posterior border of the disk on mouth closure.

## Medially Displaced Disks

Recent reports and results of clinical studies demonstrate evidence that TM joint disks may be more medially displaced than anterior medially displaced. Medial displacement is demonstrated in fresh, unembalmed cadavers in two ways.[24] In one type of displacement, the disk is located at the medial pole of the condyle when the mouth is closed. Degenerated, lateral retrodiskal tissue is positioned between the condyle and the fossa. As the condyle translates forward, the disk deflects laterally onto the moving condyle. This medially displaced disk is "recaptured" during opening. The clinical sign of this type of medially displaced disk is that palpation reveals rapid medial deflection of the condyle and lateral deflection of softer tissue just superior to the condyle at the instant of the opening click.

In the second type of disk displacement, the disk is in place, on the condyle, when the mouth is closed. When the condyle begins to translate, the disk deflects directly medially and the condyle rapidly deflects laterally. The clinical sign of this type of click is the rapid "jumping" of the condyle lateralward against the palpating finger at the instant of the opening click. These medially displaced disks were observed only in the joints in fresh cadavers in which the lateral joint structures were removed. Findings of MRI studies, however, confirm the medially displaced disk, and the authors have observed the clinical signs of condylar rapid lateral or medial displacement at the instant of an opening click. In our lim-

ited experience, these two types of clicks do not respond to ARS therapy and an operation is often required to plicate and reposition the disks if the pain is intractable.

## Determination of Responsiveness to Therapy

A series of simple tests help to determine if the disk can be "recaptured" by ARS therapy: the cotton roll test, the protrusive-retrusive test, the condyle-disk manipulation or romancing test, and the instant malocclusion test.

### Cotton Roll Test

For this test (Fig. 10–23), the patient opens the mouth wide to make certain the opening click occurs. Cotton rolls are then placed along the central fossae of the lower teeth from the second molar to the canine. The operator holds the cotton rolls with thumb and forefinger and the middle finger is placed on the face as close to the condyle as possible. The patient is instructed to close straight up into the cotton. If no click occurs on the first closure, the patient is instructed to rest a few seconds and then bite harder into the cotton rolls. If no clicking occurs when biting into cotton rolls, an ARS may also hold the condyle under the disk. If the clicking does occur, ARS therapy will likely fail.

### Protrusive-Retrusive Test

In the protrusive-retrusive test, the patient closes the mouth until the teeth are in maximum intercuspation. The operator makes certain that the closing click occurs. The patient

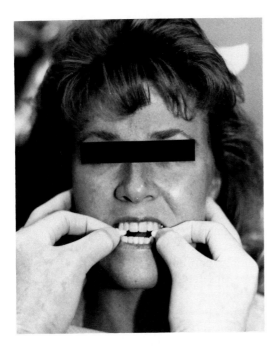

*Fig. 10–23.* Cotton roll test: patient bites on cotton rolls as the clinician's third finger palpates face near the TM joint to detect a click.

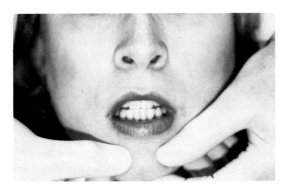

*Fig. 10–24.* Patient making protrusive movement gliding on the anterior teeth in the protrusive-retrusive test.

is instructed to hold the anterior teeth in contact while pushing the mandible forward, with the reminder to make the lower anterior teeth glide against the back of the upper anterior teeth. The operator keeps the index fingers over the condylar lateral poles during this maneuver to detect any meniscus-condyle deflection (Fig. 10–24). If a deflection (click) occurs in either joint, the protrusive click is usually farther forward than the retrusive click, just as the opening click occurs at wider opening than the closing click. This hysteresis or lag in the clicking results as the

disk is pushed farther forward on protrusion before the click occurs and is pushed farther backward on retrusion before "clicking" off the disk. This hysteresis produces a figure eight axiographic tracing as the condyle translates forward, deflecting into the central zone of the disk on one pathway, then sliding posteriorward on a different pathway, until it snaps back off the disk (Fig. 10–25). In this test, if the protrusive and retrusive clicks are within the functional range and the retrusive click is only a few millimeters forward of the maximum intercuspation position, recapture of the disk is feasible. If no clicking is noted or if the protrusive click is anterior to the edge-to-edge position of anterior teeth, an ARS is not likely to recapture the disk. Also, the muscles will not tolerate the excessive protrusive position established by the ARS to orient the condyle under the disk and hold it in place.

### Condyle-Disk Manipulation (Romancing) Test

In this test, the clinician positions the fingers under the inferior border of the mandible bilaterally, with the thumbs on the symphysis below the lower lip (Fig. 10–26). No pressure is applied as the patient opens beyond the opening click. The patient stops opening at the click and the clinician applies pressure upward on the angle of the mandible and

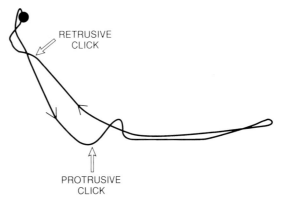

*Fig. 10–25.* Axiographic tracing showing figure 8 shape because of the hysteresis, or lag, of the disk snapping onto and off the condyle. Note that the protrusive click occurs forward on the eminence, and the retrusive click occurs as the condyle moves up into the fossa.

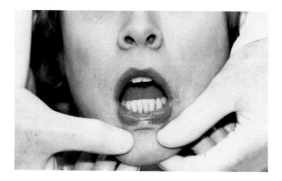

**Fig. 10–26.** Patient with mandible being bimanually manipulated back up into the fossa after the opening click in the romancing test. The operator does not apply elevating pressure on the condyles until after the opening click.

downward with the thumbs on the symphysis. This maneuver seats the condyle superiorly into the disk that was "recaptured" at the opening click. The patient is then instructed to relax and allow the clinician to slowly manipulate the condyles back up into the fossae while supporting the condyles upward into the disks continuously. If the condyle-disk assemblies can be manipulated all the way back into the fossae without clicking, the disks likely could be recaptured. If such manipulation is not possible, the disk may no longer have a thickened posterior band to hold the condyle in its central zone. The disk then has undergone morphologic change such that no central zone or "pocket" remains to fit over the condyle. Another reason for failing the romancing test is that the retrodiskal tissue has converted from a variable volume vascular tissue to a fixed volume of scar (collagen). This tissue becomes packed up in the fossa as the condyle-disk assembly is manipulated upward, blocking the posterior band of the disk until the condyle snaps behind it. If the condyle-disk assembly cannot be manipulated back into the fossae without clicking, the possibility that an ARS will recapture the disk is unlikely.

### Instant Malocclusion Test

This test is applicable only if the romancing test shows the disks are recapturable and the condition is unilateral. This maneuver is performed after the condyle-disk assemblies are romanced up into the fossae. While maintaining the superior pressure at the angle of the mandible, keeping the disks wedged above the condyles, the patient is reminded again to relax. The clinician then rotates the mandible up and down to lightly tap the teeth. The patient is asked to note where teeth are touching as they are lightly tapped. If the internal derangement is unilateral, the condyle is displaced downward on the affected side by the posterior band of the disk that is wedged above the condyle. This action prevents the posterior teeth on that side from contacting, allowing the opposite posterior teeth to contact first. The clinician releases the patient's mandible and the patient reports where the teeth were touching. With the mandibular movement of speech, the condyle usually slips back off the disk in a closing click. The clinician then instructs the patient to close the teeth together and repeats the manipulation of the mandible, lightly tapping the teeth with the condyle on the affected side now positioned behind the disk. This position is that to which the teeth have accommodated during the period of disk displacement, so the posterior teeth typically contact simultaneously. When the clinician can demonstrate this immediate change in tooth contact with the disk in place and then anteriorly displaced, the patient will understand that the disk slips into and out of the joint space so as to lower and raise the condyle and open or close tooth contact on the affected side. The clinician can also be more certain that the disk is, indeed, anteriorly displaced.

### Anterior Repositioning Splint (ARS) Therapy

When one considers the various types of joint pathofunction that can occur, the fact that ARS therapy is often not indicated becomes clear. The clinician must make an accurate diagnosis before designing a treatment plan. A trend in recent years has been to use fewer ARS than in previous years. Oral and maxillofacial surgeons report that in patients in whom ARS therapy failed to relieve pain and pathofunction, the fossa fills with vascular connective tissue that actually prevents the condyle from seating back up into the fossa. It now seems important to reduce the duration of ARS therapy to approximately 3 months. Quick positioning of the condyle back up in the fossa does not allow the formation of vascular connective tissue that blocks its repositioning.

The authors institute ARS therapy only in the event of short-term, painful, reciprocal clicking that responds to the cotton roll test with cessation of clicking; that clicks only a few millimeters forward of the intercuspal position with retrusion in the protrusive-retrusive test; that does not click with manipulation of the condyle and disk up in the fossa in the romancing test; and demonstrates opening of the posterior occlusion of the affected side in the instant malocclusion test. We try to limit the duration of ARS therapy to 3 months.

## References

1. Thilander B.: The structures of the collagen of the temporomandibular disc in man. Acta Odontol Scand, 22:135, 1964
2. Mathews M.P. and Moffett B.C.: Histologic maturation and initial aging of the human temporomandibular joint (Special issue). J Dent Res, 53:246, 1974
3. Toller P.A.: Opaque arthroscopy of the temporomandibular joint. Int J Oral Surg, 3:17, 1974
4. Choukas N.C. and Sicher H.: The structure of the temporomandibualar joint. Oral Surg Oral Med Oral Pathol, 13:1203, 1960
5. Findlay I.A.: Mandibular joint pressures. J Dent Res, 43:140, 1964
6. Griffin C.J. and Sharpe C.J.: The structure of the adult human temporomandibular meniscus. Aust Dent J, 5:190, 1960
7. Batson O.B.: The anatomist looks at the temporomandibular joint. Trans Acad Ophthalmol Otolaryngol, 60:413, 1956
8. Blackwood H.J.J.: Vascularization of the condylar cartilage of the human mandible. J Anat, 99:551, 1965
9. Helmy E., et al: Osteoarthrosis of the temporomandibular joint following experimental disc perforation in Macaca fascicularis. J Oral Maxillofac Surg, 46:979, 1988
10. Schneider K., et al: Modeling of jaw-head-neck dynamics during whiplash. J Dent Res, 68:1360, 1989
11. Pinto O.F.: A new structure related to the temporomandibular joint and middle ear. J Prosthet Dent, 12:95, 1962
12. Burch J.C.: The cranial attachment of the sphenomandibular (tympanomandibular) ligament. Anat Rec, 156:433, 1966
13. Loughner B.A., et al: Discomalleolar and anterior malleolar ligaments: Possible causes of middle ear damage during temporomandibular joint surgery. Oral Surg Oral Med Oral Pathol, 68:14, 1989
14. Sicher H. and DuBrul E.L.: Oral Anatomy. 6th Ed. St. Louis, C.V. Mosby, 1975
15. Thilander B.: Innervation of the temporomandibular joint capsule in man. Trans Roy School Stock Umea, 7:1, 1961
16. McNamara J.A.: The independent functions of the two heads of the lateral pterygoid muscle. Am J Anat, 138:197, 1973
17. Mahan P.E., et al: Superior and inferior bellies of the lateral pterygoid muscle EMG activity at basic jaw positions. J Prosthet Dent, 50:710, 1983
18. Gay T., et al: The acoustical characteristics of the normal and abnormal temporomandibular joint. J Oral Maxillofac Surg, 45:397, 1987
19. Baumgarten M., et al: Normal human synovial fluid: Osmolality and exercise-induced changes. J Bone Joint Surg (Am), 67:1336, 1985
20. Westesson P.L.: Double contrast arthrography and internal derangement of the temporomandibular joint. Swed Dent J, 13(Suppl):1, 1982
21. Luckerath W.: Personal communication, 1989
22. Tyndall D.A. and Matteson S.R.: Radiographic appearance and population distribution of the pneumatized articular eminence of the temporal bone. J Oral Maxillofac Surg, 43:493, 1985
23. Coffey J.P., et al: A preliminary study of the effects of tooth guidance on working-side condylar movement. J Prosthet Dent, 62:157, 1989
24. Westesson P.L.: High speed cinematography of condylar clicking movements in dissected TMJ autopsy specimens. Option C videotape (BK-0020B), Continuing Dental Education, University of Washington, School of Dentistry, Seattle, WA., 1987

# 11

# *Temporomandibular Joint Arthritides*

**Degenerative Arthritis**
  Pathogenesis
  Juvenile Degenerative Arthritis
  Reversible Degenerative Arthritis
  Irreversible Degenerative Arthritis
  Physical, Imaging, and Laboratory
      Evaluations
  Pathophysiology
  Considerations for Therapy
**Rheumatoid Arthritis**
  Juvenile Rheumatoid Arthritis
  Adult Rheumatoid Arthritis
**Psoriatic Arthritis**
**Infectious Arthritis**
  Staphylococcal Arthritis
  Streptococcal Arthritis
  Gram-Negative Bacillary Arthritis
  Arthritis Caused by Mycobacteria and
      Fungi
  Viral Arthritis
  Lyme Disease
  Gonococcal Arthritis
**Traumatic Arthritis**
  Sprains
  Acute Hypertranslation
  Acute Traumatic Arthritis
**Synovial Chondromatosis**
**Neuropathic Joint Disease (Charcot
  Joints)**
**Other Maladies**
  Tumors
  Familial Mediterranean Fever
  Mitochondrial Myopathy
  Systemic Lupus Erythematosus-
      Induced TM Joint Arthritis
  Hemarthrosis Secondary to
      Anticoagulant Therapy

The continuing quest for etiologic factors leading to arthritic conditions, a quest that will lead to accurate nomenclature, has been a continuum of concern for researchers, clinical investigators, and clinicians for the past century. The chronicles reflect that those who have a primary interest in the temporomandibular (TM) joint have engaged in a parallel quest, especially in the last few years.

Nothing about the TM joint is occult; often multifactorial pathophysiologies afflict a patient, and the challenge is to establish the diagnosis or diagnoses for each individual. Therefore, the descriptors used in this chapter are based on the nomenclature used for joints elsewhere in the body. Maladies of the TM joint should be accurately diagnosed and should receive care as dictated by the ever-unfolding basic life sciences.

## Degenerative Arthritis

Degenerative arthritis of the TM joint has several other names, including: temporomandibular arthropathy,[1] osteoarthrosis, osteoarthritis, and mandibular stress syndrome.[2] DeBont, Boering and associates concluded that although the pathogenesis of degenerative arthritis is not completely understood, it does involve matrix alterations, disintegration of the collagen network, and fatty degeneration of the articular cartilage, which could be the initial features of the disease.[3] They wrote, "It is assumed that a breakdown of articular tissues occurs whenever a joint is subjected to repetitive overload in excess of its functional capacity, or when it is subjected to normal loads while the functional capacity is reduced as a part of aging or idiopathically."

The osseous, soft tissue, and functional changes of the TM joints and contiguous tissues were well described by Toller.[1] Nickerson and Boering expanded on Boering's earlier thesis, reported in the literature of the Netherlands, in which the natural course of TM joint osteoarthrosis was described.[4,5] The Toller report, the reports by Boering and his colleagues, and other observations interpreted natural courses of osteoarthritis in the TM joints.[1-7] For the majority of the patients, the course of the disease ended in approximately 18 to 36 months without direct or significant indirect treatments to the TM joints. Often there was a residual alteration of the condyle.

Quinn utilized arthroscopic and histologic observations to show that, though there were cartilaginous differences, the TM joint functioned and responded the same as other synovial joints of the body.[8] He observed many points of similarity between the pathologic lesions of chondromalacia of the patella and the TM joint, and he concluded that chondromalacia of the patella and of the TM joint are the same disease process. Each area had a generation of cartilage with the resultant bone loss of osteoarthritis.

For purposes of clinical clarity, we have identified four age-group-related TM joint degenerative arthritides. These age-related groups of patients are identified for the purpose of the following discussion and for descriptions of treatment objectives: 8 to 15 years, 15 to 25 years, 25 to 40 years, and 40 years and older. Juvenile degenerative arthritis, usually monoarticular and afflicting children 8 to 15 years, may cause permanent changes to the condylar process and ramus.[5] Reversible degenerative, usually monoarticular, arthritis may afflict the TM joint of patients 15 to 25 years, typically female patients. Patients in the 25 to 40-year age group can have, in our experience, either reversible or irreversible types of TM joint degenerative arthritis. The irreversible type affects the TM joint of patients 40 years of age and older in a manner similar to other joints.

### Pathogenesis

Repair may occur at any point in the disease process. The earlier repair occurs in the course of the disease, the more likely the final form of the condyle will appear normal. Compared to other joints, the TM joint has great remodeling potential.[9] Clearly, the younger the patient, the greater the likelihood of repair, except with juvenile degenerative arthritis as described by Boering.[5]

Degenerative joint changes of the TMJ are ". . . directly related to the aging process and functional abuse of the joint. Initial remodeling changes of the mandibular condyle occur within physiologic limits."[10] If the physiologic limits of remodeling are surpassed or unfavorably influenced by concurrent metabolic alterations, degenerative changes may develop. Examples of surpassing physiologic limits are evident in individuals with less sturdy muscular and ligamentous support of the TM joint, in overloading of a TM joint by inadequate occlusal support, as described in Chapter 9; and examples of metabolic alterations in female patients undergoing hormonal alterations.

Regardless of the etiology, cartilaginous cells in the condylar articular fibrocartilage become necrotic and a proliferation of fibrous connective tissue occurs in an attempt to maintain a smooth articular surface. This proliferation results in a loss of elastic compressibility of the articulating surface, and a transfer of stress occurs to the underlying bone, resulting in trabecular hypertrophy. Osteoclastic activity occurs on the subcondylar bone with the formation of medullary compartments or Ely's cysts. The vascular mesenchyme converts to granulation tissue, which may proliferate from the subchondral medullary spaces through fragmentation defects in the condylar surface to become contiguous with the lower joint space. Denuding of the bone eventually occurs, with fracturing defects on the condylar articulating surface. As free bodies of the cartilaginous matrix migrate into the inferior joint compartment, chronic inflammatory cells respond producing synovitis.

Concurrently, the multipotential cells of the periosteum proliferate reactive bone and cartilage, which forms at the insertion of the capsule and produces severe lipping and eburnation. The exposed subarticular bone undergoes pathologic regressive remodeling as the degenerative process continues, producing cratering and osteophyte formations on the articular surface of the condyle (Fig. 11–1).

The meniscus undergoes degenerative changes owing to the function of the altered condyle against its lower surface. The meniscus may undergo hyperplasia, hyaline degeneration, fracturing, and perforation (Fig. 11–2).

The accumulated stresses, usually confined to the lateral and anterior slopes of the mandibular condyle, may be transferred to the posterior slope of the articular eminence of the temporal bone, which may lose its collaginous surface followed by loss of the subsurface bone.

## Juvenile Degenerative Arthritis

Boering,[5] an oral surgeon from the Netherlands, identified a degenerative arthritis in children that may manifest as early as 8 years of age, but usually is first diagnosed between 12 and 15 years.[4] The chief complaint is TM joint pain on a lateral mandibular movement. A crossbite relationship is noted, as are loud crepitant sounds in the TM joint. On the affected side, antegonal notching is observed, and the condylar neck is situated posteriorly and horizontally. The condyle becomes elongated and flattened on the anterior superior surface, and the patient develops a crossbite on the affected side. The contralateral side appears normal.[11,12]

The panoramic radiograph of a patient first examined during adulthood may display the antegonal notching, the horizontal angulation of the neck of the condylar process, flattening of the condyle, and a deficiency in the height of the ramus from the condyle to pogonion of 6 to 10 mm on the affected side. An adult patient may respond to a question during the medical history as follows, "I remember that, when I was 12 years old, I had my teeth cleaned and I had pain in front of my ear for the next week. I thought everybody had that type of pain when they went to the dentist."

## Reversible Degenerative Arthritis

Degenerative arthritis has a predilection for female patients in the first 10 or 15 years after the beginning of menarche. This monoarticular degenerative disease is associated with bony changes of the condyle and myospasms.[9,10] Patients often experience concurrent muscle contraction (tension) or vascular headaches. Overlapping and reinforcing factors at this time of life may produce myofascial pain: mixed dentition with the expected occlusal disharmonies that deflect the condyles from their normal functioning posi-

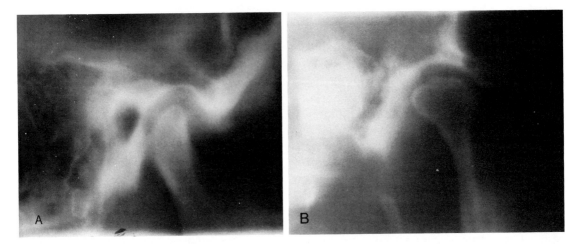

*Fig. 11–1.* A. A 26-year-old woman with unilateral painful subluxation of a TM joint meniscus. The lateral projection of corrected polycycloidal tomogram disclosed loss of the condylar cortex as seen in the second stage of degenerative arthritis. The patient was treated with temporary intraoral splints and simple analgesics for 12 months when the process subsided. B. An 18-year-old woman with unilateral transient painful dislocation of a TM joint meniscus. The frontal projection of corrected polycycloidal tomogram disclosed osteophytic changes on the condylar cortex as seen in the third stage of degenerative arthritis. The patient was treated with temporary intraoral splints and simple analgesics for 18 months when the process completed its cycle and the condylar head remolded.

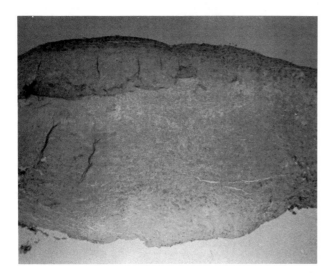

*Fig. 11–2.* Fibrovascular hyperplasia of a meniscus removed from a 43-year-old female patient with a 10-year history of unilateral degenerative arthritis with signs and symptoms of meniscus dislocation. The previous treatments included a variety of nonsurgical methods such as splint therapy and procedures to the occluding surfaces of the teeth.

tions, peer pressures to conform or to not conform, the necessary social and intrafamily adjustments that occur during the transition from childhood to adulthood, and experimentation with lifestyles that often include being malnourished on an occult basis, even though large quantities of fad and "quick" foods are ingested.

The disease rarely affects male subjects who have the same life factors just summarized. Stewart and Standish[13] studied 23 patients who were 19 years old or younger. Six patients had osteoarthritis. They observed that most of these patients had acute symptoms that lasted about 9 months. They recommended nonsurgical management as the first line treatment. Studies involving female primates yield findings that indicated hormonal changes are associated with the TM joint maladies.[14] A combination of the hormonal changes and the fact that females have less sturdy muscles and ligaments as compared to young males are probably the major factors in the constellation of etiologies that may lead to monoarticular degenerative arthritis of the TM joint.

The osteoarthritic process may be observed in association with the ingestion of oral contraceptives.[15] It reverses, with cessation of signs and findings and the return of normal functioning capabilities, if the use of this form of contraception ceases.

## Irreversible Degenerative Arthritis

Degenerative arthritis of the TM joint that develops in concert with aging or other catabolic changes is usually irreversible. Degenerative joint disease is common in all individuals, to a greater or lesser degree, after the third or fourth decades of life. In one report, 40% of 400 TM joints of individuals 40 years of age and older had evidence of degenerative joint disease.[16] In a study of 69 cadavers, 87% showed degenerative histopathologic changes.[17] Results of other studies of cadavers confirm the expected findings of TM joint changes in the elderly that include degenerative fibrocartilage hyperplasia, abnormal retrodiskal changes, and myxomatous degeneration.[18,19]

An interesting correlation involves the incidence of degenerative joint disease in young women at a stressful time of their lives who may have reversible degenerative changes of the TM joint and the incidence of TM joint degenerative arthritis in women 35 to 50 years of age, the time of life associated with menopause. We observed that these women are often individuals who demand and expect much from themselves and their loved ones or persons who have had to cope with a major business, social, or family change in their lives.

## Physical, Imaging, and Laboratory Evaluations

Physical examination reveals decreased motions of the mandible owing to muscular spasms associated with the diseased TM joint. The joint is typically sensitive to palpation. The combination of a monoarticular diseased TM joint and muscular spasms causes limitation at opening and restriction on lateral movements away from the affected side. On the rare occasions that the degenerative arthritis is bilateral, movements in both joints are restricted. In either case, unilateral or bilateral, subluxating clicks of the menisci may be noted, either audibly, by palpation, or by auscultation. One or both menisci may be dislocated, causing a closed locked condition impeding the opening and lateral movements of the mandible. Although the disease is typically unilateral, the function of both TM joints is affected.

Imaging of the TM joint hinges on radiographs selected from various techniques: transcranial, transpharyngeal, transorbital, and corrected polycycloidal tomography. The findings include, depending on the severity of the condition and the stage of the arthritis: normal appearance of the condyle; narrowing of the joint space; loss of part (usually the anterior-superior lateral surface) or all of the cortex of the condyle by cratering; subchondral sclerosis that may resemble marbleized bone; subchondral cyst formations, the microvascular osseous spherical areas labeled Ely's cysts; buttressing of the condyle to produce an appearance of an anterior lip or beak; single, groups, or generalized osteophyte formation on the condylar articular surface; and, in the irreversible classification, osseous changes to the articular eminence of the temporal bone.

Although not a primary diagnostic tool, a radionuclide bone scan may be indicated. Increased uptake is often demonstrated in those patients with TM joint arthritides. If the disease is in the subchondral sclerotic state or is remodeling, the radionuclide localizes to the condyle. Separation of images may occur with TM joint movements in patients with involvement of the articulating surfaces of the temporal bone as well as the expected changes in the condyle. Diffuse uptake is indicative of synovitis.

Arthroscopic evaluation may be of value if a question arises regarding the diagnosis. Arthroscopic examination of the superior joint space may reveal an irregular superior surface of the disk, with fraying and an overall more yellowish red appearance than the normal whitish, smooth disk. Brawny-red focal areas usually are indicative of pathologic irregularity of the condyle; perforations of the disk or the retrodiskal tissues may be present, with and without osteophytes arising from the condyle. Loss or stretching of the posterior fibrous attachment also may be evident.

The diagnosis of degenerative arthritis is usually established by assessing the findings from the history, physical examination, and imaging. Generally, laboratory tests of the sparse synovial fluid of the TM joint are usually not reasonable nor are they helpful in establishing the diagnosis. In the event of effusion in the TM joint of a patient with degenerative arthritis, an aspirated sample of the synovial fluid is similar to an egg white and is a colorless, clear, highly viscous fluid. If the patient exhibits clinical evidence of inflammation, the synovial fluid sample may contain abundant leukocytes.

## Pathophysiology

Degenerative arthritis of the TM joint, although expressed as a disease entity, may be described by using the words of Sokoloff, when he discussed osteoarthritis as, ". . . not so much a single disease as a pattern of reaction of articular tissues to mechanical and biologic events."[20] This pattern was described by Toller in four stages.[1]

### Stage One

Stage one, as described by Toller, begins with a fibrillation of the fibers on the articular surface of the condyle in the area of the greatest articular contact. Synovial fluid passes between the fibers and they fray or fibrillate, as with other diarthrodial joints, into joint space. Immediately below the fibrillated articular fibrous surface, the cartilaginous area hypertrophies and mineralizes. Denudation and eburnation of the fibrous articular surface continues until all of the fibrous tissue is lost, and the mineralizing cartilaginous zone develops into a thickened bony surface; the medullary bone of the condyle appears normal at this stage.

In the first stage of the process, the patient has myospasms, tenderness of the TM joint area to palpation, subluxation, and possibly dislocation of the meniscus, if predisposed. Radiographic changes may include only a minimal loss of joint space. Many patients, especially those in younger age groups, ex-

perience a resolution of the process with a return to normal function.

The bony surface articulates with the inferior surface of the meniscus, which probably is relatively uninvolved in the disease process at this point, aside from becoming unstable and producing clicking and, occasionally, a closed lock condition, if predisposed. It seems reasonable to avoid meniscectomy and other open joint surgical procedures, instead prescribing intraoral splint therapy and simple analgesics, 325 mg of acetylsalicylic acid every 2 hours during painful exacerbations and continuing for 1 day after cessation of the pain. Splint therapy to relieve intrajoint pressures and indicated occlusal therapy may be instituted.

### Stage Two

This stage represents a progression of degeneration of the cortical covering of the condyle. The condylar articular cortex becomes thinned and perforated. The medullary spaces of the condyle are invaded by synovial fluid and become fibrotic. The radiographic images may display localized areas of the lack of cortex, which are represented as irregular radiolucencies of the articular surface.

The pathophysiology of stage two may feature the production of small pressure cysts, Ely's cysts,* in the medullary space. These fibrous-walled, highly vascular cysts form in

---

*Dr. Leonard Wheeler Ely, 1868–1944, was Professor of Surgery, Stanford University School of Medicine, 1913–1934. He had great concern for accuracy of nomenclature and believed that degenerative arthritis, osteoarthritis, hypertrophic arthritis, and other terms, ". . . almost without number . . ." were misnomers. Until the etiologies were better defined, he elected to use the term, "the second great type of chronic arthritis," with the first being rheumatoid arthritis. He observed in his laboratories, by radiographic imaging, and at surgery, cavities in bones associated with the second great type of chronic arthritis. He first described these in 1916, then in 1920, and gave a definitive description in his textbook of 1923 in which he wrote, "Upon sectioning the bone, one finds larger and smaller places in which the bone tissue is lacking. These spaces may be filled with fibrous marrow, or they may be the seat of cysts, large and small. Sometimes fibrous tissue and cysts are intermingled . . ."

1. Ely L.W.: A study of 100 dry bones sawn in the laboratory; bone and joint studies 1. Palo Alto, Stanford University, 1916.
2. Ely L.W.: The second great type of chronic arthritis. Arch Surg, 1:158, 1920.
3. Ely L.W.: Inflammation in Bones and Joints. Philadelphia, J.B. Lippincott, 1923.

response to punctate openings in the cortex that are associated with microfractures, and the intracapsular pressures apparently induce the small cysts. If the cysts collapse, a generalized erosion of the articular surface of the condyle occurs.

Attempts by the body at bony repair may be successful and represent another route of classifying the disease as reversible. We have observed 13- to 25-year-old women with monoarticular degenerative joint disease in whom eventual repair of the condyle after this stage of localized articular surface cortex perforations was determined radiographically.

Treatment continues as described previously: the long-term prescription of nonsteroidal anti-inflammatory drugs (NSAID) as indicated; shorter duration, 2 to 6 days, prescription of 325 mg of aspirin every 2 hours during waking hours; and splint therapy combined with indicated temporary occlusal therapy for pain relief.

### Stage Three

Stage three is a continuation of the erosion that followed the microcyst-associated fractures and loss of the articular surface of the condyle. Pain is not a prominent feature of this stage, although the patient and family remark on the crepitant sounds. A large erosive defect is a prominent radiographic finding.

We observed in many older patients that the process may stabilize at this erosive stage for many years, with no associated disabling problem. Pharmacotherapeutic care, as for the earlier, painful stages, is not usually necessary. Consideration is warranted for continued stabilization of the occlusal table to relieve pressures on the TM joint, because the ramus of the mandible tends to move laterally and superiorly toward the affected side owing to the loss of height by the erosion.

### Stage Four

Stage four, the repair stage, occurs 18 months to 3 years after the onset. Although radiographs may show a deformed condyle, it serves the patient well without pain. The condyle, although deformed, has a cortex and a new growth of a fibrous articular surface that arises from and is in continuity with the synovium. The presence of the meniscus is influential in enabling the TM joint to survive the degenerative arthritis process and to arrive at the stage of repair as a usable and useful structure.

## Considerations for Therapy

### Assessing the Etiologies of TM Joint Degenerative Arthritis

The major complaint, pain, may have different etiologies in TM joint degenerative arthritis. The pain may arise from periarticular structures, synovial membrane inflammation, osteophyte production, and the degenerative bony disease process itself.

The muscles and ligaments, perhaps lax before the onset of the active arthritic process, may become unstable because of the degenerative arthritic structural changes within the TM joint. Myospasms and stretching of these structures produce pain, especially at their insertions. A self-defeating cycle of events ensues, consisting of the instabilities and spasms causing more spasms and instabilities as the joint itself undergoes destabilizing pathologic changes, thus perpetuating the multifaceted cycle of painful, deleterious events.

The active growth of osteophytes is a source of acute pain evidenced on mandibular movements and by palpation. Pain occurs when the disease process affects the subchondral bone; this layer of bone is innervated, in contrast to cartilage.

The synovial membrane is a source of pain in arthritic changes elsewhere in the musculoskeletal system, but it is often overlooked in the TM joint. The lack of access for circumferential palpation of the TM joint and the prominent role other structures play in health and disease may lead the clinician to overlook the synovium.

### Types of Therapy

Active therapy to relieve pain of degenerative arthritis must include, first, understanding the pathophysiology of the process by not only members of the treating team, but also the patient and the patient's support group of family and friends. Active therapy includes physical therapy, pharmacotherapeutic agents, and surgical intervention.

**Physical Therapy.** Physical therapy takes several inter-related factors into consideration: exercises, muscle spasm relief, and support of the joint.

Active isometric and isotonic exercises to strengthen the supporting musculature and to maintain the range of motion of the mandible may be prescribed or provided. Physical therapy may include, with great effectiveness, ultrasound, surface heat, and transcutaneous nerve stimulation. Physical therapy is directed toward the neck and shoulder girdle when they become involved.

The use of splints to support the mandible in a corrected anatomic relation to the TM joint and to relieve pressures within the joint must be carefully monitored. A patient, experiencing relief with the use of an intraoral splint, may simply disappear from a doctor's practice. Clearly, a splint that is not adjusted apace with joint changes may have a deleterious effect on the joint and the dentition.

To determine whether splint therapy is indicated, a provocation test is helpful. The patient bites forcefully on the posterior teeth in intercuspal position and notes the amount of pain and discomfort. Cotton rolls are then placed on the lower posterior occlusal table, and the patient bites forcefully into the cotton, noting the amount of pain. If biting on the cotton rolls reduces the pain, the patient should benefit from use of a muscle relaxation splint. The dentition supporting the splints is carefully monitored, however, to prevent damage by the splints. Permanent restorative, prosthodontic, orthodontic, or occlusal therapy is delayed until the process has either resolved or stabilized.

**Pharmacotherapeutic Therapy.** The use of aspirin continues to be a reliable and effective agent for relieving arthritic pains. Ingested on a short-term basis as is required for most patients with degenerative arthritis in the TM joint, the side effects of alterations of the role of platelets in the coagulation mechanism is not a contraindication to the use of the agent. We recommend two or three 325-mg tablets as the initial dose, with one 325-mg tablet every 2 hours during waking hours for no more than 6 days per series for acute exac-

erbations. Aspirin is more effective and produces only minimal irritations to normal gastric mucosa if it is ingested as a powder accompanied by a minimum of 6 ounces of water. If the aspirin has an odor of vinegar, it has probably hydrolyzed. In this form, it is ineffective as an analgesic and is potentially damaging to the gastrointestinal tract.

Other NSAID, such as ibuprofen (Motrin), sulindac (Clinoril), diflunisal (Dolobid), indomethacin (Indocin), piroxicam (Feldene), and naproxen (Naprosyn), are used if aspirin is not effective. The NSAID form an unusual class in that when one agent loses its effectiveness, another may control the pain well. The clinician can switch and often keep the arthritis pain under control for an extended period. If the patient has gastric ulcer disease or experiences such signs and symptoms as heartburn, a change in gastrointestinal tract function, or tarry stools, either the NSAID is discontinued or a histamine H-2 inhibitor, such as cimetidine (Tagamet), or a gastric mucosal protectant, such as sucralfate (Carafate), is added to the NSAID regimen. If the NSAID is discontinued, acetaminophen (Tylenol) may be prescribed.

The manufacturer's warnings, cautions, indications, and dosages should be reviewed before administration of pharmacotherapeutic agents. Cimetidine may cause gynecomastia, and it provides a systemic histamine H-2 inhibition. Sucralfate is so poorly absorbed it provides, in effect, a local histamine H-2 inhibition. Aspirin may inhibit platelet aggregation and cause gastrointestinal hemorrhage, especially with long-term, high-dose usage. Prescribing acetaminophen is sometimes necessary as a substitute for aspirin, but it provides only an analgesic effect; it is not as effective as aspirin in reducing joint inflammation and the potential for liver damage is a concern.

Steroids are not often indicated in the treatment of degenerative arthritis of the TM joint. Oral steroid preparations are ineffective in pain relief when administered in reasonable doses, and their long-term use for pain relief is avoided in favor of the prescription of aspirin or NSAID.

The intra-articular injection of steroids in the TM joint is used on only one or two occasions for the entire 1½ to 3-year cycle, during especially severe episodes. The continued use of intra-articular injections may lead to deterioration of the condyle on a chemical basis in addition to the disease process. Kopp and associates described the short- and long-term effects of intra-articular injections of sodium hyaluronate and of corticosteroid solutions;[21,22] they found that hyaluronate (Hylatril) had fewer side effects than corticosteroids and produced decreases in intra-articular adhesions and in the incidence of synovitis. They administered 0.5 ml in the superior joint space with two injections, 2 weeks apart. They concluded that hyaluronate use is reasonable for patients with TM joint inflammation, especially for those individuals with advanced osteoarthritis for whom corticosteroids seemed less effective.

Hydrocortisone may be considered as a phosphoresis application in which hydrocortisone acetate is mixed with a carrying agent, such as petrolatum, and is spread over the preauricular area. An ultrasound transducer is moved over the TM joint area, with increasing intensities, until the patient reports a warm sensation. One treatment per day for 10 to 14 days may decrease myofascial pain related to exacerbations of osteoarthritis.

Tricyclic antidepressants stimulate endogenous endorphins and enkephalins in addition to their role as psychotropic agents.[23] These opioids, thus stimulated, are of value in relief of chronic pain associated with myospasms. We recommend an initial dosage of one 10-mg tablet of amitriptyline three times daily for 30 days. This level may be increased to 75 mg per day until the desired effect is obtained. As a monitor, when the patient feels a drying in the mouth, the level of ingestion is maintained, with no further increase in doses. Other antidepressant drugs that, like amitriptyline, elevate brain levels of serotonin are trazodone (Desyrel) and doxepin (Sinequan, Adapin).

**Surgical Intervention.** Various procedures, such as partial condyloplasty, condylotomies, meniscus repair, and meniscectomy, are indicated in highly selected cases when the pain is overwhelming on a true somatic basis. In general, the placement of alloplastic condylar or glenoid fossa implants is not indicated. Clinicians show a growing interest and capability in using dermal or other biologic materials as a graft to repair defects in the meniscus and to cover the surface of the condyle or the glenoid fossa after meniscectomy. The most conservative surgical procedures warrant consideration with due regard for the cyclic nature of the disease: it progresses from pathologic changes that occasionally accompany the surpassing of physiologic limits and proceeds through a cycle of events that usually leads to repair.

## Rheumatoid Arthritis

The oral and maxillofacial manifestations of rheumatoid arthritis include a progressive apertognathism (anterior open bite) as the condyle and necks are affected by the disease (Fig. 11–3). The disease usually involves the TM joints bilaterally and symmetrically, but it can be unilateral. The disease is a chronic, incurable disorder that afflicts 2 to 3% of the population.

The incidence of TM joint involvement is the same in edentate and dentate patients.[24] When these joints are involved, the disease typically begins at their periphery, as the synovial tissues are converted into pannus cells. These cells release enzymes that erode the condyle and temporal bone from the periphery inward toward the center of the articular surfaces. The marrow spaces beneath the eroding bone become acutely inflamed. The pannus cells are converted into fibroblasts; as the condyles erode, the remaining condylar process moves superiorly into the glenoid fossa and produces a fibrous ankylosis. The radius of the closure arc shortens so that the last pair of molars contact on mandibular closure with the creation of an anterior open bite. A progressive loss of posterior teeth usually follows the open bite deformity. As the apertognathism and the fibrous ankylosis progress, the range of motion of the mandible becomes negligible. In addition to the loss of teeth, loss of mandibular function by ankylosis, and the orthognathic deformity, the patient may have difficulty in swallowing and may experience sleep apnea because of the encroachment of the upper airway as the

that may occlude the external auditory meatus. The cartilage on the lateral one half of the anterior wall of the external auditory meatus is flexible and mobile enough that the swelling may occlude the meatus. Findings in the oral cavity usually include altered posterior occlusion related to the accumulation of the products of the acute and chronic inflammatory processes within the joint space. The facial nerve is located enough inferiorly that no palsy is usually noted. Cervical lymphadenopathy is an inconsistent finding.

Infectious arthritis of the TM joint is difficult to diagnose, because the symptoms are similar to those of tumor and of rheumatoid arthritis in this region.[29] Radiographs of the joint usually show an enlarged joint space and, if the infection is chronic, erosion of the condyle. The infection may destroy the disk and involve the temporal bone. An additional impetus for an early diagnosis and treatment is the often significant morbidity and possible mortality associated with infectious arthritis of the TM joint.

Aspiration and examination of joint fluid is helpful in establishing the definitive diagnosis, but it is difficult because of the small amount of synovial fluid in the TM joint. Infection in the overlying parotid gland is ruled out before aspiration to avoid contamination of a previously normal joint. Drainage, debridement, and irrigation of the joint with antibiotic solutions are recommended. General systemic supportive antibiotic therapy should be vigorous and prolonged.

Infectious arthritis of the TM joint is usually monoarticular, suggesting a local rather than a systemic etiology. Local etiologic factors may be related to invasion of the joint by external trauma, extrinsic from an ear infection, or sequelae of a surgical procedure (Fig. 11–4). Infectious arthritides are treated as may be appropriate with due regard for the etiology and possible subsequent ravages. In a young person who does not have skeletal maturity, a facial skeletal growth deformity may arise as the result of an infection of the TM joint.

### Staphylococcal Arthritis

Staphylococci reside in and on all the oral, nasal, and maxillofacial tissues. These per-

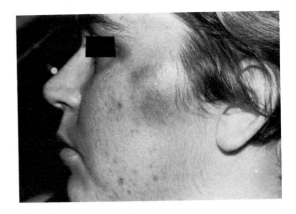

**Fig. 11–4.** Postoperative TM joint acute inflammatory process. The inflammation dissected anteriorly from the surgical site and was overlying the zygomatic arch. This inflammation was treated with incision, drainage, and antibiotic therapy.

sistent bacteria can be or become resistant to penicillin, tetracycline, erythromycin, and, even, chloramphenicol, and they may produce large quantities of penicillinase. Septic staphylococcal arthritis occurs as acute involvement of a joint after a primary infection elsewhere in the body. The usual signs and symptoms of an acute inflammation are warm, reddened, swollen overlying tissues and a severely painful joint with limitation of motion. On the rare occasion when staphylococci attack the TM joint, the treatment consists of identification of the organisms, incision and drainage, supportive care, and antibiotic therapy. Before positive identification of the microorganisms, the antibiotic to prescribe for adults is nafcillin (250 to 500 mg every 4 to 6 hours for a minimum of 3 weeks).

### Streptococcal Arthritis

Pneumococcal arthritis from *Streptococcus pneumoniae*, a normal inhabitant of the nasopharynx, may be preceded by an underlying metabolic or disease process, such as alcoholism or multiple myeloma. This type of septic arthritis rarely affects the TM joint. Initial treatment consists of incision and drainage with supportive antibiotic therapy (5 million units of penicillin G intravenously per day).

Streptococcal infections may arise from the hemolytic *Streptococcus pyogenes* or the anerobic *Streptococcus viridans*, and produce arthritis by a toxic or sensitivity reaction within a TM joint. Treatment consists of incision and drainage and a course of penicillin G (250,000 U/kg/day in 4 doses for 2 weeks) for *Staphylococcus pyogenes*. For a *Streptococcus viridans* infection, ampicillin is effective (250 mg four times daily for 3 weeks).

## Gram-Negative Bacillary Arthritis

*Hemophilus influenzae* arthritis occurs predominantly in children. The attack produces an immunity, and thus this gram-negative coccobacillus is rarely seen in adults.[17] The treatment consists of incision and drainage and combined therapy of ampicillin (100 mg/kg/day orally) and chloramphenicol (50 mg/kg/day intravenously, divided into four doses per day). As results of culture and sensitivity studies become available for a given patient, one or the other of these antibiotics may be discontinued.

*Escherichia coli* is the third most common microbial pathogen in wound infections after staphylococci and streptococci. *Pseudomonas aeruginosa* infections occur in individuals with cardiopulmonary disease, lymphoma, or severe burns, or who are receiving immunosuppressive agents. *Klebsiella pneumoniae*, a saprophyte of the upper respiratory tree, and the widely distributed *Proteus* bacilli have the potential to produce septic arthritis. *Pseudomonas aeruginosa*, along with *E. coli*, are responsible for the greatest number of gram-negative septic arthritic infections. Treatment of such infections includes incision and drainage, supportive care, and administration with monitoring and dose adjustments as necessary, of gentamicin (3 to 5 mg/kg/day intramuscularly in 3 doses for 3 weeks).

Bacterial arthritis produced by gram-negative rods most often occurs in debilitated individuals, especially those with urinary and bowel sepsis. Characteristically, the arthritis is monoarticular and is associated with pain, inflammation, and edema. The progress of the treatment of the affected joint is usually slow because of the background illness. Antibiotic therapy is initiated promptly and vigorously and is changed as indicated by identification of the responsible organism. Appropriate antibiotics include gentamicin, tobramycin, amikacin, chloramphenicol, and ampicillin.

## Arthritis Caused by Mycobacteria and Fungi

*Mycobacterium tuberculosis* can invade the joints by either hematogenous or lymphatic metastasis or by reactivating a latent lesion. Articular destruction begins at the periphery and proceeds centrally at a slow pace when compared to pyogenic infections. Articular tuberculosis is often a combination of osteomyelitis and arthritis.

In about 50% of patients with skeletal tuberculosis, the disease affects the spine, with the larger weight-bearing joints (hip and knee) being the next most often infected. Tuberculosis arthritis is initially a monoarticular, chronic disease with a peak incidence in the fourth and fifth decades of life. The most useful immunologic test for a differential diagnosis is the skin test.

Septic joints may be produced by leprosy; coccidiomycosis, a fungus most often found in the semi-arid areas; blastomycosis and histoplasmosis, primarily, in the United States, in the middle Atlantic states and the Ohio and Mississippi River valleys; and candida, usually in individuals with concurrent disease. Actinomyces israelii, an anaerobic bacteria-like obligate, is a normal inhabitant of the oral cavity; skeletal involvement may occur, usually secondary to the adjacent soft tissue infections, with the spinal column most frequently affected. Treatment involves long-term penicillin and tetracycline use.

## Viral Arthritis

Bilateral arthralgia of the joints of the limbs is common in patients afflicted with rubella (German measles). Monoarticular joint involvement occurs in 20 to 25% of patients. The TM joint may be the focal point, beset by arthritis of either gradual or sudden onset. No standard radiologic changes are discernible. Treatment consists of the usual management of systemic diseases.

## Lyme Disease

Lyme disease gained its name from Lyme, Connecticut, one of the communities in which the disease was first identified. A spirochete, *Borrelia bergdorferi*, was isolated as the causative organism for the production of Lyme disease. The spirochete is carried in the nymphal stage deer tick, *Ixodes dammini* in the northeastern United States and *Ixodes pacificus* in California and Oregon. The vector animals are both wild animals and family pets.

At the point of bite by the tick, an erythematous rash develops, erythema chronicum migrans, as do such signs and symptoms as malaise, chills, fever, and either polyarticular, oligoarticular, or monoarticular arthritis. In an excellent review of the disease, Harris reported a case involving a 35-year-old white woman with a dull ache in the right jaw that was aggravated by mandibular movements.[30] A tentative diagnosis of Lyme disease was made based on her history of being an active gardener living in a wooded area and the presence of erythema. Harris wrote, ''The currently accepted (treatment) regimen is tetracycline 1 g daily in divided doses for 10 to 20 days for adults and penicillin, 1 to 2 g daily in divided doses for the same period for children.'' If indicated, these doses may be doubled or supplemented with intramuscular administration of benzathine penicillin.

## Gonococcal Arthritis

*Neisseria gonorrhoeae* appears to have a strong affinity for synovial fluid. As early as the 14th century, and continuing for 500 years of medical writing through the 19th century, an association between arthritis and urethritis was noted. The factors responsible for the arthrotropic properties of gonococci are not yet defined, but in a small percentage of patients, arthritis is a complication of urethritis owing to gonococcal infections. The clinical features suggestive of gonococcal arthritis include fever, polyarthritis, skin lesions, joint fluid containing white blood cells, and diagnosis by cultures of the blood. The treatment consists of systemic management of the microbial infection and management, as indicated, for the residuals of the disease in the TM and other joints.

## Traumatic Arthritis

Traumatic arthritis may occur from a single or repetitive episodes of trauma. The various clinical manifestations include sprains, acute traumatic synovitis, post-traumatic osteoarthritis, chronic monoarticular arthritis, rapid bone atrophy, osteochondritis dissecans, bursitis, injuries to muscles and tendons, and arthropathy.

### Sprains

When a joint is forced beyond its normal range, the resulting stretching or tearing of the supporting ligaments is a sprain. The capsular ligament and, possibly, the meniscus and its attachments may be disrupted, with resulting edema; hemorrhage and hemarthrosis also may occur. Usually, the patient complains of severe pain centered in the TM joint area. Early treatment consists of ice packs for 10 minutes every 3 hours, compression dressings, simple analgesics, and, perhaps, an anesthetic block of the auriculotemporal nerve to control the pain. Examination of the occlusal relations and radiographs obtained in the open and closed mandibular positions allows identification of any condyle and condylar neck fractures.

Patients experience an initial limitation of motion of the mandible, with a controlled return of the mandible to full use, providing a fairly immobile osseous base for repair of the injured soft tissues. This type of injury is usually self-limiting, with full return to function.

The analgesic may be aspirin (two 325-mg tablets stat, then one tablet every 2 hours during waking hours for 3 or 4 days. In the evening, a Timed-Release, 650-mg tablet is prescribed). Nonnarcotic analgesics, especially aspirin, are extremely effective in pain control when taken on a regular basis. Ibuprofen (one 400- or 600-mg tablet three times daily) may be prescribed for patients for whom aspirin is contraindicated.

Regional anesthetic agents, procaine, lidocaine, and mepivacaine, may be used for both pain control and diagnostic purposes, i.e., if pain is relieved by injecting a local anesthetic in the area of the lateral TM joint ligament, the injury is probably extracapsular.

The authors examined a 21-year-old man who had received a lateral blow to the mandible while playing touch football. He was experiencing severe pain in the left TM joint and held his hand across his left preauricular region. Examination revealed resistance to any mandibular movement, simultaneous posterior stops on closure, and no anterior or posterior opened bite. The left auriculotemporal nerve was anesthetized with 3% mepivacaine without a vasoconstrictor, and the pain was relieved in approximately 3 minutes. We gave the patient an ice pack to apply to the left preauricular region and prescribed ibuprofen (600-mg tablet three times daily). Twenty-four hours later, the patient reported that the pain did not return when the anesthetic wore off, and he had discontinued the ibuprofen medication. The patient experienced no postinjury problems from the time of the 24-hour postoperative visit to a recall examination 3 years later.

A 22-year-old man had right preauricular pain of 60-minutes duration. The history revealed he had had an occlusal gold foil restoration placed in his lower left first premolar and the pain began on completion of the procedure. When he closed his mouth, the left posterior teeth contacted prematurely. When he forced the right teeth into occlusion, he had a sensation of swelling or fullness in the right preauricular region, and the pain increased. Lateral transcranial radiographs revealed no abnormal bony contours, but the right TM joint space was slightly wider than the left. A regimen of ice packs and moist heat alternately at 5-minute intervals for 30 minutes every 2 hours was recommended. Indomethacin (25-mg capsule, three times daily with meals, was prescribed). Twenty-eight hours later, the posterior teeth closed into simultaneous occlusion, and the soreness was minimal. The patient had no TM joint-related signs or symptoms to report at a routine 3-month postoperative recall appointment.

## Acute Hypertranslation

So-called whiplash injuries of the TM joint and associated soft tissues are possible, likely related to a sudden and violent hypertranslation of the condyle. The translation occurs as the head is rapidly extended and discordant movements of the major and accessory muscles of mastication may not stabilize the TM joints. These movements distract the condyles down and forward, producing a transient joint sprain. In a rear-end impact automobile injury, many sensory clues and physical energy-absorbing buffers protect against and prevent discordant movements, including the sounds before impact of a vehicle following closely that cause the patient to tense the musculature involuntarily and protect the TM joints. Buffering the TM joint from the impact is from the absorption of energy by the automobile's bumpers, chassis, body, and seats. At greater risk than the TM joints, which are designed for extreme movements, is damage to the spinal column, nerve roots, or spinal cord by violent hyperextension; these spinal column and nervous system injuries were described by Gay and Abbott as whiplash injury.[31] They noted the compounding effect of emotional stress.

We have seen hundreds of patients who incurred maxillofacial trauma,[32] but so-called TM joint whiplash injury was the source of referral only in the past 15 years, and all of these instances involved slow-moving motor vehicular accidents in which the patients were seeking legal, not medical, benefits. We are impressed that patient awareness of a clicking sound or other actual internal derangement of a TM joint and a history or a memory of an episode of trauma may be combined with a hope of a psychologic benefit or legal recourse. One is reminded of the observation of the orthopedic surgeon H.M. Frost, "In my time I have seen for diagnosis and/or treatment, more than 10,000 patients with unresolved liability from a real or imagined injury. Yet in the same period, I have seen only three patients desiring help or advice for such injury after liability was closed!"[33]

Weinberg and Lapointe identified 28 patients with post-whiplash TM joint symptoms of internal derangements that were confirmed arthrographically in 22 patients and in 10 of the 22 patients who elected to have surgery. There was no follow-up data.[34]

## Acute Traumatic Arthritis

Swelling and pain may occur after a direct blow to the TM joint or from injury to the TM joint transmitted by the mandible, which was the recipient of trauma. Clinical evaluation indicates an effusion within the joint and, assuming no maxillofacial skeletal fractures occurred, the patient may note that the posterior teeth feel "pushed out" of occlusion. The effusion within the joint space usually contains some blood; the greater the hemarthrosis, the greater the level of pain. Initial treatment may consist of cold packs and compression dressings.

The prognosis is excellent, providing the return to function, in graded exercises, occurs as soon as possible. As a practical approach to function, the patient is instructed to use one half a piece of sugarless chewing gum and, over 10 days, increase the size of the chewing gum to two or three pieces. Physical therapy exercises may be indicated.

If, however, the mandible is immobilized as part of the treatment, prognosis may be less favorable. The lack of movement enhances the possibilities of fibrosis, ossification of the hematoma, and ankylosis. Such immobilization may be unavoidable, however, the need dictated by concurrent injuries.

Synovial chondromatosis may be a long-range result of trauma to the synovial tissues. It manifests years after the original trauma, and the solution is surgical removal of "joint mice."

## Synovial Chondromatosis

Synovial chondromatosis is a condition of unknown etiology in which foci of cartilage develop in the synovial membrane of a joint, apparently through metaplasia of the sublining connective tissue of the synovial membrane.[35] The joint capsule originates, embryologically, from the same primitive tissue that creates periosteum and perichondrium. Hyaline cartilage islands, usually microscopic, are found in the synovial membrane and produce nests of chondrocytes that grow into cartilaginous bodies. These bodies may become dislodged into the joint space as free bodies that survive in synovial fluid (Fig. 11–5). The free cartilaginous bodies acquire a perichondrium and, through proliferation, layers of chondrocytes are added to the periphery and

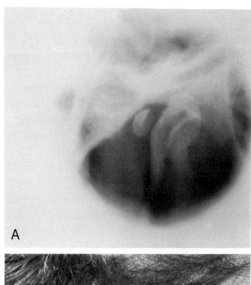

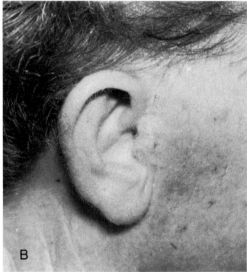

*Fig. 11–5.* A. Cartilaginous particles of synovial chondromatosis removed from a unilateral superior TM joint space of an adult woman. These freely floating bodies were in the superior joint space and were interfering with mandibular movements on an erratic and unpredictable basis. B. Incision line one week postoperatively.

produce synovial chondromatosis, often referred to as "joint mice."

Synovial chondromatosis may produce pain with movement of the TM joint, but often the presenting complaint is limitation of motion, usually in an irregular and unpredictable manner, depending on the location and the number of the synovial chondromatosis bodies. It is more common in men than in women and is usually first diagnosed in middle-aged adults, although the condition has been present for years. The disorder is found in association with the arthritides, and the history does not always include previous acute trauma to the TM joint. Thompson and associates described a patient in whom the synovial chondromatosis had extended beyond the confines of the joint capsule, encompassing the condylar neck and extending into the parotid gland.[36] The lesion resembled a benign mixed tumor.

The treatment is surgical removal of the usually free-floating masses.[37] During the operation, the synovium is inspected for areas of cartilaginous transformations, and these, too, are excised.

## Neuropathic Joint Disease (Charcot Joints)

A variety of neurologic disorders may result in arthropathy as a complication. Eichenholtz recounted the J.M. Charcot 1868 report on the clinical manifestations of neuropathies that produce joint problems either as a consequence of diseases of the nervous system or from a congenital absence of pain perception.[38]

The neuropathic arthropathy follows a loss of proprioceptive or nociceptive activity, which leads to a relaxation of the supporting soft tissues and instability of the joint. Severe and cumulative injury to the skeleton and the joints results in degeneration of the cartilaginous and osseous structures.

The pathologic changes may advance to changes similar to non-neuropathic degenerative joint disease. The changes include fibrillation and erosion of the articular surfaces, destruction of the menisci, formation of local bodies within the joint capsule, and growth of osteophytes. The joints may continue to be hypermobile, and the osteophytes become large and irregularly shaped.

The onset may be insidious, with greater destruction of the joint than is indicated by the concurrent clinical signs and symptoms. In some cases, therefore, the first indication of the problem may be an intracapsular or juxtacapsular fracture.

Early clinical examination reveals hypermobility and warmth to palpation. Later, findings include a loss of the articular surfaces and formation of intracapsular loose bodies.

A variety of disorders of the central and peripheral nervous systems may produce sensory impairments that could produce Charcot joints: acromegaly, leprosy, amyloid neuropathy, peripheral nerve injury, and hereditary sensory neuropathies. Repeated intra-articular injections of cortisone have been implicated as a cause. In order of incidence for producing Charcot joints are: syphilitic tabes dorsalis, diabetic neuropathy, alcoholic neuropathies and avitaminosis, pernicious anemia, and syringomyelia. In a study of 68 patients with neuropathic joint disease, Eichenholtz reported that 35% of the patients had painful swelling while 41% had painless swelling of the affected joints.[38]

Treatment includes temporizing surgical approaches to remove all cartilage, debris, and poorly vascularized sclerotic bone. The synovia and capsule are debrided. Total joint replacements may be necessary.

## Other Maladies

Many functional maladies have TM joint manifestations, including tumors, genetic and hereditary disorders, systemic lupus erythematosus, and hemarthrosis secondary to medications.

### Tumors

When the evidence from physical evaluation and imaging techniques is suggestive of a tumor in the TM joint, often if the tumor is benign, the joint moves freely, with expected alterations owing to the presence of the tumor. If the lesion is malignant, the joint likely is fixed or has limited range of motion.

A common tumor is an osteochondroma. Marks and associates observed that osteochondromas usually appear at the metaphyseal region of long bones and, in the mandible, they may manifest in the condylar process, the coronoid process, and the parasymphyseal area.[39] The lesion is asymptomatic but may lead to myofascial pains, meniscal painful or painless subluxation (clicking), or dislocation (closed lock). The presenting complaint is often facial asymmetry. The treatment usually involves surgical excision, including the surrounding periosteum. Each case is different, and repair of the meniscus may be indicated, as described by Schweber and Fensilli.[40] If the excision includes the entire condylar process, individuals can function without a replacement, but the usual course of therapy is to reconstruct the condylar process with an alloplastic condyle or a costochondral graft.

Malignant neoplasms may arise from the mandibular or temporal aspects of the TM joint or are a metastatic presentation. The signs and symptoms of myofascial pain or dysfunction may be the problem that prompts the patient to seek care from a dentist, and a metastatic adenocarcinoma in the condylar region is not an unusual finding. Hecker and associates[41] and Owen and Stelling[42] described a 63-year-old woman and a 68-year-old man, respectively, who received therapy directed toward an expectation that the patients had TM joint maladies; both patients had adenocarcinomatous metastatic lesions.

### Familial Mediterranean Fever

Familial Mediterranean fever (periodic disease, recurrent polyserositis) is a genetic disorder affecting the Middle Eastern population of Sephardic Jews, Armenians, and Arabic individuals. The etiology is unknown, but the disease begins in childhood regardless of gender and involves the serous membranes, including the synovial tissues. Patients experience intermittent and recurring attacks of abdominal, chest, and joint pain, which are nonpainful, except for the involved joints, between exacerbations. The TM joint is rarely involved. Tovi and associates, however, described a patient with TM joint involvement that began with ". . . joint effusion without bony changes . . . Later, severe arthritic changes with marked reduction in the volume of the condyle . . . simulating aseptic necrosis."[43]

### Mitochondrial Myopathy

Van Sickels and associates described three patients with TM joint pain and dysfunction who proved to have a hereditary disorder, mitochondrial myopathy.[44] The presence of this muscular systemic myopathy in a patient

population underlines the heterogeneity of the population of many Western nations.

### Systemic Lupus Erythematosus-Induced TM Joint Arthritis

Systemic lupus erythematosus is a many faceted connective tissue disorder producing fever; skin and visceral lesions; hematologic abnormalities, such as anemia, thrombocytopenia, and leukopenia; and involvement of joints. Autoimmune phenomena are noted and management is complex. If the signs and symptoms of TM joint pain and dysfunction are present, the TM joint may undergo aseptic necrosis; radiographic views display one or more bone fragments in the area. In view of the ongoing autoimmune phenomena associated with this connective tissue disorder, treatment directed toward the TM joint includes conservative surgical removal of the fragments. The major treatment thrust for the facial pains is nonsurgical management of the occlusal table.

### Hemarthrosis Secondary to Anticoagulant Therapy

Hess and Baart reported a case involving a patient who had an open bite deformity of rapid onset.[45] The 17-year-old female patient was receiving anticoagulant therapy. The hemarthrosis was unilateral and responded to aspiration of 3½ ml of blood from the joint space. This case emphasizes the fact that not only is the TM joint subject to general systemic influences, but also the integrity of the joint space is an anatomic fact. The capsule of the joint space is a physical barrier and gives practical meaning to the adjectives intracapsular and extracapsular.

### References

1. Toller P.A.: Osteoarthrosis of the mandibular condyle. Br Dent J, 134:223, 1973
2. Ogus H.: Degenerative disease of the temporomandibular joint in young persons. Br J Oral Surg, 17:17, 1979
3. DeBont L.G.M., Boering G., Liem R.S., and Havinga P.: Osteoarthritis of the temporomandibular joint: A

We appreciate the review of this chapter by Dr. David A. McLain, rheumatologist, of Birmingham, Alabama.

light microscopic and scanning electron microscopic study of the articular cartilage of the mandibular condyle. J Oral Maxillofac Surg, 43:481, 1985

4. Nickerson J.W. and Boering G.: Natural course of osteoarthritis as it relates to the internal derangements of the temporomandibular joint. Oral and Maxillofac Surg Clinics of N Am, 1:27, 1989

5. Boering G.: Arthrosis deformans van het Kaahgewricht. Leiden, Stafleu en Tholen, 1966

6. Stegenga B., DeBont L.G.M., and Boering G.: Osteoarthrosis as the cause of craniomandibular pain and dysfunction: A unifying concept. J Oral Maxillofac Surg, 47:249, 1989

7. Rasmussen O.C.: Temporomandibular arthropathy, clinical, radiologic, and therapeutic aspects, with emphasis on diagnosis (thesis). Int J Oral Surg, 13:365, 1984

8. Quinn J.H.: Pathogenesis of temporomandibular joint chondromalacia and arthralgia. Oral and Maxillofac Surg Clinics of N Am, 1:47, 1989

9. Ogus H.D. and Toller P.A.: Common Disorders of the Temporomandibular Joint. Bristol, John Wright & Sons, 1981

10. Kreutziger K.L. and Mahan P.E.: Temporomandibular degenerative joint disease, part I. Anatomy, pathophysiology and clinical description. Oral Surg Oral Med Oral Pathol, 40:297, 1975

11. Dibbits J.M.H.: Juvenile Temporomandibular Joint Dysfunction and Craniofacial Growth: A statistical analysis. Leiden, Stafleu en Tholen, 1977

12. Dibbits J.M.H.: Symptoms of TMJ dysfunction: Indicators of growth patterns? J Pedodont, 9:265, 1985

13. Stewart C.L. and Standish S.M.: Osteoarthritis of the TMJ in teenaged females: Report of cases. J Am Dent Assoc, 106:638, 1983

14. Aufdemorte T.B., et al: Estrogen receptors in the temporomandibular joint of the baboon (Papio cynocephalus): An autoradiographic study. Oral Surg Oral Med Oral Pathol, 61:307, 1986

15. Spiera H. and Plotz C.M.: Rheumatic symptoms and oral contraceptives. Lancet, 1:571, 1969

16. Blackwood H.J.J.: Arthritis of the mandibular joint. Br Dent J, 115:317, 1963

17. McAllister A.D.: A microscopic survey of the human temporomandibular joint. N Z Dent J, 50:161, 1954

18. Castelli W.J.: Histopathologic findings in temporomandibular joints of aged individuals. J Prosthet Dent, 53:415, 1985

19. Akerman S., Kopp S., and Rohlin M.: Histologic changes in temporomandibular joints from elderly individuals. Acta Odontol Scand, 44:231, 1986

20. Sokoloff L.: The Biology of Degenerative Joint Disease. Chicago, University of Chicago Press, 1969

21. Kopp S., Wenneberg B., and Carlsson G.E.: The short-term effect of intra-articular injections on temporomandibular joint and dysfunction. J Oral Maxillofac Surg, 43:429, 1985

22. Kopp S., Carlsson G.E., Haraldson T., and Wenneberg B.: Long-term effect of intra-articular injections of sodium hyaluronate and corticosteroids on the temporomandibular joints. J Oral Maxillofac Surg, 45:929, 1987

23. Blumer D. and Heilbronn M.: Second year follow-up study on systemic treatment of chronic pain with antidepressants. Henry Ford Hosp Med J, 29:67, 1981

24. Larheim T.A., Storhaug K., and Tveito L.: Temporomandibular joint involvement and dental occlusion in a group of adults with rheumatoid arthritis. Acta Odontol Scand, 41:301, 1983

25. Kent J.N., Carlton D.M., and Zide M.F.: Rheumatoid disease and related arthropathies. Oral Surg Oral Med Oral Pathol, 61:423, 1986

26. Haanes H.R., Larheim T.A., and Nickerson J.W.: Discectomy and synovectomy of the temporomandibular joint in the treatment of rheumatoid arthritis: Case report with three-year follow-up study. J Oral Maxillofac Surg, 44:905, 1986

27. Lowery J.C.: Psoriatic arthritis involving the temporomandibular joint. J Oral Maxillofac Surg, 33:206, 1975

28. Baetz K. and Klineberg I.: Psoriatic arthritis of the temporomandibular joint. Case report. Aust Dent J, 31:335, 1986

29. Bounds G.A., Hopkins R., and Sugar A.: Septic arthritis of the temporomandibular joint—a problematic diagnosis. Br J Oral Maxillofac Surg, 25:61, 1987

30. Harris R.J.: Lyme disease involving the temporomandibular joint. J Oral Maxillofac Surg, 46:78, 1988

31. Gay J.R. and Abbott K.H.: Common whiplash injuries to the neck. JAMA, 152:1698, 1953

32. Alling C.C. and Osbon D.B.: Maxillofacial Trauma. Philadelphia, Lea & Febiger, 1988

33. Frost M.M.: Musculoskeletal Pain. In Facial Pain. 2nd Ed. Edited by C.C. Alling and P.E. Mahan. Philadelphia, Lea & Febiger, 1977

34. Weinberg S. and Lapointe H.: Cervical extension-flexion injury (whiplash) and internal derangement of the temporomandibular joint. J Oral Maxillofac Surg, 45:653, 1987

35. Alling C.C., Rawson D.W., Staats O.J., and Middleton R.A.: Synovial chondromatosis of the temporomandibular joints. J Oral Maxillofac Surg, 31:691, 1973

36. Thompson K., Schwartz H.C., and Miles J.: Synovial chondromatosis of the temporomandibular joint presenting as a parotid mass. Possibility of confusion with a benign mixed tumor. Oral Surg Oral Med Oral Pathol, 62:377, 1986

37. Davis C., Davis W.H., DiTraglia R., and Kaminish R.M.: Synovial chondromatosis of the temporomandibular joint. J Prosthet Dent, 60:5, 1988

38. Eichenholtz S.N.: Charcot joints. Springfield, C.C Thomas Pub., 1966

39. Marks R.B., Carlton D.M. Jr., and Carr R.F.: Osteochondroma of the mandibular joint. Oral Surg Oral Med Oral Pathol, 58:30, 1984

40. Schweber S.J. and Fensilli J.A.: Osteochondroma of the mandibular condyle: Report of case and review of literature. J Am Dent Assoc, 113:269, 1986

41. Hecker R., Noon W., and Elliott M.: Adenocarcinoma metastatic to the temporomandibular joint. J Oral Maxillofac Surg, 43:629, 1985

42. Owen D.G. and Stelling C.B.: Condylar metastasis with initial presentation as TMJ syndrome. J Oral Med, 40:198, 1985

43. Tovi F., Barmeir E., Peist M., and Bar-Ziv J.: Protracted temporomandibular joint arthritis in familial Mediterranean fever. J Oral Maxillofac Surg, 43:466, 1985

44. Van Sickels J.E., Gruber A.B., Kagan-Hallet K.S., and Dowd D.C.: Mitochondrial myopathy presenting as a TM dysfunction. J Oral Maxillofac Surg, 45:168, 1987

45. Hess J., and Baart J.A.: Sudden open bite resulting from hemarthrosis: Report of a case. J Oral Maxillofac Surg, 46:513, 1988

# 12

# *Temporomandibular Joint Surgery*

Facial pain patients usually have a summation of anatomic, physiologic, and psychologic factors that put the temporomandibular (TM) joint and the associated musculature and ligaments at risk. Some individuals, usually women, exhibit a lack of sturdiness of the TM joint. Additionally, in young women, metabolic factors may play a role in producing TM joint arthritis, usually monoarticular, which undergoes a painful degenerative phase.

Chronic, repetitive, unremitting trauma to inherently unstable TM joints may result in intracapsular instabilities, such as subluxation and dislocation of the menisci; in limitation of mandibular movements owing to myospasms of the cervical and the major and accessory muscles of mastication; and in strains of the ligaments. Such trauma may arise from one or more anatomic factors that change posteriorly the locus of vectors of the muscles of mastication that tend to overload the TM joints. These factors may be a steep occlusal plane, mandibular retrognathism, maxillary prognathism, or other orthognathic facial skeletal abnormalities.

The habitual posturing of the mandible in abnormal positions may damage the musculoskeletal system associated with the TM joints. Examples of noxious habits are positioning the mandible in strained isometric open occlusion, in full clenched occlusion, in bruxing activities, in a forward position for esthetic reasons, and other habits detrimental to stability of the TM joints.

To ensure a successful outcome of TM joint surgery to correct intracapsular instabilities, control of the anatomic factors just mentioned must be considered. In many instances of internal derangement of the TM joint produced by psychologic factors, correction or control of the abnormal anatomic relationships by facial skeletal surgery and by orthodontic treatments and other occlusal therapy may permit the patient to recover from the myospasms and intra-articular instabilities without TM joint surgery. Similarly, in many patients with internal derangements of the TM joint, correction of the abnormal anatomic relationships by orthodontic treatments and other occlusal therapy, and by facial skeletal surgery, may obviate surgical intervention into the TM joint. These somatic treatments, which alter the facial skeleton in some patients and the occlusal relations in all patients, achieve the best results when accompanied and followed by physical therapy designed to increase muscular mobility and strength. In many cases, the somatic treatments must be supported with psychophysiologic care.

The report by Okeson and Hayes is indicative of the high success rate produced by nonsurgical treatment of TM joint disorders.[1] They mention their 80% success rate may not have been totally due to the modalities used, and that lower levels of emotional stress may have contributed to the 80% success rate of pain reduction. Green and Laskin indicated that TM joint internal derangements may produce a variety of accommodative responses, that arthritic lesions may repair, and bone surfaces remodel in response to function; they emphasized the initial treatment of internal derangements should be nonsurgical.[2]

Patients with meniscus dislocations (closed lock) may have a treatment history that is similar to those with a painful meniscus subluxation (clicking). (Not to be confused with condylar dislocation and subluxation, meniscus dislocation is synonymous with closed lock; meniscus subluxation is synonymous with a clicking TM joint.[3]) If nonsurgical medical therapy is not effective, either open or arthroscopic TM joint surgery may be indicated. Meniscus repositioning, meniscorrhaphy, diskoplasty, disk repair, ligament and capsular procedures, meniscectomy, eminence contouring, condylar repositioning procedures, and placement of temporary or permanent alloplastic devices may be considered.

Fortunately, controversy still exists about the etiology of the various manifestations of TM joint maladies. With parallel clinical and pathologic descriptions of internal derangements associated with degenerative arthritis, for example, some doctors believe there is a disorder that tends to be progressive in its course.[4] Other doctors note a cycle course that includes a possible resolution or reasonable accommodation for some patients. Impressive success rates may be cited for a wide variety of surgical and nonsurgical modalities and techniques.[1,5–9] These successes in managing patients who may be desperate with pain and disabilities have led to an occasional opinion that emphasizes limited aspects of the overall problem or of a given technique.

After violent and acute trauma, an injured meniscus is usually treated successfully by rest, and, possibly, physical therapy and occlusal therapy; for patients with a residual disability that is unresponsive to nonsurgical approaches, intracapsular repair is considered. On rare occasions, so-called whiplash injuries and other events featuring a temporary dislocation of the TM joint manifest as subsequent painful subluxation or dislocation of the meniscus. If nonsurgical care is unsuccessful, a TM joint surgical procedure may be indicated.

Chronic mandibular dislocations are amenable to surgical intervention, and the need for an accurate, etiologically based diagnosis is imperative. A completely successful surgical solution for a dislocating mandible in a patient afflicted with Parkinson's disease may not be possible or reasonable.

This chapter is a discussion of TM joint surgery for patients disabled by nonresolving arthritic changes, painful meniscus subluxations, meniscus dislocations, and chronic mandibular dislocations. The surgical approaches to the TM joint are the preauricular, modifications of the preauricular, postauricular, modifications of the postauricular, arthroscopic, and transoral and extraoral approaches for osteotomies of the posterior mandibular ramus and condylar process.

## Preoperative Considerations

Appropriate imagery, to confirm clinical impressions, is necessary. There is a temptation to utilize multiple imagery modalities for defensive legal reasons and for scientific inquiry. Lessin and Gross in a review of 50 TM joint surgeries emphasized confirming accuracy of clinical findings at surgery without preoperative arthrograms, CT scans, or MRI modalities.[10]

Preoperative considerations include obtaining the maximum potential from intraoral manipulations by using, when indicated, splints and physical therapy. Physical therapy modes, ranging from iontophoresing to muscle strengthening, are designed to relieve myofascial pains and spasms and to stabilize the TM joints.

Nonresolving, irreversible arthritic changes of the TM joint are differentiated from the typically monoarticular, self-limiting, reversible degenerative arthritis associated with the metabolism of women in the second and third decades of life. Fortunately, in regard to reversible degenerative arthritis, the manifestations are cyclic, and although painful, usually resolve. Management involves simple analgesics and possibly splint therapy. Crepitation may be severe in a joint with degenerative arthritis, yet if pain sensory nerve endings are not involved, the patient experiences no pain, and mandibular movements are reasonable, the indications for surgery are not strong. If, however, limitation of motion increases over a period of 12 months, then a surgical solution may be considered. Painful and irreversible degenerative arthritis, proven by data from a history and imaging techniques, may be relieved by surgery.

Painful meniscus subluxations are tempting in terms of considering a surgical solution. Often the patient has had multiple types of dental therapy performed and says, "Nothing has worked, but I am agreeable to having you do whatever you want, and I have 'good' insurance." In fact, many of these patients are referred to the surgeon with the expectation of all concerned—the referring doctor, the patient, and the patient's family—that an operation is forthcoming. We have had patients in the preceding circumstances who benefitted from our instruction to have the first movement of the mandible involve a hinge rather than a protrusive movement, thus eliminating an annoying early clicking sound. Many patients have responded successfully to splint and occlusal related therapy, others to physical therapy exercises, and a few patients came to realize that they were discharging mental stresses by tensing the masticator primary and associated cervical muscles. Clearly, the etiology must be established before surgical intervention or institution of another form of therapy.

## Preoperative Preparation

Antibiotic therapy begins the night before the operation and continues for 7 to 10 days.

Cephalosporins are the usual agents. The preoperative preparation of the patient includes two surgical soap shampoos the night preoperatively, three for long-haired individuals; the morning of the operation the hair is shampooed again. Control of the hair includes removal of the temporal tuft for the preauricular approaches and removal of a 2-cm radius around the posterior and superior area for the postauricular approaches. In our self-conscious society, the patient may prefer being shaven when friends and family are not present, i.e., hair removal is performed in the operating room after the establishment of the nasoendotracheal general anesthesia. Large adhesive pads are used to blot the entire lateral side of the face and hair to pick up stray wisps. Cotton is placed in the external auditory meatus before the hair is removed to prevent small strands of hair from falling against the ear drum and producing a persistent cough that results from irritation of the ninth cranial nerve.

The hair is swept and combed away from the surgical site and is slathered with an antibiotic ointment to keep it in place. The surgical scrub includes the lateral side of the neck and face superiorly from the clavicular area and includes the external auditory meatus. A cellulose sponge or a ball of absorbent cotton saturated with an antibiotic ointment is placed in the external auditory meatus.

Drapes are stapled or sutured in place to expose the ear, the lateral canthus of the eye, and the angle of the mandible. Adhesive, transparent plastic drapes provide occlusion from microbes and permit visibility of the lateral facial and forehead areas. A modified towel clip is placed through the skin, engages the angle of the mandible, and provides a means of mobilizing the mandible intraoperatively. If the anatomy of the patient precludes towel clip placement, either a screw or pin is placed in a manner as is used for application of external skeletal fixation fracture devices or a dissection is performed to give access to the angle of the mandible for placement of a bone clamp or other device. One risk associated with the preceding techniques is penetration of the inferior alveolar neurovascular structures.

## Approaches for Intracapsular Surgery

The surgical approaches to the TM joint are designed to provide surgical access for an intracapsular operation, to minimize the risk of encountering branches of the facial nerve (CV VII) or of influencing the postoperative activity of the facial nerve branches, to avoid the delays necessary to manage branches of the transverse facial artery and the superficial temporal blood vessels, and to provide an esthetic incision line (Fig. 12–1).

### Preauricular Approaches

The preauricular approaches begin by an incision with either a No. 15 blade or an electric hot blade in the depression, fold, or crease at the junction between the anterior cartilage of the ear and the broad planes of the facial

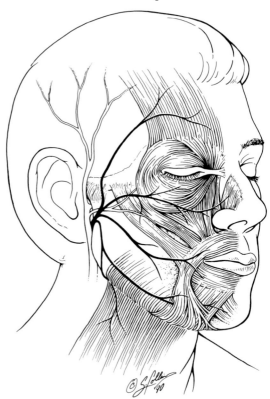

*Fig. 12–1.* Preauricular neurovascular anatomy. One of the many variations of the branches of CN VII is shown as solid black lines. Three branches of the external carotid artery are demonstrated: the superficial temporal artery passing vertically and laterally to the zygomatic process of the temporal bone; the maxillary passing medially to the condylar neck; and the transverse facial artery passing laterally to the condylar neck.

tissues. The incision may begin at the area of the superior-anterior helix and must terminate at the level of the tail of the inferior helix that is palpable through the ear lobe (Fig. 12–2).

The approach may feature a two-level flap. The cutaneous and subcutaneous tissues are elevated by blunt dissection anteriorly for 2 or 3 cm using small, curved dissection scissors. The cutaneous flap is sutured anteriorly with a 3-0 or 2-0 black silk horizontal mattress suture. A small cylinder of moistened gauze is positioned to produce a curve rather than a fold as the flap is turned anteriorly. The cutaneous flap is gently massaged occasionally during the operation to encourage circulation. Sharp and blunt dissection continues through the preauricular tissue above the zygomatic process to the temporal fascia. This medial flap is reflected anteriorly, with the base of the surgical site in the temporal fascia. The periosteum overlying the process is left intact until the tissues lateral to the capsule are dissected and elevated.

Major trunks of the tortuous superficial temporal artery and vein or the transverse facial artery are ligated with 3-0 or 4-0 silk sutures, and arterioles and venules are ligated with absorbable sutures. For small vessels, the use of surgical diathermy is possible if no facial nerve branches are in the immediate vicinity.

The use of a nerve stimulator, set on 2 mA, precedes the dissections to identify branches of the facial nerve and to protect them from damage. Instead of five major branches of the pes anserinus of the facial nerve, a wide variety of nerve trunks may be noted, including an abundance of filaments distributed to the muscles of facial expression. Normal retraction of tissues sometimes incapacitates the transmitting capabilities of the branches of the facial nerve in the vicinity, and with regard to TM joint surgery, the temporal branch is at greatest risk.

Modifications of the approach to this point are in extensions of the superior aspect of the incision anteriorly, either as a straight line, which provides the appearance of an upside-down hockey stick, or an anterior curve of the incision line. Hall and associates compared the effect of two different incisions on the incidence of the loss of function of the frontalis muscle and orbicularis oculi muscle;[11] the hockey stick incision produced loss of function in 22 of 88 patients (all but 1 patient had a return of normal function within 2 to 12 months); a short incision extending from the pinna to the midtragus region and with no skin dissection produced loss of function of

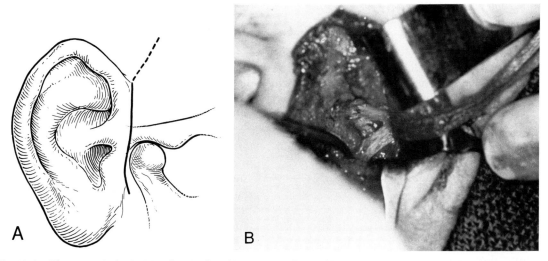

**Fig. 12–2.** The preauricular incision line is placed in a crease (if available). It may have an extension on the superior aspect. The extension may be at an angle as a curved extension, or resemble the blade of a hockey stick. A. Diagram of a preauricular incision; B. Dissection toward the TM joint via a preauricular incision. Note the lateral temporomandibular ligament and the beginning of the zygomatic process of the temporal bone.

the frontalis muscle and none of the orbicularis oculi musculature in 2 patients.

The initial dissection usually is directed to the level of the temporal fascia superior to the zygomatic process of the temporal bone. This tissue is reflected en bloc down to the superior rim of the zygomatic process.

After the preauricular dissection is completed to the zygomatic process of the temporal bone, it proceeds medially, parallel to the long axis of the cartilaginous canal. The lateral head of the condyle is palpable, and moving the mandible helps in identifying and localizing the condyle.

The surgeon makes an incision to bone through the periosteum overlying the zygomatic process of the temporal bone as far forward as the posterior aspect of the arch of the zygomatic process. Blunt dissection is used to raise the soft tissues lateral to the TM joint from the neck of the condyle. A new blade is used to incise lightly through the tissues lateral to the capsule and boldly through the periosteum on the neck of the condyle.

Surgical exposure of the capsule often reveals glistening, firm, sometimes taut, whitish tissue. One may see the lateral ligament, the temporomandibular ligament, as a separate structure, although it is usually a thickened portion of the capsule.

At this juncture, a self-retaining retractor is placed and the operation proceeds with use of either a macroscopic or microscopic approach. When the intracapsular procedure is completed, the preauricular surgical site is closed by layers, with absorbable acid sutures used for the deep structures and polyethylene or monofilament nylon sutures used in the cutaneous areas. Sutures of the latter types give an esthetically acceptable result, as occurs with most atraumatic suturing techniques (Fig. 12–3). Pressure packs are used for 24 to 48 hours postoperatively.

## Direct Lateral Approach

The surgeon incises and dissects directly to the lateral aspect of the condyle. Although more direct and away from the superficial temporal vessels, this approach may not be as esthetically satisfying, may limit access, and is in the area of the upper zygomatic and

the temporal branches of the facial nerve (Fig. 12–4).

## Endaural Approaches

Variations of preauricular approaches include passing the incision line posterior to the tragus. The cartilaginous tragus remains in place, and the flaps are developed, as described previously, either as en bloc elevation to the temporal fascia or by first developing the cutaneous flap, as is associated with the preauricular incision (Fig. 12–5).

A true endaural approach features the incision line sweeping medially through the anterior notch between the cartilage of the external auditory meatus. Anterior dissection is performed, which leads into the same location of the TM joint as from the lateral preauricular approaches. The endaural dissection passes directly to the TM joint in a plane that is medial to the superficial temporal artery and vein, the transverse artery, and branches of the facial nerve.[12] A modified endaural incision described by Nishioka and Van Sickels was placed posterior to the tragus with subsequent retraction of the skin over the tragus.[13]

## Postauricular Approaches

Preoperative preparation is as summarized previously. A tuft of cotton, about 1 to 1.5 cm in diameter, that is impregnated with antibiotic ointment is placed carefully at the junction of the cartilaginous and bony portions of the external auditory meatus to avoid an atmospheric pressure pumping action against the ear drum. A regional anesthetic with a vasoconstrictor is infiltrated into the postauricular and superior auricular areas. A curved incision is made 5 to 10 mm from the posterior junction of the auricula to the cutaneous tissues overlying the mastoid process. The incision extends from near the tip of the mastoid process of the temporal bone to the superior curvature of the auricula (Fig. 12–6).

Kreutziger described a superior extension of the incision that passes, in a curvilinear manner, superior and anterior to the external ear.[14] This incision provides broader superior access to the surgical site.

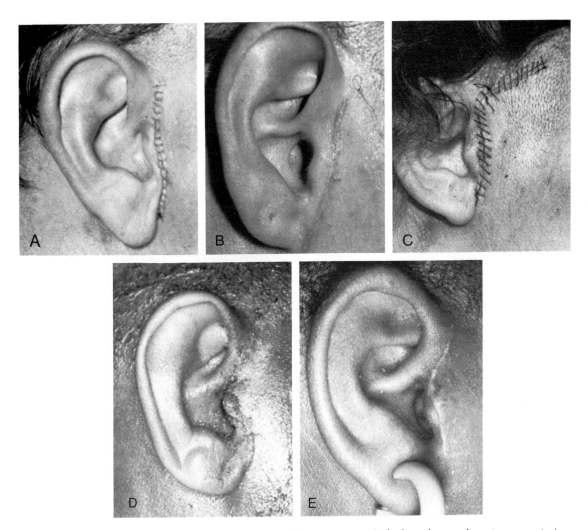

*Fig. 12–3.* Examples of preauricular incisional lines at 48 hours postoperatively. In each case, the cutaneous suturing material was monofilament nylon or (for subcutaneous continuous technique) polypropylene suture. A. Closure using continuous loop intermittently locked technique; B. Subcutaneous continuous technique; C. Preauricular suture with an oblique extension arm that provided access for an extensive reconstruction of the TM joint; D. Combined preauricular and endaural incision line and approach; E. Preauricular incision line that produced a hypertrophic scar. The patient had other operations and incurred lacerations that did not produce the hypertrophic areas. In retrospect, a posterior auricular approach would have been preferable.

Blunt dissection from the superior aspect of the incision proceeds lateral to the temporal fascia to the zygomatic process of the temporal bone. Concurrent with the dissection to the zygomatic process, the lateral 10- to 15-mm part of the external auditory meatus is dissected free. At the medial aspect of the external auditory meatus, just before the point at which the osseous portion begins, the posterior aspects of the canal lack cartilage and intermittent fissures of cartilage are evident on the anterior aspects. The canal is flexible because of the dissection and must be

supported with a finger or an instrument. The posterior and then the anterior halves of the canal are divided with dissection scissors. The proximal aspect of the divided canal is closed with a 3-0 black silk suture to provide protection from foreign particles and solutions that might enter the canal. The posterior aspect of the condyle is palpable, especially with manipulations of the mandible, and the soft tissue approach continues toward the middle of the posterior roll of the condylar head. Dissection then proceeds immediately lateral to the condyle, placing the superior

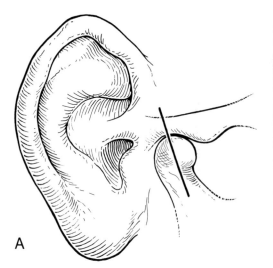
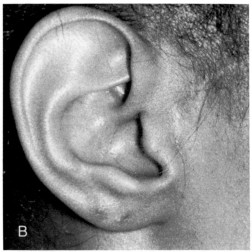

Fig. 12–4. Direct lateral approach. A. A direct dissection to the TM joint passes through a linear incision line and then directly to the lateral pole of the mandibular condyle; B. A twelve-month postoperative view of a patient who had a direct lateral approach with an oblique extension arm at the superior margin of the incision.

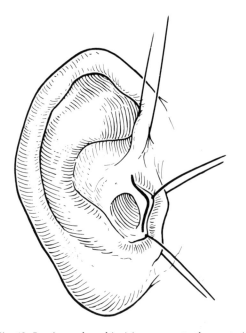

Fig. 12–5. An endaural incision passes to the posterior aspect of the TM joint.

lobules of the parotid gland, the superficial temporal and transverse facial vessels, the auriculotemporal nerve, and branches of the facial nerve in the lateral flap.

The periosteum over the zygomatic process of the temporal bone, as far forward as the articular eminence, is incised to bone. A vertical incision, as described previously, is made lightly over the capsule and then firmly on the neck of the condyle to divide the periosteum. Reflection of the tissues reveals the capsule, and the surgeon prepares to enter the joint for either microscopic or macroscopic procedures.

After completing the intracapsular surgery, closure by layers begins by removing the sutures temporarily closing the divided ear canal, and 4 to 6 4-0 absorbable sutures are used to approximate the fibrous membranes of the posterior and the cartilaginous portions of the anterior halves of the external auditory meatus. Sutures are used as necessary to stabilize the flap superiorly and posteriorly, and 4-0 to 6-0 polyethylene or other cutaneous sutures stabilize the external incision line. Pressure dressings, as used for otoplasties, are applied for 24 to 48 hours.

## Circumaural Approach

A circumaural incision to expose the TM joint begins midway between the inferior and superior aspects of the posterior attachments of the auricula, extends anteriorly and superiorly to the external ear, and continues inferiorly in the preauricular area. The external auditory meatus is not divided, as occurs with the posterior auricular approach. With this technique, the surgeon avoids the facial nerves and the major branches of the superficial temporal artery, and gains direct access

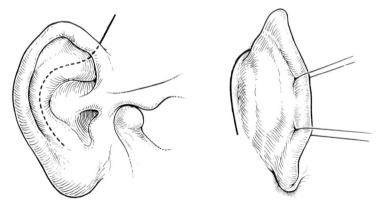

*Fig. 12–6.* Posterior auricular incision provides excellent access to the TM joint.

to the joint space, as with the endaural and posterior auricular approaches (Fig. 12–7).

### Arthroscopic Approaches

Lavaging, inspecting, and performing some surgical procedures, especially in the superior joint space, may be performed with arthroscopic instrumentation. This procedure may be separate and distinct or an intraoperative step of a planned intracapsular operation. Some surgeons frequently use the arthroscope intraoperatively as part of the overall surgical plan; it is rare that inspection of the superior joint space arthroscopically adds information that was not known by preoperative clinical assessment and imaging.

### Comment on Approaches to the TM Joint

When using a preauricular approach, postoperative transient weakness of activity of the temporal branch of the facial nerve infre-

quently occurs, more often when use of a superior extension arm or en bloc elevation of the tissues down to the temporal fascia is involved than when the shorter preauricular incision with a two-layer flap is used. The forward folding of the thicker block of tissues tends to impinge on the facial nerve as compared to a two-level retraction. The preauricular incision and the use of the array of TM joint surgical instruments that now abound provide adequate access to the joint, and this type of incision is acceptable from an esthetic standpoint. The postauricular, the intrameatal variation of the preauricular, and the endaural approaches give outstanding access to the joint. These incisions require dividing, reapproximation, and repair of auricular structures, and access to the anterior aspects of the TM joint articular eminence area, as with the placement of joint prostheses, may be restricted in some patients.

## Intracapsular Procedures and Surgery

Intracapsular procedures include arthroscopic lavaging and surgery, eminence con-

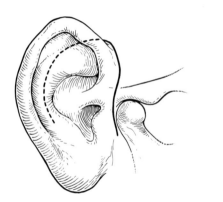

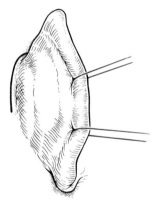

*Fig. 12–7.* Circumaural incision and approach combines the dissection beneath the superficial temporal vessels with the posterior auricular approach without dividing the external auditory fibrocartilage canal.

touring, meniscoplasty, meniscorrhaphy, diskectomy or meniscectomy, condyloplasty, and placing alloplastic devices, autogenous grafts, and allogeneic materials. The meniscus consists of the articular fibrocartilage disk and the posterior zones of connective tissue. Therefore, the usual procedure that is commonly labeled meniscectomy more accurately should be referred to as diskectomy, unless the contents of the bilaminar zone also are removed.

Access is a problem in all types of surgery, and an age-related reduction of the TM joint space occurs in patients with loss of posterior teeth.[15] To ensure adequate access, manual maneuvers in the oral cavity or with instruments applied to the gonial angle or the condylar neck may be necessary to move the condyle inferiorly.

### Arthroscopic Lavaging and Surgery

Fibrotic adhesions within the joint space may appear in several variations, as viewed with arthroscopic examinations. The entire joint space may have dense tentacles of fibrosis; in other cases, only the synovium is covered with cicatricial formations. If necessary, one means by which to obtain greater intraarticular surgical access is the instillation of Ringer's solution or normal saline under slightly higher pressures to increase the joint space. Arthroscopic instruments are used to release adhesions by manipulation and incision, and to obtain biopsy specimens, either directly or by centrifuging the outflow of irrigating fluids (Fig. 12–8). Producing a posterior control to an anteriorly displaced disk is possible by performing a myotomy at the anterior aspect of the disk with a microknife and creating a groove, with cauterization, at the junction of the disk and the bilaminar zone. This process permits the disk to move posteriorly, where it is held in place during 7 to 10 days of immobilization of the mandible. Thus, the disk is moved posteriorly and is stabilized with the scar contracture produced by the cauterization.

Sanders, in a well-documented and well-illustrated report, described the lysis of adhesions, lavage of the joint space, partial meniscectomy, synovectomy, and steroid placement procedures.[16] Montgomery and colleagues reported that arthroscopically-delivered lysis and lavage in the superior joint space, for patients referred with unsatisfactory results from nonsurgical therapy, resulted in significant improvement in mandibular movements, masticatory ability, and decreased pain. There was no improvement in the incidence of TM joint sounds and the position of the disk was unchanged in the majority of the patients.[17] After arthroscopic procedures, we prescribe physiotherapeutic measures for several months of controlled, gradually increasing mobilization of the mandible.

Arthroscopic surgical techniques may be considered a variation of low magnification microsurgical procedures. The instrumentation, measured in diameters of a few millimeters, is enlarged on the television screen monitors. One limiting factor of surgical procedures is the size of the instruments; in the minds of patients and of referring doctors, arthroscopic surgery of the TM joint may be considered as versatile as that of the knee, without appreciating that the larger volume of the intracapsular area of the knee permits the use of larger instruments. Therefore, although we expect increasing versatility with the application of arthroscopic techniques in the TM joint, we must temper our expectations because of the realities of the diminutive instrumentation.

The means to inspect the inferior joint space and the perfection of instrumentation to permit effective alterations of the meniscus and the condylar head will make arthroscopic procedures ever more useful.

### Eminence Contouring

Eminence contouring, usually combined with an intracapsular operation, may be performed as a separate operation. The articulating surface of the temporal bone articular eminence is a part of the lining of the joint space; if the articulating surface is removed, bone repair may be erratic. As Weinberg described, the excision or reduction of lateral aspects of the articular eminence decompresses the intracapsular area by creating a larger anterior recess in the superior joint

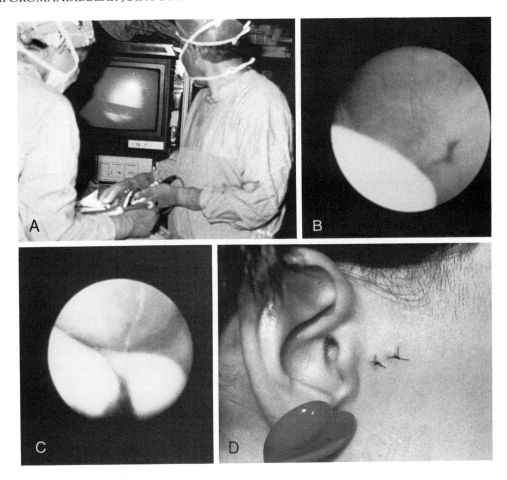

*Fig. 12–8.* Arthroscopic techniques provide highly magnified images on television monitors of the intracapsular structures. The technique features a thorough lavage of the superior joint space; surgical procedures utilizing small curets and knives. Surgical diathermy may be performed. A. Operating team performing arthroscopic procedure using a television monitor; B. View of intracapsular tissue showing a normal superior space of a TM joint with a slight hyperemia; and C, a linear perforation of a disk (Courtesy of Dr. A. Thomas Indresano); D. Closure of the two puncture sites used to insert the arthroscopic instruments at 24 hours postoperative.

space.[18] Eminence contouring, if carried far enough medially, removes the superior articular surface from the TM joint and may result in future problems related to irregularities in the repair of the articular surface.

The temporal articulating fossa, the glenoid fossa, extends too far medially under the middle cranial fossa to permit removal or contouring of the entire slope of the articular eminence; the amount contoured is limited to the lateral one half or one third. Preoperative review of laminographic radiographs permits assessment of a possible lateral and inferior extension of the middle cranial fossa into the articular eminence. These images may reveal an anterior extension of the mastoid air cells invading the articular eminence, and med-

ullary spaces within the eminence may be apparent; these findings do not constitute absolute contraindications to surgery, but they warrant consideration in terms of protecting the patient from untoward sequelae involving the mastoid air cells. Tyndall and Matteson reported that 2.6% of the population have pneumatized articular eminences of the temporal bone.[19] Kraut reported the obturation of pneumatized articular eminences with a gelatine sponge and the use of methylmethacrylate resin for the articulating surface.[20]

The eminence is scored with a fissure bur across its base as a continuation of the inferior border of the zygomatic arch. An osteotome is inserted into the groove created by the bur, and the lateral one third to one half of the eminence is removed. The osseous surgical site is smoothed with files.

In some cases, the partial decrease in anterior osseous restrictions of the joint space, produced by the eminence contouring, is sufficient, and further surgical intervention is not necessary to increase the space for condylar and meniscal movements. The usual indication for the reduction of the steep articular eminence is to gain access to the TM joint area for intra-articular TM joint surgical procedures.

## Meniscoplasty

A variety of procedures are available to reposition a meniscus that is displaced or requires recontouring. After entering the superior joint space, manipulation of the mandible demonstrates the relative movements of the articular disk and the condyle, which should confirm the preoperative clinical findings suggestive of subluxation or dislocation of the meniscus. Inspection of the superior surface of the meniscus discloses any perforations, tears, or cracks; the extent of possible elongation or detachment of the posterior fibers is estimated.

An inverted L incision over the posterior-lateral aspect of the condyle opens the inferior joint space. The meniscus is freed from its attachment to the lateral pole of the condyle. The articular surface of the condyle is in-

spected, and irregularities of the condylar surface are removed by shaving with an osteotome, or, if necessary, a file. Changing the condylar articular surface should be avoided if possible and minimized if necessary.

The meniscoplasty is performed by removing a wedge of tissue at the bilaminar-diskal junction and closing the triangular defect with sutures. The entire width of the posterior attachment of the meniscus is transsected and reattached.

We have reattached the lateral aspect of the disk either by suturing to close periostial and capsular tissue or by placing drill holes in the lateral condylar pole area (Fig. 12–9). With the development of this procedure came the reminder that too firm an attachment of the disk prevented the condyle from passing freely through the inferior joint space; a concurrent condyloplasty provided additional space, but sometimes produced the expected complications of an irregular repair of the condyle. Stern reported securing the posterior aspect of the disk with a mattress suture through a transverse hole in the condylar process.[21]

A section from the lateral pterygoid muscle superior belly (the sphenomeniscus muscle) may be removed when a muscular restriction is encountered in moving the disk posteriorly to its corrected position on the condyle. The rationale for the procedure is as follows. After an anteriorly displaced disk dislocates, a

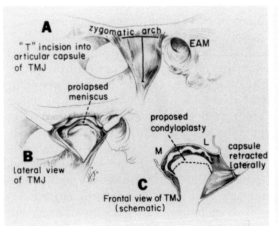

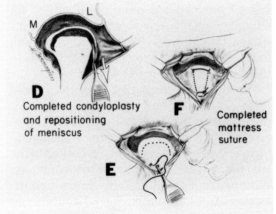

*Fig. 12–9.* Concept described in 1972 for attaching the lateral aspect of the disk to the lateral pole of the condyle. Experience has taught that the reattachment of the disk to the lateral pole should not be as tight as shown in this artist's concept.

closed lock situation, the anterior-posterior length of the disk is shortened and prevents the superior 15 to 20% of the lateral pterygoid superior belly muscle fibers to stretch to their normal physiologic length. In time, this fixation at a shortened length causes a decrease in the number of sarcomeres in the superior aspect of the muscle. The inferior 80 to 85% of the muscle fibers stretch to their normal length or greater, because they are attached to the condyle.

Contouring of the disk is performed if abnormal waves or irregularities are present. The instrumentation consists of laser, scalpel blades, and shaving devices, some of which are used with arthroscopic procedures.

The meniscus is usually displaced anteriorly, although a posterior dislocation is possible.[22,23] It is replaced on the condyle and is stabilized by a meniscoplasty.

## Meniscorrhaphy

This procedure permits the junctional tissues of the meniscus to remain intact. The meniscus is freed of adhesions within the superior and inferior joint spaces and any necessary condyloplasties are completed. The lateral border of the meniscus is sutured to the posterior-lateral capsule by using polyglycolic acid sutures. As with the meniscoplasty operations, the inferior joint space is closed by firm suturing of the vertical or L-shaped capsular incision.[18]

## Diskectomy (Meniscectomy)

Diskectomy, usually referred to as meniscectomy, is the oldest of the intracapsular operations. It was performed in the first half of the 20th century for meniscus dislocations that were disabling. The reintroduction of meniscectomy in the 1950s met with an unfavorable reaction to the procedure by health care professionals because of an apparent return of symptoms in many patients. The procedure often was performed to correct conditions roughly defined as pain dysfunction, not necessarily disabling conditions caused by structural defects that were amenable to a surgical solution. During the 1970s and 1980s, meniscectomies were often performed in con-

junction with the placement of a mandibular fossa alloplastic or biologic implant; in many instances, the implants, especially the alloplastic implants, have produced secondary problems.

Diskectomy often produces deformation of the condyle, an adaptive remolding that occurs in the first 1 or 2 postoperative years and then stabilizes. Eriksson and Westesson described 15 patients who received meniscectomies between 1947 and 1960 and had a mean follow-up of 29 years.[24] All patients were free of pain, none had subjectively experienced dysfunction, no facial nerve deficits were noted, and all but one had a range of motion of greater than 39 mm. The basis on which results were judged as successful involved pain relief and improved function. Crepitation of a TM joint without pain and a reasonable or normal range of motion of the mandible were a successful result. Radiologically, all of the joints had structural hard tissue changes, osteophytes, and flattening of the articular eminence and condyle. They wrote, "The clinical and radiologic findings may therefore be regarded to be the result of functional rebuilding of the joint after surgery or an asymptomatic stage of arthrosis."

Usually, diskectomy results in a decrease of translational movement of the condyle that is not disabling; the long-term postoperative opening range of motion of the mouth is expected to be decreased slightly, but a useful 30- to 45-mm anterior opening has usually been achieved in our patients. Only the superior fibers of the lateral pterygoid muscle, the sphenomeniscus muscle, which stabilize the meniscus in conjunction with the posterior bilaminar zone fibers, are affected by the diskectomy. The inferior belly of the lateral pterygoid muscle remains intact and available to move the mandible anteriorly. The decreased translational motion is probably the result of scars anterior to the condyle.

The loss of the meniscus results in a decrease in vertical height of the ramus area, and adjustments to occlusion, owing to posterior prematurities, may be necessary. A variety of alloplastic and biological implants are available for use in the mandibular fossa to restore the lost structure and compensate for the loss of vertical height. However, bioengineering of the postoperative translational and compressive forces of the condyle have not been defined for the wide variations of the condyle and the implant interfaces and, for that matter, of the condyle with no implant in place. The translational and compressive forces have led to disruption of the implants and adaptive distortions of the condyles.

### Condyloplasty

Altering the shape of the condyle removes the effects of degenerative diseases and has been a part of a regimen to increase the joint space in patients with meniscus subluxation and dislocation and in the management of persistent mandibular dislocation. The amount of condyle removed varies with the complete condylectomy, the removal of the superior one half of the condyle, the shave of the condyle, and, most recently, the selected removal of diseased portions. After condylectomy or condyloplasty, many surgeons do not place a device and many others routinely use a temporary or permanent alloplastic replacement.

Walker and Kalamchi reviewed cases involving 50 patients who had undergone condyloplasties of 2 to 4 mm, freeing of the disk, and secure suturing of the disk to the condylar stump and to the lateral capsule.[25] All patients received 3 months of postoperative physiotherapy. The 50 patients had the preoperative signs and symptoms of internal derangements that were resolved postoperatively with no recurrences. The authors reasoned that the success was related to the increase in the intra-articular joint space produced by the condyloplasty and the postoperative physical therapy. The condyloplasty permitted unrestricted movement within the joint space and eliminated compression of the bilaminar zone. The physical therapy, which included daytime use of the mandible and nighttime immobilization, was designed to provide progressively increasing range of motion of the mandible, thus preventing painfully tethering scar contractures in the extracapsular tissues.

### Meniscus and Disk Perforations

Meniscus perforation is not an indication that the perforation should be repaired; for example, a perforation noted as an incidental finding on an arthrogram may not represent a pathophysiologic finding. Historical and clinical findings of a disability of the TM joint, usually with an osseous change on the condyle associated with the perforation, are indications for repair of a perforation with an implant of biologic tissue or by direct surgical closure. If there are minimal to no osseous changes, then a disk perforation may be successfully treated through open or arthroscopic TM joint surgery by mobilizing the disk, freeing it of adhesions, and smoothing irregular margins. As Quinn pointed out, the TM joint is not a weight-bearing joint; therefore, an opening in the disk should not be a significant biomechanical problem in itself.[26]

### Condylar, Meniscal, and Glenoid Fossa Devices and Materials

Different devices and materials have been inserted after diskectomy with and without condylectomy and condyloplasty, including silicone rubber alloplastic caps or bumpers wired to the condylar process; either temporal fascia or temporalis muscle turned into the operated space and, usually, attached to either the condylar process or the glenoid fossa; dermal graft, cartilage, including ear cartilage, or other fresh or preserved biologic materials attached to the condylar head or the glenoid fossa; silicone rubber sheets inserted into the surgical site and removed in 30 to 90 days; reinforced silicone rubber sheets attached to the glenoid fossa; metallic fossa implants; dense plastic implants; and polytetrafluoroethylene implants (Fig. 12–10).

The placement of glenoid fossa alloplastic implants as part of the correction of intracapsular maladies has not produced reliable results. The condylar head often undergoes a flattening deformation because of an alteration of proprioception from the TM joint regardless of whether an alloplastic device is placed. The implants wear and fragment, including those in TM joints with normal physiologic pressures, and deteriorate, producing foreign body reactions that erode surrounding mandibular and temporal bone structures.

With regard to polytetrafluoroethylene im-

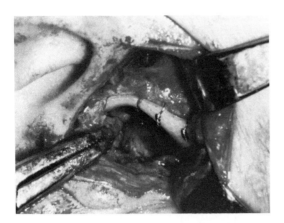

*Fig. 12–10.* Placement of a reinforced silicone rubber glenoid fossa implant during the 1970s. This is a procedure that is no longer in vogue in 1990 as a permanent implantation following TM joint diskectomy. (Courtesy of the archival records of Drs. Edward L. Mosby and Eugene J. Messer.)

plants, Heffez and associates observed that, "The risks of displacement and fragmentation of the laminate outweigh benefits . . . "[27] and, in a retrospective study, Florine and associates found, "The severity of change found . . . in treated joints . . . was greater than that previously reported with other surgical implants."[28] A giant cell granulomatous response may occur in the presence of polytetrafluoroethylene; the condyle may be engulfed and disappear and portions of the glenoid fossa may be destroyed. We recommend removal of the implants at the first sign of any untoward clinical or radiographic finding, with or without signs and symptoms of inflammation (Fig. 12–11).

Silicone rubber implants in the glenoid fossa show fragmentation from normal occlusal and mandibular movement forces. Dolwick and Afdermorte reported surgical and histopathologic observations of patients who required the removal of silicone rubber implants.[29] They found granulomatous and multinucleated giant cells associated with the silicone material as well as the presence of material in lymph nodes consistent with fragmented silicone, and these findings are consistent with our experience (Fig. 12–12).

The breakdown observed in some of the silicone rubber and polytetrafluoroethylene implants is not related to therapeutic misadventures or lack of interocclusal therapy. We

observed, for example, the destructive granulomatous process occurring without a break, tear, or disruption of the Teflon articulation surface. In some patients, the problem induced by alloplastic implants is on the same order as the new pressures sensed by the mandible when meniscectomy is performed and postoperative deformation of the condylar head is observed.

The placement of a removable silicone rubber sheet is designed to produce a biologically acceptable surface to help guide the early repair of bone and to produce an area for articulating movements between the condyle and the glenoid fossa. A silicone rubber cap may be placed on the head of the condyle after a condyloplasty, and it is stabilized with wire sutures. A fibrotic capsule forms around the superior circumference of the cap and movements of articulation are well preserved. As fibrosis invades the area between the cap and the recipient site, however, the device, maintained only by the wires, becomes unstable and must be removed. Removal is fairly simple; after the cap is located, it lifts easily out of its fibrotic nest.

Newer applications and uses for polytetrafluoroethylene and silicone rubber have been developed. DeChamplain and Marshall reported the use of autopolymerizing silicone rubber as an interpositional material.[30] They observed that it was quickly constructed during an operation and accurately adapted to the bony architecture at the temporal bone and condylar process. Feinberg and Smilack, in a series of 21 TM joint operations, sutured a soft patch of polytetrafluoroethylene over the incision line of the capsule after intracapsular surgical procedures.[31] This measure reduced tension and restriction of capsular tissues and assisted in the postoperative translational movements of the condyle after intracapsular surgical procedures.

For many years, autogenous biologic implants—fascia, muscle, cartilage, and dermal grafts—have been placed after meniscectomy and condyloplastic procedures, with the dermal grafts and ear cartilages being the latest additions. The temporalis fascia and the lateral pterygoid muscle fibers are in the area of the operation and are readily accessible to be placed over the condyloplastic area or in the

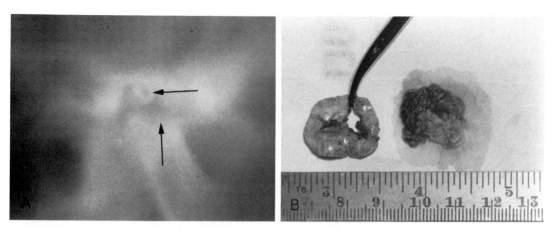

***Fig. 12–11.*** Giant cell tumor destruction of a condyle by a polytetrafluoroethylene implant. A. Corrected polycycloidal imagery displayed loss of condyle (vertical arrow) in the presence of a nonpathologic retaining wire (horizontal arrow); B. The implant with a perforation and the tumor.

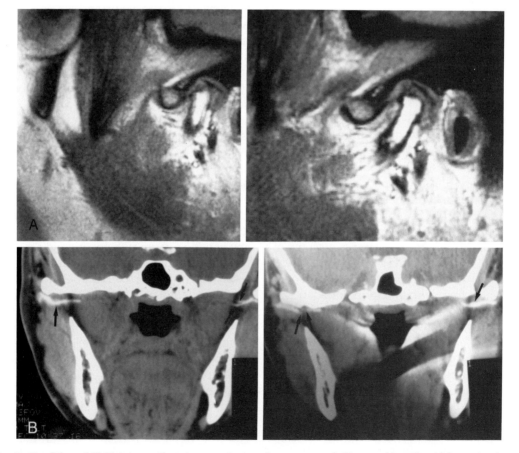

***Fig. 12–12.*** Bilateral TM joint granulomatous reactions to the presence of silicone rubber glenoid fossae implants in a 47-year-old female patient. The implants had been placed 5 years earlier, because nonsurgical care had not been successful in managing painful anterior displacements of the TM joint disks. The following views are of the right; both sides were similar. A. Left and right: At 2 years postoperative, MRI studies show the implant encapsulated in fibrous connective tissue, deformation of the condyle, and a disruption of the implant; B. Left and right: At 5 years postoperative, the patient was referred to us, and CT studies revealed both implants to be tortuous and disrupted (arrows).

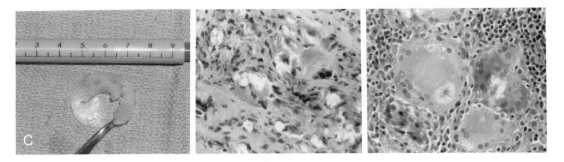

*Fig. 12–12. Continued.* C. Left: Following removal, the silicone rubber implants were found to be thinned, friable, and perforated. Center: The fibrous connective granulation tissue totally encapsulating the implant. Right: A preauricular lymph node showed vascular granulation tissue, double refractile foreign material, and a diffuse foreign body granulomatous reaction with numerous large multinucleated histiocytes. (Courtesy of Dr. Robert E. Jones, Jr., Pathologist, Brookwood Medical Center, Birmingham, Alabama.)

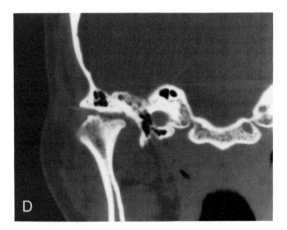

*Fig. 12–12. Continued.* D. Following removal of the implants, a CT frontal view of the right condyle displayed the changes commensurate with condylar deformation that follows TM joint diskectomy.

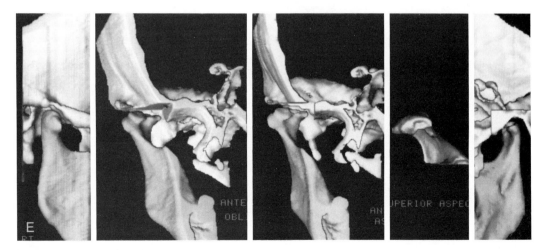

*Fig. 12–12. Continued.* E. Using the information from the preceding CT, a reconstructed 3-D CT study of the right ramus and condyle was made. Correlations are evident with the original CT as the anatomy is viewed from (left to right) the direct lateral, anterior oblique, anterior, superior, and medial aspects. (The reconstructed 3-D CTs are courtesy of ISG Technologies, Inc., Mississauga, Ontario, Canada.)

region of the diskectomy as pedicle grafts, thus maintaining their own life-support viability.

In 1962, Georgiade reported the use of dermal grafts during TM joint operations.[32] Recently, the versatility of dermal grafts has been further explored. They are used for repair of meniscus perforations, as glenoid fossa implants, to construct disk-like structures between the lateral pterygoid muscle and the retrodiskal tissues, and as caps over condyles after meniscectomy or condyloplasty (Fig. 12–13). In an experimental study with monkeys, Tucker and associates reported, "Dermal tissue is similar to discal tissue in that it is composed primarily of dense fibrous connective tissue and has an elastin component."[33] Stewart and associates noted, in repairing perforations in an experimental study with monkeys, a gradual process of incorporation of the dermal graft into the meniscus, termed a functional bandage for the meniscus; after continued physiologic function, the dermal graft was completely assim-

ilated and the meniscus gradually returned to a more normal architecture.[34] Six months after the grafting procedure, they noted a synovial migration to the repaired area and a thickening of the central part of the meniscus to resemble a normal configuration.

## Extracapsular and Combination Procedures

### Condylotomy

This procedure has a high rate of success in relieving painful intracapsular maladies. The procedure, described by Ward, involves division of the condylar neck with a Gigli saw (Fig. 12–14).[35] The condyle is permitted to seek a new relationship with the meniscus and the glenoid fossa, with neither intraosseous nor intermaxillary fixation. Modifications of the procedure include a preauricular approach to minimize the possibility of injury to the facial nerve, maxillary artery, and inferior alveolar neurovascular structures.[36]

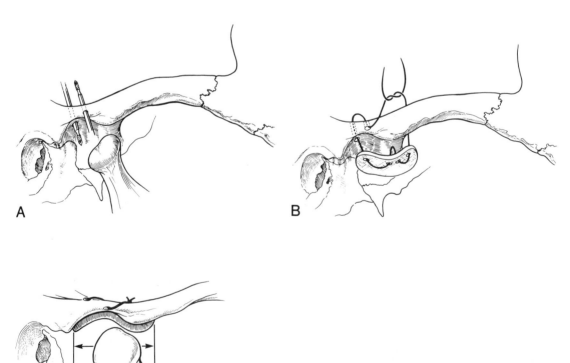

*Fig. 12–13.* A, B, and C show a diagram of an attachment method of implants to the glenoid fossa. This technique has been used for the attachment of dermal grafts. (The suturing technique was described to us by Dr. Michael F. Nealis, San Antonio, Texas.)

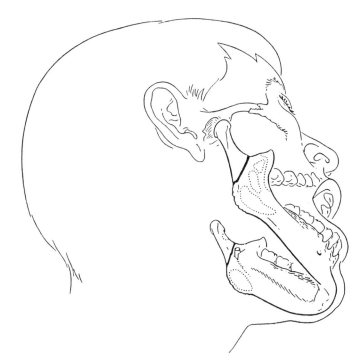

*Fig. 12–14.* Division of the ramus from the gonial angle area through the mandibular notch (sigmoid notch) with a Gigli's saw. Diagram of osteotomy lines for Gigli's wire saw when using Tarsitano and Gossman's variation. The technique we used was described by Drs. John J. Tarsitano and J. Rudolph Gossman, Jr. (Tarsitano J.J. and Gossman J.R. Jr: Doctor Gigli's saw and the closed mandibular osteotomy: an appraisal, a variation, and a report of a case. J Oral Maxillofac Surg, 29:409, 1971.)

Emboldened by the success of the Ward procedure, we performed an open oblique osteotomy of the mandible in five patients during which we moved the posterior mandible inferiorly an arbitrary distance of 3 mm. These patients were referred to our practice after appropriate nonsurgical care of more than 12 months duration to correct either painful subluxation or dislocation of the meniscus; no intracapsular osseous changes were noted. All patients had postoperative posterior prematurity of the occlusion, as would be expected in patients with a mandibular condylar fracture dislocation. This result was anticipated and did not constitute a management problem. One patient had a nonunion that required subsequent bone graft repair. Five years later, three patients had continuing cessation of symptoms, and two continued with intermittent, recurring, nearly nonpainful subluxation of the meniscus (Fig. 12–15). In this series, we used postoperative intermaxillary fixation for 6 to 8 weeks, with the objective of giving the TM joint a period of rest rather than using bone-plate rigid fixation of the osteotomies. Helfrick, with similar indications, performed transoral oblique osteotomies without fixation of the posterior segment and has excellent results 5 years postoperatively (Fig. 12–16).[37]

## Manipulations and Operations for Mandibular Dislocations

### Acute Dislocation

A normal anterior mandibular dislocation that is self reducing may follow wide opening movements of the mandible. Occasionally, the condyle does not return to its normal position in the glenoid fossa and, accompanied by muscular spasms, may become locked in the open position with either a bilateral or unilateral anterior dislocation of the condyle onto a position on the infratemporal surface of the squama of the temporal bone.

Reduction of dislocations of the mandible usually involves the method that has been advocated for centuries. According to a translation from the Edwin Smith papyrus, 1600 B.C., "If thou examinest a man having dislocation in his mandible, shouldst thou find his mouth open and his mouth cannot close for him, thou shouldst put thy thumbs upon the ends of the two rami of the mandible inside his mouth and thy two claws under his chin,

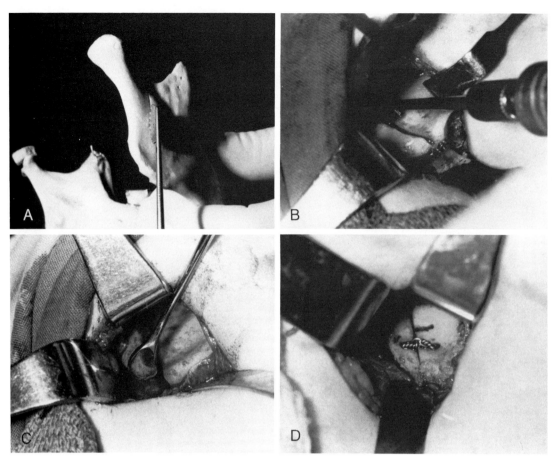

**Fig. 12–15.** Surgically moving the condyle inferiorly. A. Osteotomy line on a dried specimen; B. Osteotomy being completed at the gonial angle; C. Freeing the posterior segment; D. Posterior segment positioned 3 mm inferiorly as measured between the horizontal line anterior to the osteotomy and the transosseous wire. The drill hole on the posterior segment was aligned with the horizontal line before moving the posterior segment inferiorly.

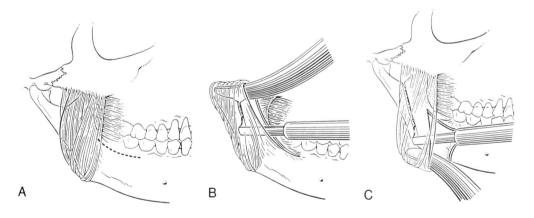

**Fig. 12–16.** Transoral vertical osteotomy of the ramus. A. The incision through the mucoperiosteum should be placed low; B. A retractor designed for the right mandibular (sigmoid) notch is placed. With the mandible in the closed position, and with due regard for anatomic variations, the shaft of the saw is approximately parallel to the maxillary dentition, and the osteotomy is performed; C. If needed to visualize the inferior aspects of the osteotomy, a retractor designed for the left mandibular (sigmoid) notch is placed at the inferior border of the right mandible and the osteotomy is completed.

and thou shouldst cause them to fall back, so they rest in their places."

Because the anterior aspect of the articular eminence has a gentle slope, if any, and the dislocation of the condyle(s) persists because of muscular spasms, we find the following technique is anatomically and physiologically logical. The patient is upright with the head firmly against a rest. The clinician stands in front of the patient and grasps the mandible with the thumbs intraorally along the base of the mandible and supports the body of the mandible, bilaterally, with the other fingers. With a rapid, gentle, persistent, firm left and right translational vibrating movement to the mandible, the muscles usually relax and the condyles return to the glenoid fossae.

If the mandible is not reduced with the first 5-minute attempt with the horizontal vibratory technique, a local anesthetic agent is introduced into the lateral and medial pterygoid muscles, either extraorally or transorally. In the event the reduction of the dislocation still cannot be effected, a local anesthetic is placed intracapsularly and the manipulation, if still necessary, is repeated. Additional muscular relaxation is achieved by the administration, usually intravenously, of a tranquilizing agent, diazepam or midazolam; in rare, extremely resistant cases, a general anesthetic is necessary.

After the mandible is reduced, especially in the extremely resistant cases, immobilization of the mandible by intermaxillary fixation is necessary for 14 days to enable the periarticular soft tissues to repair.

### Recurrent and Chronic Dislocations

Table 12–1 is a classification of the etiologies of recurrent dislocations. In many cases, recurrent dislocations are secondary to or are accompanied by systemic or psychologic etiologies. Regional and local treatment must address the background problem.

In patients with recurrent dislocation that results from regional TM joint disease or anatomic abnormalities, nonsurgical management is recommended as the first approach. The nonsurgical regimens are occlusal therapy to remove local stimuli to bruxism and physical therapy with external heat, shortwave diathermy, and, most importantly, ex-

**TABLE 12–1.** *Etiologies of Recurrent Mandibular Dislocations*

| |
|---|
| Hereditary |
|    Ehlers-Danlos syndrome |
| Developmental |
|    Flattened articular eminence |
|    Steep articular eminence and deep glenoid fossa |
|    Abnormal mandibular condyle |
| Trauma |
|    After acute trauma |
| Functional |
|    Uncoordinated neuromuscular activity |
|    Habits |
| Psychiatric Illness |
|    Hysteria |
|    Anxiety |
| Drug Therapy |
|    Prochlorperazine |
|    Perphenazine |
|    Reserpine |
| Neurologic Disease |
|    Parkinson's disease |
|    Epilepsy |
|    Multiple sclerosis |
| Degenerative maladies |
|    Senile muscle and collagen atrophy |
|    Loss of intraoral vertical dimension |

Courtesy of Dr. Robert Ord of England.

ercises to strengthen the masticatory muscles and pericapsular ligaments. If the nonsurgical methods are not successful, surgical intervention is considered.

### Soft Tissue Surgery for TM Joint Dislocations

A common denominator to soft tissue surgery is the production of scarring, which, in a matter of months or years, may prove to be an unreliable method of correcting a recurrent or chronic mandibular dislocation problem.

Surgical approaches to the soft tissues include the injection of sclerosing solutions into the joint spaces. The resultant fibrosis is nonspecific in location and, after a time of limiting the motion of the mandible, may resolve and permit the recurring or chronic dislocation to return. Plication of the capsule with either absorbable or nonabsorbable sutures can successfully limit the unrestricted forward movement of the condyle.

In 1887, Annandale reported the logical procedure of repositioning a dislocated meniscus and suturing it to the capsule to assist in management of a chronically recurring dislocating mandible.[38] Other approaches to the mandibular dislocation include meniscectomy, meniscectomy combined with a partial or complete detachment of the lateral pterygoid muscle, and myotomy of the lateral pterygoid muscle.[39] Maw and McKean[40] and Gould[41] described scarification procedures designed to shorten the temporalis tendon and produce a transverse scar of the oral mucosa overlying the anterior aspect of the mandibular ramus.

## Hard Tissue Surgery for TM Joint Dislocations

Perceived impediments to retruding movements of dislocated mandibles could be removed by the performance of reduction condyloplastic procedures and articular eminence contouring. In our experience, however, reduction condyloplasties are not reliably successful and often result in both a recurrence of the dislocation as well as posterior occlusal prematurities. With eminence contouring procedures, scarring is likely produced anterior to the lateral aspect of the track of the condyle and may successfully prevent recurring anterior displacement of the condyle.

Operations to raise the height of the articular eminence logically impede the forward progress of the condyle.[42] Autogenous or freeze dried bone grafts to the articular eminence may be considered. The height of the lateral aspect of the articular eminence may be accentuated by a down-fracturing and transposing of the root of the zygomatic process of the temporal bone, as popularized by Gosserez and Dautrey.[43] The use of alloplastic materials to raise the height of the articular eminence has included placing chrome-cobalt meshes, small orthopedic bone plates, and, in our practice, miniplates for midfacial orthognathic and facial trauma surgery.

## Hypomobilities

Hypomobilities of the TM joint may result from bony (true) ankylosis or fibrous (false) ankylosis, myospasms secondary to local anesthetic injections and agents, hematomas,

infection, coronoid process hypertrophy, neoplasms, and arthritides.

## Bony Ankylosis

Correction of a bony ankylosis involves removing the uniting bone or leaving it in place and creating a new articulating surface. The decision regarding which of these two techniques to use depends on the location and the extent of the ankylosis. If the bony ankylosis is within the confines of the TM joint space, it may be amenable to correction via a preauricular or postauricular approach.

If the bony ankylosis is beyond the confines of the TM joint area, the surgical approach is usually through a posterior subgonial angle incision, which permits access for sectioning the condylar neck at the level of the mandibular (sigmoid) notch or higher on the condylar process and placement of an interpositional autogenous, homogeneous, or alloplastic material (Fig. 12–17).

The sigmoid notch is identified via a gonial angle submandibular approach, and the condylar neck is sectioned from the notch posteriorly; the soft tissues on the medial aspect of the area are protected with a metallic retractor, guarding against laceration of the maxillary artery. If placing a metallic instrument on the medial side of the osteotomy site is impossible, the bony cut may be best performed with a power-driven, fine-tooth saw, which tends to displace soft tissues. If a bur is used, the surgeon may wish to estimate the depth of the osteotomy and complete it with a chisel. If the mandible is not freed after sectioning of the condylar neck at the level of the sigmoid notch, the osteotomy is carried anteriorly across the base of the coronoid process to the anterior border of the mandible. At this juncture, the osteotomy line is converted to an ostectomy by placing a parallel osteotomy and removing the intervening bone, thus producing a gap after the ostectomy.

The interpositional homogeneous and autogenous materials consist of fascia obtained from the patient, temporalis fascia, fascia lata, and muscle.[44–47] Total and partial alloplastic TM joint replacements and costochondral grafts have been used to reconstruct joints

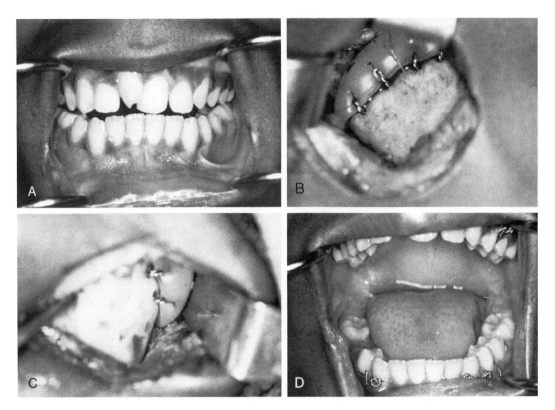

*Fig. 12–17.* Common denominators in managing mandibular ankylosis are to remove the fibrous or osseous bridging and to produce a gap to prevent reattachment. Silicone materials have been versatile at time of operation, but often the silicone must be removed as it becomes mobile and encapsulated; however, an effective gap remains that serves as a flail joint. A. Preoperative view of limitation of opening in a young man with bilateral mandibular ankylosis; B and C. Silicone implants following bilateral ostectomies of the mandibular rami via a subgonial angle approach; D. Postoperative range of motion. Unfortunately, in this young patient, reossification occurred over the ostectomy sites that encased the silicone implants and further surgery was indicated.

lost by surgery to correct ankylosis, trauma, oncologic surgery, and persistent arthritic diseases in the TM joint.[48,49]

Immobilization of the mandible is frequently indicated for 36 to 48 hours postoperatively, but early and continuous physical therapeutic movement is mandatory. Vigorous, wrenching movements are not as effective as continuous, steady, moving pressures. Connole described an intraoral device consisting of a continuous circle of vinyl material prepared to fold on itself and engage the maxillary and mandibular dentition, providing positive but gentle opening pressures;[50] other devices for extraoral pressures may be devised. In the early postoperative period, physical therapy is beneficial, and long-term evaluations and controls by the surgeon and physical therapist are indicated. Mechanical,

portable devices are available to provide continuous motions to repairing TM joints. The movement exercises must be pursued for years.

### Fibrous Ankylosis

Fibrous ankylosis is evaluated to ensure that the predisposing condition is controlled to avoid recurrences postoperatively. The earliest form of treatment includes physical therapy. In the event such therapy does not achieve adequate range of motion, surgical intervention is indicated, with use of the approaches just described.

In both bony and fibrous ankylosis, use of a subgonial angle approach is common. This approach necessitates a subperiosteal elevation of the masseter muscle mass, and a post-

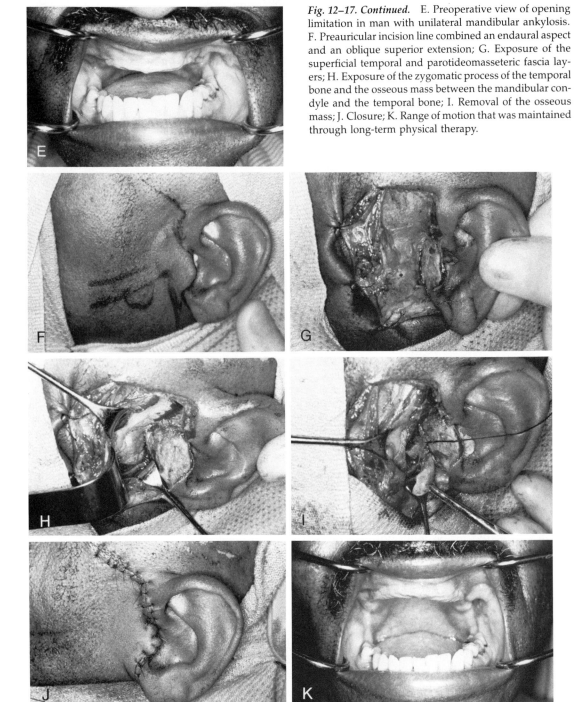

*Fig. 12–17. Continued.* E. Preoperative view of opening limitation in man with unilateral mandibular ankylosis. F. Preauricular incision line combined an endaural aspect and an oblique superior extension; G. Exposure of the superficial temporal and parotideomasseteric fascia layers; H. Exposure of the zygomatic process of the temporal bone and the osseous mass between the mandibular condyle and the temporal bone; I. Removal of the osseous mass; J. Closure; K. Range of motion that was maintained through long-term physical therapy.

operative sequela may be a reossification process originating in the periosteum that may well encase the surgical site in bone and effectively nullify the treatment. The postoperative course of physical therapy may help to prevent the new bone formation, which, radiographically, appears as a shower of bone. Reossification may appear despite correct surgical and physical therapeutic methods, however, and the informed consent by the patient should acknowledge accepting the possibility of this complication.

## Myospasms

Myospasms of the medial pterygoid muscle may occur immediately after an anesthetic injection involving the inferior alveolar nerve. The etiology of the problem is a small area of degeneration of the muscle that results from the anesthetic solution. The hypomobility usually persists for 48 to 60 hours, followed by progressive improvements in mandibular movement, with a return to normal function in about 2 or 3 weeks as muscle repair takes place.

Another muscle-related hypomobility typically occurs in heavy-muscled individuals after long dental appointments and is progressive, becoming completely established in 3 to 5 days postoperatively. The trismus is painless, and the prognosis is guarded. The treatment consists of forced opening of the mandible while the patient is under a full general anesthetic. The forced opening is accompanied by a tearing sensation and sounds from within the muscle masses as the blocked muscle bundles are moved. Maximum opening to be achieved by the forced maneuver is in the 35- to 40-mm range, probably the preoperative range of the patient. The treatment plan involves long-term opening exercises accompanied by physical therapy and deep heat applications. In some individuals, the condition is treated by using bite opening devices, as described previously with the postoperative care of bony and fibrous ankyloses (Fig. 12–18).

A complicating factor with both of the above mentioned muscle-related hypomobilities is TM joint internal derangements that were present before the onset of the hypomobility or were predisposed to occur when the muscular imbalances were established. Appropriate therapy for the TM joint malady must be instituted; however, definitive treatment, permanent alterations of the coronal surfaces, and direct surgical approaches into the joints, in most cases, should await normalization of the muscles.

## Infection

Infection of the masticator space produces trismus and is treated by incision and drainage of acute inflammatory products, antibiotic therapy, and supportive care. Exercises, as mentioned previously, may be necessary when the inflammation accompanying the infection is chronic. The infection may result from odontogenic etiologies, especially the mandibular third molar maladies wherein the ramus and body of the mandible intersect anterior to the retromolar trigone, the class 3

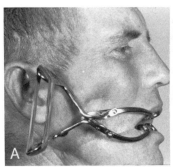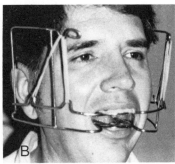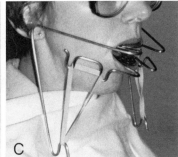

*Fig. 12–18.* Bite opening exercising devices that use extraoral elastic pressures to move the mandible. Self-curing acrylic trays are prepared to support and protect the dentition. A. Unilateral device; B and C. Versatile device that may be prepared by local instrument manufacturers.

relationship of Gregory and Pell.[51] In this anatomic arrangement, the masticator space is both medial (medial pterygoid muscle) and lateral (masseter muscle) to the third molar. An inflammation associated with a maxillary third molar, likewise, may produce a crippling trismus owing to eruptive phenomenon into the attachment of the lateral pterygoid muscle (Fig. 12–19). The offending third molar is removed with the usual supportive care provided for patients undergoing oral and maxillofacial surgical procedures.

An inferior alveolar injection may be accompanied by aspiration of blood, which is possible because of pooling of extravasated blood in the pterygomandibular space and not because the needle orifice is located within a blood vessel. The pooled blood in the pterygomandibular fossa could form a hematoma that is susceptible to microbial invasion from either a hematogenous route or by direct inoculation at the time of the injection. If the infection remains chronic, the patient has no pain and the vital signs remain normal. The treatment consists of antibiotic therapy, exercises for the mandible, and reassurance. If the infection produces an acute inflammatory process, then more direct care to the area, including incision and drainage, is necessary.

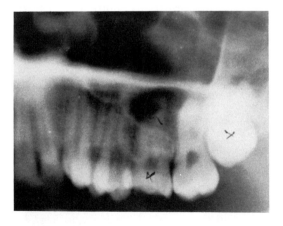

**Fig. 12–19.** The eruption of the maxillary third molar in this patient affected the pterygoid muscles and produced limitation of the opening of the mandible with a resultant subluxation of the TM joint meniscus. All other etiologic factors were eliminated. After removal of the third molar, a normal range of motion returned and the signs and symptoms of an internal derangement of the TM joint subsided.

## Elongated Coronoid Processes

Elongated coronoid processes produce mechanical hypomobility at about 20 to 25 mm maximum opening. The elongation may be a developmental phenomenon or it may be acquired in individuals who have had prolonged intermaxillary traction. As a developmental problem, individuals with tapered facial skeletons and posterior constriction of the oral cavity seem predisposed. In these patients, interferences between the posterior tuberosities of the maxillae and the coronoid processes may restrict lateral, protrusive, and opening mandibular movements. Impediments by the coronoid processes in opening movements also may be secondary to fracture displacement of the osseous structures of the zygomaticomaxillary complex.

The removal of coronoid processes involves a transoral approach. An osteotomy is performed, usually with a reciprocating powered saw, from the depth of the sigmoid notch from either the medial or lateral side of the mandible, although the lateral approach provides greater access owing to the hypomobility. The process is allowed to remain attached to the temporalis muscle fibers and the process retracts superiorly. The temporalis muscle attaches inferiorly to the anterior aspect of the osteotomy and, therefore, remains an effective elevating and rotating muscle for the mandible. The possibility exists that reossification will occur with the production of an even longer process, necessitating dissection of the entire coronoid process from the temporalis muscle.

## Neoplasms

Malignant neoplasms tend to produce hypomobilities of the TM joint. Benign neoplasms tend to deviate but not immobilize the joint. Treatment of the neoplasia may result in widespread loss of normal structures, and surgical reconstruction of the TM joint may be indicated.

## Complications

### Nerve Dysfunction

An annoying complication associated with TM joint surgery is the rare postoperative facial nerve dysfunction. Nerve dysfunction may occur even though the surgical approach to the TM joint was routine and without apparent complication and was performed with deft, delicate, gentle, and accurate management of the soft tissues. Many variations exist in the pattern of distribution and in the number of branches of the facial nerve as it passes to the muscles of facial expression. As a prognostic point, we observed that if the corrugator muscle is still functioning in patients with postoperative loss of function of the facial nerve, the return of the nerve to complete activity usually follows. In a review of approximately 200 TM joint operations, two patients had lack of function of the temporal branch—persistent, probably permanent loss in one patient and possibly permanent loss in the other. With one of the patients, the use

of surgical diathermy for hemorrhage control in the vicinity of the nerve produced an immediate, probably permanent paralysis (Fig. 12–20). With the other patient, normal and usual retraction of the flap produced nerve dysfunction with a resultant paralysis that persisted for 2 years postoperatively, when the patient was lost to follow-up observation.

A report that is not in the chronicles concerns a surgeon who was not trained in TM joint surgical techniques and used a "hockey stick"-shaped incision. The oblique arm of the incisional line was placed at the inferior line of the vertical preauricular incision, severing all of the facial nerves.

An unusual complication of TM joint surgery is inferior alveolar nerve sensory dysfunction related to the placement of a modified, large towel clip or other instrument

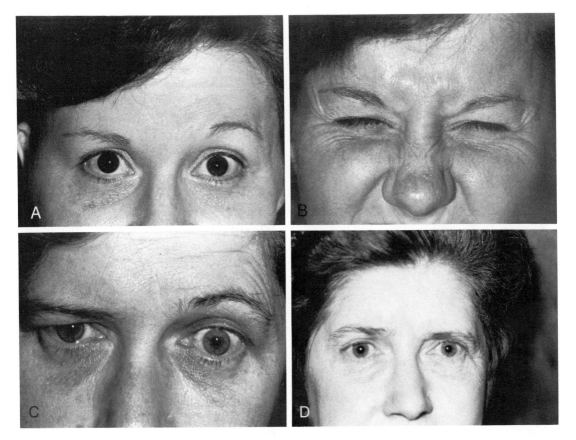

*Fig. 12–20.* Postoperative TM joint surgery dysfunction of the temporal branch of the facial nerve. A. Patient demonstrates inability to raise the right eyebrow 3 months postoperatively; B. The patient demonstrates that the corrugator muscles were intact, and nearly complete function returned to the temporalis nerve over the course of 2 years postoperatively; C. At 5 years postoperatively, another patient demonstrates an inability to raise the right eyebrow after the probable application of a surgical diathermy in the vicinity of the temporal branch of the facial nerve; D. At 10 years postoperatively, the patient underwent soft tissue plicating and tucking involving the right superior eyelid.

through the mandibular ramus. The instruments allow the use of inferior traction, but penetration of the inferior alveolar canal is possible.

## Infection

Infection is a rare complication. We have had only one case, and it was associated with the overlying soft tissue. Management consisted of incision, drainage, and antibiotic therapy, with no untoward sequelae (Fig. 12–21).

## Deafness Secondary to Providing Surgical Access

Access is both a problem and a principle in all surgical endeavors. In procedures involving the TM joint, the lack of access may be of greater concern in individuals who have a loss of posterior teeth and an age-related reduction in joint space.[15] To gain access, instruments and manual procedures are used to move the condyle inferiorly. A loss of hearing may result from forced movement of the condyle inferiorly. Unpublished reports cite incidences of dislodging of the stapes out of the oval window and of tearing of the posterior-superior quadrant of the tympanic membrane producing deafness, without penetration into

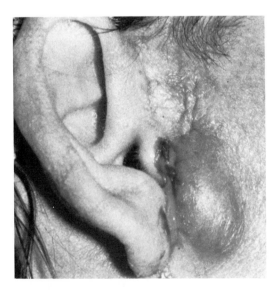

**Fig. 12–21.** Postoperative TM joint surgery infection of subcutaneous soft tissues, responded promptly to incision, drainage, and antibiotics.

the middle ear. The dislodging and tearing result from depression of the condyle in a patient with an enlarged anterior malleolar ligament that is displaced when its continuation, the sphenomandibular ligament, is forced inferiorly. The downward force on the nonelastic ligament may pull inferiorly on the anterior malleolar ligament and pull the malleus downward and forward.[52]

## Reactions to Alloplastic Devices

The largest number of complications are associated with alloplastic implanted devices producing destructive giant cell granulomas, failing of the implants by erosion and fraying, and displacement of the devices. At present, the placement of alloplastic devices has given way to the use of biologic materials: fascia, muscle, and dermal grafts.

## Anomalous Anatomy and Misdirection of Instruments

With open dissection or with the placement of arthroscopic instruments into the joint space, the external auditory canal is a landmark. The usual medial course of the canal is an S-shaped curving tube; the lateral part is directed superiorly and anteriorly, the central part is directed posteriorly, and the inner part is directed anteriorly and inferiorly. From the concha to the tympanic membrane, the external meatus is between 2 and 3 cm in length. The cartilaginous portion comprises incomplete circles of cartilage interspersed with fibrous connective tissues.

If the curvatures of the canal are beyond the nominal locations or if the soft tissue between the fibrous connective tissues of the canal and the TM joint are dense, the canal may be penetrated, usually between the cartilaginous plates. This complication occurs because either the location of the canal is anomalous or it is retracted forward by the dense soft tissues. In these cases, the external auditory meatus is entered and the tympanic membrane may be visualized. Because of either unusual anatomy or misdirection of an arthroscopic instrument, penetration past the tympanic membrane and into the middle ear is possible.[53]

We observed a case in which the surgeon who was not familiar with TM joint surgical procedures identified an extremely heavy bony outer rim of the osseous portion of the external auditory meatus as the concavity of the glenoid fossa. Confusion regarding the anatomy was clarified before the tympanic cavity was entered, and the operation was redirected to the TM joint without auditory impairment.

## Auriculotemporal Syndrome

Auriculotemporal syndrome may follow surgical manipulations of preauricular soft tissues as in parotidectomies and TM joint surgeries. In a report of the syndrome occurring following TM joint surgery, Kryshtalskyj and Weinberg observed the onset may be a matter of weeks, as with their patients, to months or years following parotid surgery and radical neck gland dissections.[54] The syndrome appears with sweating over the area of cutaneous innervation by the auriculotemporal and great auricular nerves in response to gustatory stimuli. It is caused by an aberrant cross regeneration of nerve fibers between the postganglionic secretomotor parasympathetic fibers of the auriculotemporal nerve and the cervical plexus joining the severed postganglionic fibers that supply the cutaneous sweat glands.

## Invading the Foramen of Huschke

During early childhood, a foramen may be present on the anterior osseous tympanic plate, just anterior to the TM joint. The foramen may persist into adulthood and the retrodiskal tissue that normally originates on the tympanic plate will originate in the subcutaneous tissue of the auditory meatus. Inspection reveals a bulging caused by the movements of the condyle in the meatus. This structural defect could put the middle and inner ear structures at risk by open TM joint surgery exposure, arthroscopic penetration, TM joint implant migrations, or associated inflammations.[55,56]

Appreciation is extended to Drs. Robert Ord, Keith Kreutziger, Simon Weinberg, Michael Nealis, Eugene Messer, and Thomas Indresano for giving so freely of their time and resources for the development of this chapter.

## References

1. Okeson J.P. and Hayes D.K.: Long-term results in treatment of temporomandibular disorders: An evaluation of patients. J Am Dent Assoc, 112:473, 1986
2. Greene C.S. and Laskin D.M.: Long-term status of TMJ clicking in patients with myofascial pain and dysfunction. J Am Dent Assoc, 117:461, 1988
3. Dolwick M.F., et al: Arthrotomographic evaluation of the temporomandibular joint. J Oral Maxillofac Surg, 37:793–799, 1979
4. Wilkes C.H.: Internal derangements of the temporomandibular joint. Arch Otolaryngol Head Neck Surg, 115:469, 1989
5. Dunn M.J., et al: Temporomandibular joint condylectomy: A technique and postoperative follow up. Oral Surg Oral Med Oral Pathol, 51:363, 1981
6. Mercuri L.G., et al: Intra-articular meniscus dysfunction surgery. Oral Surg Oral Med Oral Pathol, 54:613, 1982
7. Leopard P.J.: Anterior dislocation of the temporomandibular disc. Br J Oral Maxillofac Surg, 22:9, 1984
8. Feinberg S.E. and Smilock M.S.: Technique of functional disc repositioning in internal derangements of the temporomandibular joint. J Oral Maxillofac Surg, 45:825, 1987
9. Eppley B.L. and Defino J.J.: Surgical treatment of internal derangements of the temporomandibular joint: Evaluation of two techniques. J Oral Maxillofac Surg, 46:721, 1988
10. Lessin M.E. and Gross P.D.: Temporomandibular joint disorders: Discussion of a rational approach to surgery and a retrospective analysis of surgeries performed. Oral Surg Oral Med Oral Pathol, 67:374, 1989
11. Hall M.B., et al: Facial nerve injury during surgery of the temporomandibular joint. A comparison of two dissection techniques. J Oral Maxillofac Surg, 43:20, 1985
12. Dias A.D.: A truly endaural approach to the temporomandibular joint. Br J Plast Surg, 37:65, 1984
13. Nishioka G.J. and Van Sickel J.E.: Modified endaural incision for surgical access to the temporomandibular joint. J Oral Maxillofac Surg, 45:1080, 1987
14. Kreutziger K.L.: Extended modified postauricular incision of the temporomandibular joint. Oral Surg Oral Med Oral Pathol, 63:2, 1987
15. Rieder C.E. and Martinoff J.T.: Comparison of the multiphasic dysfunction profile with lateral transcranial radiographs. J Prosthet Dent, 52:572, 1984
16. Sanders B.: Arthroscopic surgery of the temporomandibular joint: Treatment of internal derangement with persistent closed lock. Oral Surg Oral Med Oral Pathol, 61:361, 1986
17. Montgomery M.L., et al: Arthroscopic TMJ surgery: Effects on signs, symptoms, and disc position. J Oral Maxillofac Surg, 47:1263, 1988
18. Weinberg S.: Eminectomy and meniscorrhaphy for internal derangements of the temporomandibular joint. Oral Surg Oral Med Oral Pathol, 57:241, 1984
19. Tyndall D.A. and Matteson S.R.: Radiographic appearance and population distribution of the pneumatized articular eminence of the temporal bone. J Oral Maxillofac Surg, 432:493, 1985

20. Kraut R.A.: Methyl methacrylate obturation of the pneumatized articular eminence of the temporal bone. J Oral Maxillofac Surg, 43:554, 1985

21. Stern N.S.: An alternative procedure for repositioning the anteriorly displaced TMJ disc. J Craniomand Disord Facial Oral Pain, 2:13, 1988 ,

22. Blankestijn J. and Boering G.: Posterior dislocation of the temporomandibular disc. Int J Oral Surg, 14:437, 1985

23. Gallagher D.M.: Posterior dislocation of the temporomandibular joint meniscus: Report of three cases. J Am Dent Assoc, 113:411, 1986

24. Eriksson L. and Westesson P.L.: Long-term evaluation of meniscectomy of the temporomandibular joint. J Oral Maxillofac Surg, 43:263, 1985

25. Walker R.V. and Kalamchi S.: A surgical technique for management of internal derangements of the temporomandibular joint. J Oral Maxillofac Surg, 45:299, 1987

26. Quinn J.H.: Letter to the editor: TMJ articular disc perforation, a new perspective. J Oral Maxillofac Surg, 47:1348, 1989

27. Heffez L., et al: CT evaluation of TMJ disc replacement with Proplast-Teflon implant. J Oral Maxillofac Surg, 45:657, 1987

28. Florine B.L., et al: Tomographic evaluation of temporomandibular joints following discoplasty or placement of polytetrafluoroethylene implants. J Oral Maxillofac Surg, 48:183, 1988

29. Dolwick J.F. and Afdermorte T.B.: Silicone-induced foreign body reaction and lymphadenopathy after temporomandibular joint arthroplasty. Oral Surg Oral Med Oral Pathol, 59:449, 1985

30. DeChamplain R.W. and Marshall E.T. Jr.: Autopolymerizing Silastic for interpositional arthroplasty. J Oral Maxillofac Surg, 46:572, 1988

31. Feinberg S.E. and Smilack M.S.: Lateral capsular ligament reconstruction in temporomandibular joint surgery. J Oral Maxillofac Surg, 46:6, 1988

32. Georgiade N.: Surgical correction of TMJ dysfunction by means of autogenous dermal grafts. Plast Reconstr Surg, 30:68, 1962

33. Tucker M.R., et al: Autogenous dermal grafts for repair of temporomandibular joint disc perforations. J Oral Maxillofac Surg, 44:781, 1986

34. Stewart H.M., et al: Histologic fate of dermal grafts following implantation for temporomandibular joint meniscal perforation: A preliminary study. Oral Surg Oral Med Oral Pathol, 62:481, 1986

35. Ward T.: Surgery of the temporomandibular joint. Ann R Coll Surg Engl, 28:139, 1961

36. Tasanen A and von Konow L.: Closed condylotomy in the treatment of idiopathic and traumatic pain-dysfunction syndrome of the temporomandibular joint. Int J Oral Surg, 2:102, 1973

37. Helfick J.: Personal communication. 1989

38. Annandale T.: Displacement of the inter-articular cartilage of the lower jaw, and its treatment by operation. Lancet, 1:411, 1887

39. Sindet-Pedersen S.: Intraoral myotomy of the lateral pterygoid muscle for treatment of recurrent dislocation of the mandibular condyle. J Oral Maxillofac Surg, 46:445, 1988

40. Maw R.B. and McKean T.W.: Scarification of the temporal tendon for treatment of chronic subluxation of the temporomandibular joint. J Oral Maxillofac Surg, 31:22, 1973

41. Gould J.F.: Shortening of the temporalis tendon for hypermobility of the temporomandibular joint. J Oral Maxillofac Surg, 36:781, 1978

42. Randzio J. and Fischer-Brondies E.: Augmentation of the articular tubercle in treatment of chronic recurrent temporomandibular luxations. Oral Surg Oral Med Oral Pathol, 61:19, 1986

43. Gosserez M. and Dautrey J.: Osteoplastic procedure for treatment of temporomandibular luxations. Trans. of 2nd Congress of Oral Surgery. Copenhagen, Munksgaard, 1967

44. Georgiade N., et al: Experimental and clinical evaluation of autogenous dermal grafts used in the treatment of TMJ ankylosis. Plast Reconstr Surg, 19:32, 1957

45. Narang R. and Dixon R.A.: Temporomandibular joint arthroplasty with fascialatta. Oral Surg Oral Med Oral Pathol, 39:45, 1975

46. Timmell R. and Grundschober F.: The interpositional use of lyodura in operations for ankylosis of the temporomandibular joint. J Maxillofac Surg, 10:193, 1982

47. Pogrel M.A. and Kaban L.B.: The role of a temporal fascia and muscle flap in temporomandibular joint surgery. J Oral Maxillofac Surg, 48:14, 1990

48. Kent J.N., et al: Experience with a polymer glenoid fossa prosthesis for partial or total temporomandibular joint reconstruction. J Oral Maxillofac Surg, 44:520, 1986

49. Alling C.C. and Alling R.D.: Facial reconstructive surgery. In Alling C.C. and Osbon D.B. Maxillofacial Trauma. Philadelphia, Lea & Febiger, 1988

50. Connole P.W. and Obeid G.: A simple appliance for continuous jaw exercises. J Oral Maxillofac Surg, 46:520, 1988

51. Pell G.J. and Gregory B.T.: Impacted mandibular third molars: Classification and simplified technique for removal. Dent Dig, 39:330, 1933

52. Loughner B.A., et al: Discomalleolar and anterior malleolar ligaments: Possible cause of middle ear damage during temporomandibular joint surgery. Oral Surg Oral Med Oral Pathol, 68:14, 1989

53. Van Sickels J.E., et al: Middle ear injury resulting from temporomandibular joint arthroscopy. J Oral Maxillofac Surg, 45:962, 1987

54. Kryshtalskyj B. and Weinberg S.: An assessment for auriculotemporal syndrome following temporomandibular joint surgery through a preauricular approach. J Oral Maxillofac Surg, 47:3, 1989

55. Herzog S. and Fiese R.: Persistent foramen of Huschke: Possible risk factor for otologic complications after arthroscopy of the temporomandibular joint. Oral Surg Oral Med Oral Pathol, 68:267, 1989

56. Heffez L., et al: Developmental defects of the tympanic plate: Case reports and review of the literature. J Oral Maxillofac Surg, 47:1336, 1989

# Part V

# Vascular and Nervous Systems

# 13

# Vascular System

Numerous vascular problems in the head and neck may manifest as oral or dental pain. Detailed knowledge of the head and neck vasculature and its innervation is required to diagnose and treat these problems, because observations on conscious patients reveal that cranial vessels refer pain to the facial and other areas.

## Nociceptive Innervation of Arteries

Electrical stimulation and application of heat, tension, or pressure to the vessels of cooperative surgical patients can evoke pain from all of the major extracranial arteries (Fig. 13–1). Rhythmic distention by intermittent spreading of a clamp in an arterial lumen or repetitive stretching between sutures provokes throbbing discomfort. Mechanical irritation of multiple areas elicits more widespread pain, whereas continuous stimulation precipitates nausea and vomiting. Vigorous constriction of vessels by application of epinephrine causes no discomfort. Application of a local anesthetic proximal to the point of stimulation can prevent the occurrence of pain. The superficial temporal, supraorbital, and frontal arteries refer pain to facial areas

(Fig. 13–2). The arteries of the face are also involved in facial pain.

## Referral of Pain from Intracranial Vessels

The main trunks of all the intracranial dural arteries are sensitive. Irritation of the middle meningeal artery provokes deep aching in the area of stimulation and behind the eye (Fig. 13–3). Referral from the anterior meningeal arteries is limited to the forehead and eye.

The sagittal sinus refers pain to the frontal and periorbital areas, but it is usually less intense than that from the arteries (Fig. 13–4). Stimulation of the transverse sinus, the straight sinus, and the torcular Herophili (confluens) provokes referral to the forehead and eye; manipulation of the cavernous sinuses causes ocular and maxillary pain.

Stimulation of the large vessels at the base of the brain produces a deep, intense, dull

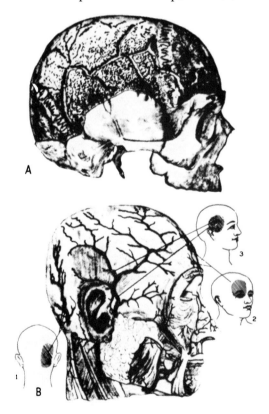

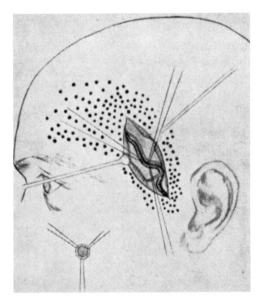

*Fig. 13–1.* Traction sutures in the superficial temporal artery. Distention induced by traction sutures with distribution of the induced pain are indicated by the stippled area. (From Ray B.S. and Wolff H.G.: Experimental studies on headache. Arch Surg, *41*:813, 1940.)

*Fig. 13–2.* Distribution of pain elicited by stimulation of the supraorbital and frontal arteries and the superficial temporal artery. (From Ray B.S. and Wolff H.G.: Experimental studies on headache. Arch Surg, *41*:813, 1940.)

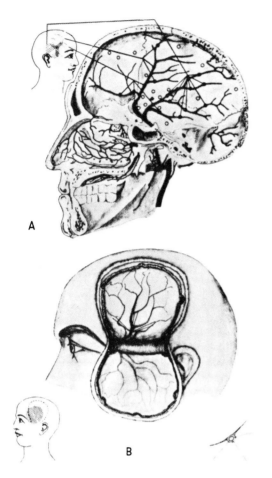

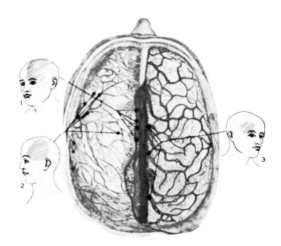

*Fig. 13–4.* Pain referral from the margin of the superior sagittal sinus (1), middle meningeal artery (2), tributaries of the superior sagittal sinus (3). O indicates the point of stimulation insensitive to pain. (From Ray B.S. and Wolff H.G.: Experimental studies on headache. Arch Surg, *41*:813, 1940.)

*Fig. 13–3.* Distribution of pain referral after stimulation of the middle meningeal artery and its branches. (From Ray B.S. and Wolff H.G.: Experimental studies on headache. Arch Surg, *41*:813, 1940.)

vation by the trigeminal nerve. Findings of a recent study demonstrated the activation of trigeminal brain stem nociceptive neurons by middle meningeal artery stimulation.[1] In this study, electrical stimulation of the middle meningeal artery of the cat evoked potentials in trigeminal subnucleus caudalis neurons. Seventy-eight subnucleus caudalis neurons could be excited by middle meningeal artery stimulation. Interestingly, 88% of the 40 neurons studied in detail were also excited by noxious stimulation of the facial skin.

## Three-Dimensional Microanatomy of Nerve Fibers on Vessels

In another recent study, investigators used scanning electron microscopy and electron probe x-ray microanalysis immunohistochemistry on cerebral blood vessels to demonstrate three-dimensional microanatomy of the nerve fibers on the cerebral blood vessels of the guinea pig.[2] Nerve fibers 2- to 8-μm in diameter form a plexus on the outer surface of the adventitia. After branching, the nerve fibers penetrate the blood vessel adventitia. Substance P-immunoreactive nerve fibers form a meshwork pattern in the outer layer of the adventitia and vasoactive intestinal polypeptide (VIP) immunoreactive nerve fibers form a spiral running pattern in the inner

ache, often with nausea; in contrast, the arteries deeper in the brain are insensitive (Fig. 13–5). Pain from the intracranial internal carotid is noted behind the eye and low in the temporal region. The proximal middle cerebral artery refers in similar fashion, whereas irritation of the anterior cerebral artery evokes pain around the eye (Fig. 13–6).

In summary, intracranial vessels with facial pain reference include: anterior meningeal arteries, intracranial internal carotid, circle of Willis and its proximal large branches, middle meningeal artery, transverse sinus, straight sinus, torcular Herophili (confluens), superior sagittal sinus, sylvian vein, and cavernous sinus.

Referral of pain to the face from these structures reflects their common sensory inner-

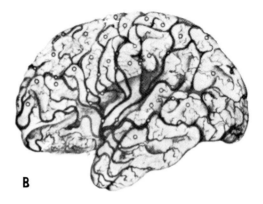

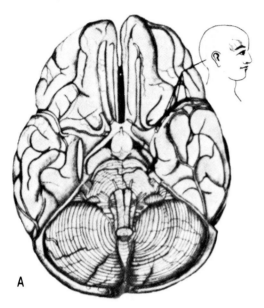

**A**

layer of the adventitia. Microapplication of VIP showed strong dilation of cerebral arteries, whereas application of substance P showed weaker dilation.[3] These findings suggest that substance P nerve fibers are not related to arterial vasomotion, but the VIP nerve fibers are vasodilative. Because substance P is involved in the mediation of pain in other tissues, one hypothesis is that the meshwork of nerve fibers in outer adventitia of cerebral blood vessels is responsible for pain of vascular origin.

Cranial bone and its diploic veins are insensitive to pain. A few areas of the floor of the cranial vault are sensitive to pain, as are the dura and pia-arachnoid, near the large meningeal arteries. The parenchyma of the cerebrum and cerebellum and the ependyma of the ventricular walls are insensitive to pain. Thrombosis of the internal carotid artery causes a unilateral, frontal headache, but thrombosis of parenchymal arteries of the cortex does not cause headache. Cases of intracranial, space-occupying lesions, such as tumors and cysts, coughing, sneezing, stooping, or straining during elimination often initiate a headache. Patients 55 years of age and older with systemic disease that alters vascular tone of intracranial vessels demonstrate a similar response.

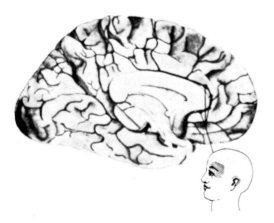

**Fig. 13–6.** Referral of pain after stimulation of the anterior cerebral artery. (From Ray B.S. and Wolff H.G.: Experimental studies on headache. Arch Surg, 41:813, 1940.)

## Temporal or Giant Cell Arteritis

Temporal arteritis occurs in patients 55 years of age and older as a diffuse, throbbing pain around the ear and temple with malaise, anorexia, weight loss, low-grade fever, and night sweats.

Findings include intimal proliferation of the arteries with disruption of the internal elastic lamina and giant cell formation (Fig. 13–7). The subclavian and vertebral arteries are often involved and all branches of the external carotid may be affected.[4] Palpation of the superficial temporal artery reveals a firm cylinder with no pulse or a flattened, fibrotic mass

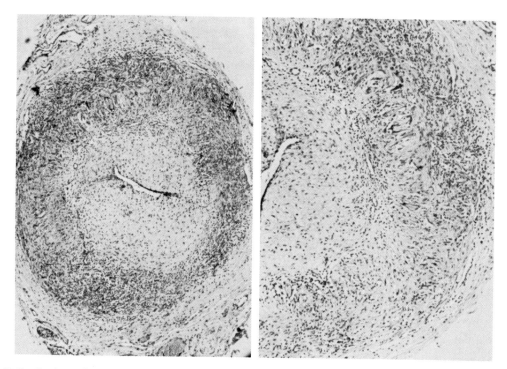

*Fig. 13–7.* Sections of temporal artery showing round cell infiltration of the adventitia and granulomatous invasion of media with giant cells, plasma cells, lymphocytes, and monocytes. Intima is thickened and lumen is narrowed. (Sections provided by Dr. Lauren Ackerman, Department of Surgical Pathology, Washington University Medical School.)

that is painful to palpation (Table 13–1). When the ophthalmic, retinal, or ciliary arteries are involved, visual defect or blindness occurs.[5] Treatment should begin promptly, with 40 to 60 mg prednisolone daily, with no delay until biopsy can be performed; visual loss may still occur 2 to 3 days after starting steroid therapy. The dose of steroid can be gradually reduced over a period of a few weeks if the symptoms do not return and the erythrocyte sedimentation rate (ESR) does not rise again. About one fourth of patients need low-dose steroid medication chronically to prevent exacerbation of symptoms. Temporal arteritis is associated with a mortality rate of 10 to 20%, even though the disease is usually self limiting over a period of 1 or 2 years.[6,7]

Muscle weakness (claudication) in mandibular muscles is common in patients with temporal arteritis, and it probably occurs because of temporalis and masseter ischemia. Arteritis of the lingual arteries has been reported.[8,9]

**TABLE 13–1.** *Temporal Arteritis*

| Disease of: | Middle and advanced age | |
|---|---|---|
| Pain: | Intense, deep, boring, facial or temporal | |
| Aggravated by: | Lying or stooping | |
| Diminished by: | Carotid compression | |
| Associated symptoms: | Fever | Visual defect |
| | Malaise | Cerebral vascular disease |
| | Anorexia | Systemic |
| Physical signs: | Temporal artery | |
| | Thick | Tender |
| | Nodular | Reddened |
| | Tortuous | Normal |
| Diagnosis: | Biopsy | |
| Therapy: | Adrenocortical steroids | |

Lingual artery involvement is demonstrated by requiring the patient to perform rapid protrusive tongue movements.[10] Tongue pain, burning dysesthesias, fatigue, and blanching of the tongue occur if the artery is involved. Because both lingual arteries are often involved, lingual infarct may occur. In one hospital, 14% of all patients with giant cell arteritis developed tongue infarction.[8]

## Case Summaries

A 63-year-old woman was referred to the authors by a dentist friend of the patient after a cursory examination of the oral cavity. The patient had upper and lower partial dentures with decayed teeth under the clasps. The patient had experienced diffuse temporal headache and malaise for 11 weeks. She was treated by two clinicians and spent 8 days in the hospital for tests. After a complete oral and occlusal examination, palpation of the superficial temporal arteries revealed a painless pulse on the left side and a painful, pulseless fibrotic mass on the right side. Her Westergren ESR was 120 mm/hr. She began taking prednisone orally at noon on the second day in our clinic and by 9:30 that evening, the pain disappeared. A biopsy of the frontal branch of the superficial temporal artery was performed the following morning. The diagnosis of giant cell arteritis was made on the basis of the biopsy results and sedimentation rate.

A 73-year-old man had dull, aching pain of sudden onset on the right side of the face of 3 weeks duration.[11] The patient thought the pain was related to his dentures. He had noted an elongated, firm, slightly movable tender mass in the lower right cheek opposite the body of the mandible just above the antegonial notch 2 weeks before examination. He had a slightly elevated temperature and findings of oral and radiographic examinations were negative. A tentative diagnosis of nonspecific lymphadenitis was made and penicillin was prescribed (6,000,000 units intramuscularly), along with instructions to use hot, moist applications four times daily. Acetylsalicyclic acid and codeine were prescribed for pain. No reduction in pain or change in his condition was evident on the third day, so the mass was surgically removed. Bleeding was heavy from what appeared to be the facial artery. The artery seemed to extend through the mass and prevented its removal. The vessel was clamped, ligated, and transected, and the mass was removed. The mass was an enlarged, coiled segment of the facial artery. The pathologist's diagnosis was transverse sections of an artery and giant cell arteritis of the facial artery. Follow-up 9 months later revealed the patient was still free of pain and had no evidence of recurrent disease.

In another case, a 77-year-old woman was admitted to the hospital with a 3-week history of pain on the right side of the head and necrosis of the skin of the temples.[12] Two teeth in the left anterior maxilla had recently exfoliated. She had an area of necrosis on the upper lip, and her ESR at the time of hospital admission was 135 mm/hr. Systemic corticosteroid therapy was started immediately, but she lost the sight in her right eye 36 hours later. Over the next 6 weeks, the ESR dropped to 55 mm/hr, the necrotic temple areas began to form a crust, and the necrotic upper lip became larger and separated, leaving a large defect. The patient died the following week. Autopsy findings revealed extensive giant cell arteritis of the arterial system.

## Polymyalgia Rheumatica and Giant Cell Arteritis

Approximately 50% of patients with polymyalgia rheumatica have associated giant cell arteritis.[13] The incidence of polymyalgia rheumatica in persons 50 years of age and older is 50 per 100,000; it is twice as common in women as in men, with a predilection for white patients.[14] Both polymyalgia and giant cell arteritis are treated with steroids. The dose is initially higher for individuals with giant cell arteritis, and the medication regimen usually must be continued for 2 to 4 years for patients with both diseases.

## Carotid System Arteritis

When patients in the 30- to 55-year age range develop diffuse, usually unilateral facial pain and palpation reveals tenderness of the carotid, facial, and superficial temporal arteries, a diagnosis of carotid system arteritis warrants consideration.[15] The authors have seen a few cases of this condition, and the patients received relief of pain after 1 week of prednisone therapy (60 mg/day). The diffuse pain returned, however, during the second week.

## Migraine Headaches

The migraine headache has plagued mankind since the beginning of recorded history. These headaches are usually severe and typically are hemicranial. Our understanding of migraine is so incomplete that universally accepted criteria for diagnosis have never been established.

### Classic Migraine

This term is used if the headache is preceded by sensory, motor, or visual symptoms. The prodrome may take the form of scotomata, nausea, sudden tunnel vision, blurring of vision, feeling of malaise, any combination of these symptoms, or other focal neurologic disturbances. The prodrome usually lasts 25 to 45 minutes, at which time the headache begins.

### Common Migraine

The common migraine headache is the same as classic migraine headache, but no prodromal symptoms occur. Common migraine is more frequent than classic migraine, and the neurologic disturbances of classic migraine prodrome often occur during the headache instead of preceding it.

### Migraine Equivalents

Focal neurologic disturbances of the prodrome without headache are common and are called migraine equivalents. Migraine equivalents often affect older patients who suffered classic or common migraine when they were younger.

Migraine often begins in childhood. By the early twenties, 50% of affected women continue to suffer the headache; most of the men stop having headaches. A parental history of migraine is obtained in 50 to 60% of patients with migraine and in 10 to 20% of headache-free subjects.[16] Evidence favors a hereditary factor in migraine, but the mode of inheritance is not clear. Seventy-five percent of adults with migraine are women, but boys account for 60% of the migraine population in children.

Emotional stress is the commonest precipitant of migrainous attacks, although no evidence exists that migraine patients are under greater stress than nonmigraine subjects. Patients tend to develop the migraine during the relaxation after a stressful event and not at the peak of stress. Migraine attacks may occur in association with asthma, hay fever, or angioneurotic edema on exposure to a specific allergen.[17]

Unilateral paresthesia is reported by one third of patients with migraine attacks. The distribution of paresthesias shows a peculiar preference for the hand and face.[18]

Typical migraine patients have one to four headaches per month. Slightly more than 50% of migraine sufferers experience symptoms on one side only. The side may vary from one headache to another, but most severe attacks tend to occur on a preferred side. The headache is usually gradual in onset, beginning over several minutes to several hours, reaching a crescendo that persists for several hours to days, and then gradually subsiding over several hours. The headache usually begins as a dull ache and becomes pulsatile when it is more severe. Some patients have a sharp jabbing pain superimposed on the dull ache. Nausea and vomiting occur in about one half of affected individuals. Most patients report blurred vision and two thirds of patients experience scalp tenderness. The superficial temporal artery sometimes is so tender that it mimics temporal arteritis.

Fluid retention occurs in most patients hours to days before a migraine attack, and the weight gain may amount to 2 to 5 pounds (as much as 2.27 kg). Polyuria begins either immediately after the onset of headache or during the period of dwindling headache intensity.

Between 10 and 20% of patients report nasal stuffiness and profuse nasal secretion as the attack terminates, which sometimes leads to a mistaken diagnosis of rhinitis or sinusitis or cluster headache. Alteration in mood, such as lethargy, fatigue, anxious irritability, or exhilaration, is often noted.

In adult women, headache occurring monthly the day before or the first day of menstrual flow, as well as at other times, is virtually pathognomonic of migraine,[19] but in young women, the onset of menarche is not related to the presence, severity, or frequency of headache.[20] The incidence of vascular headache is increased in women who use oral contraceptives.[21]

The visual hallucinations that occur during a migraine attack are usually produced by ischemia of the occipital cortex and persist when the eyes are closed. The visual hallucinations of carotid artery disease, on the other hand, result from an alteration of blood flow to the retina and typically are eliminated when the eyes are closed.[22] This information forms the basis of distinguishing migraine from carotid artery disease.

## Ophthalmoplegic Migraine

These infrequent attacks of orbital or periorbital pain usually radiate into the hemicranium, with vomiting and migraine attack. It may last 1 to 4 days. Concurrent with the headache or, more often, as it subsides, ipsilateral ptosis appears and often progresses to a complete third nerve palsy. After the headache subsides, ophthalmoplegia persists for several days. Patients with ophthalmoplegic migraine usually have a history of more common forms of migraine. This condition is easily confused with internal carotid aneurysm, Tolosa-Hunt syndrome, diabetic ophthalmoplegia, a sphenoidal sinus pathologic process, and meningitis.

## Basilar Migraine

In a recent study of 300 migraine patients, approximately 10% experienced total blindness and alteration of consciousness followed by headache. Twenty-six of 34 patients were adolescent girls, and all patients were younger than 35 years of age.[23] The attacks usually occurred in association with menstruation.

The episodes usually begin with blindness or appearance of unformed images that obscure vision, followed by vertigo, ataxia, dysarthria, tinnitus, and perioral paresthesias. Some patients lose consciousness. This phase lasts 10 to 30 minutes, at which time a severe throbbing headache, usually occipital, begins. For most of these patients, these dramatic attacks are infrequent and more common forms of migraine have occurred before and between the attacks. The attacks tend to cease with time and are replaced by common migraine.

Cerebral ischemia may serve as a precipitant of an epileptic attack in a patient with a lowered seizure threshold.[24] For many patients, it is the only circumstance under which seizures occur. These patients may fail to respond to antiepileptic agents, such as phenytoin, phenobarbital, or primidone, and their convulsive attacks can be controlled with propranolol or ergonovine maleate.[25] Patients with basilar migraine may continue in a confusional state for as long as 5 days, although it is usually of shorter duration. During this time, patients appear to be in a psychotic state with agitation, aggression, and hysterical behavior.[26] This syndrome is likely caused by brain stem ischemia.

## Periodic Migrainous Neuralgia (Cluster Headache)

Cluster headache has been described in many different ways; it is usually considered a type of vascular headache. This symptom complex has been called alarm clock headache, Sluder's headache, lower half headache, and sphenopalatine ganglion neuralgia. Given the number of variants of this syndrome and the lack of specific diagnostic criteria as described previously for migraine, attempts to classify this condition have led to great confusion.

The pain is usually severe, unilateral, and located around the orbit, temple, zygomatic or jaw region. The problem is sometimes perceived by the patient as a toothache in a maxillary molar or second premolar.[27] When taking a history, the clinician finds the pain lasts from 30 minutes to 3 hours, appears at the same time every day in one half the cases, and is accompanied by flushing (redness) or blanching of the face and conjunctiva, lacrimation, and occlusion of the nostril. These attacks frequently occur at night, during or immediately after an episode of REM (rapid eye movement) sleep. Many patients have several attacks during the night and each is associated with a REM sleep period.[28] In about 20% of patients, Horner's syndrome occurs coincident with the attack. The headaches occur daily for 2 or 3 months and then go into complete remission for months or 1 year before the next exacerbation.

The cluster headache often responds to breathing 100% oxygen, 7 liters per minute for 10 minutes. Other types of migraine do not respond to oxygen inhalation. The authors know a patient who has a small oxygen bottle for use at the office and one for home and travel use. He controls his cluster headache with oxygen. The relief from breathing oxygen may last for an hour or for days. This disease affects men more frequently than women. In one report of 95 patients, only 7 were women.[29] Most patients with cluster headache in our practice are active, high achiever, aggressive individuals.

Cluster headache or migrainous neuralgia comprises an upper syndrome, affecting the eye, forehead, and temple, and a lower syndrome, located in the cheek and jaw.[30] The lower syndrome is the type that prompts the patient to see a dentist because of suspected toothache. Another variation of the disease, chronic migrainous neuralgia, occurs in about 6% of migrainous neuralgia patients.[29] The condition is classified as chronic migrainous neuralgia when the attacks last longer than 16 weeks. These patients often benefit from the use of ergotamine tartrate and caffeine (Cafergot) or isometheptene mucate, dichloralphenazone, and acetaminophen (Midrin). Ergotamine is more effective as a suppository, but is contraindicated in patients with coronary artery disease, peripheral vascular disease, and pregnancy. When these drugs fail, methysergide (Sansert) often controls the headache. This drug should be used prophylactically, but it may cause retroperitoneal fibrosis and thus should be discontinued for a few months after 4 months of therapy. Patients who relapse during this interval often respond to lithium carbonate (250 mg tid).[31]

The histamine H2 inhibitor cimetidine (Tagamet) also controls chronic migrainous neuralgia when other drugs fail.[29] Tricyclic antidepressants, beta blockers, and calcium channel blockers are helpful in some cases.[32]

The clinician should remember that a severe headache of abrupt onset accompanied by photophobia, stiff neck, nausea, vomiting, drowsiness, delirium, or any combination of these signs is suggestive of subarachnoid hemorrhage from a ruptured intracranial aneurysm or vascular malformation. This diagnosis is more likely if the patient was straining or engaged in intercourse when the pain began.

### Pathophysiology

For many years, a common belief was that the headache phase of migrainous attacks was caused by extracranial vasodilatation and that neurologic symptoms were produced by intracranial vasoconstriction. This vascular hypothesis of migraine has given way to a belief that a neuronal phenomenon, similar to a cortical spreading depression, is responsible for the headache. Spreading depression has been demonstrated in laboratory animals and is a slow-moving, potassium-liberating depression of cortical activity, preceded by a wavefront of increased metabolic activity that spreads over the surface of the cerebral cortex.[33]

From 1981 through 1984, a method of measuring cerebral regional blood flow at 254 areas of one hemisphere by using xenon-133 inhalation and emission tomography was applied to a series of patients with classic migraine.[34,35] Findings of these studies revealed that occipital hypoperfusion (oligemia) occurs even before the symptoms begin. The decreased flow averaged 25 to 35% and progressed anteriorly in a wavelike manner at a rate of about 2 mm/min, independent of the topography of the cerebral arteries. The wave of hypoperfusion persisted for 4 to 6 hours and progressed to the frontal lobe via the insula. Subcortical perfusion remained normal during the headache and hypoperfusion was not observed at any time. A few patients with classic migraine showed no cerebral blood flow abnormalities and one patient had the wave of cortical depression in the absence of hypoperfusion. Thus, classic migraine seems to be associated with a slowly spreading, modest cortical hypoperfusion associated with local instability of vasomotor control that persists for hours. A derangement of neuronal function must cause this flow change.[36]

## Other Headaches

### Coital Headache

Men are afflicted by coital headache more commonly than women.[37] The headache occurs usually during the periorgasmic period and is a sudden excruciating, throbbing, occipital headache, sometimes with vomiting. It is not likely of psychogenic origin. If sexual activity is terminated at the onset of the headache, the latter generally subsides in minutes or within 1 to 2 hours. Many patients report previous occurrences of migrainous headaches. Ergotamine tartrate administration before sexual activity may abort the headache. No neuroradiologic abnormalities are noted in these patients.

### Altitude Headache

Altitude sickness affects many people today because of the speed with which they can travel to the mountains for skiing and recreation. The symptoms include severe pounding headache, nausea, dimness of vision, breathlessness, palpitation, anorexia, and insomnia. Evidence exists that intracranial and extracranial vasodilatation is triggered by hypoxia and/or lowered barometric pressure. The headache is aggravated by exertion, coughing, head jolting, and lying down. Temporary relief is afforded by compression of the superficial temporal arteries and by the Valsalva maneuver. Ergotamine tartrate is effective in relieving this headache.[38]

### Vitamin A-Induced Headache

Many years ago, Arctic explorers suffered violent headaches after eating polar bear liver. In 1934, analyses revealed that polar bear liver contains 15,000 IU of vitamin A per gram, and the vitamin was the agent responsible for the headaches. The acute hypervitaminosis A headache is usually frontal and retro-orbital. Nausea, abdominal pain, vertigo, and sluggishness often accompany the headache 4 to 8 hours after ingestion of the vitamin. Headaches develop after ingesting 25,000 IU of vitamin A for days or weeks, and they completely subside several days to a few weeks after vitamin A use is discontinued.[39]

## Neurovascular Odontalgia (Atypical Odontalgia)

An excruciating, annoying toothache in patients in whom no pathologic process is evident in and around the tooth or teeth is called atypical odontalgia.[40-42] This condition is believed to be a variant of cluster headache, and we have proposed a more appropriate term, neurovascular odontalgia. The sensation is often described as crawling, exploding, or pressure, not a typical toothache. The pain is localized initially to one tooth and spreads to adjacent teeth as time passes. If the teeth have large restorations or the radiographic findings are suggestive of periapical pathology, the suspected teeth often are endodontically treated, but the pain continues. The tooth is then extracted and the pain moves to the next tooth or is localized in the edentulous space. The authors have seen one case in which the pain began in the upper left first molar and slowly spread to include every tooth in the mouth during 1 year of observation. The patients are usually women ages 30 to 50 years, and they show evidence of endogenous depression. The condition usually responds well to imipramine (Tofranil) at a dosage of 10 mg tid, increasing to 25 mg tid if necessary. If tricyclic antidepressants are not effective, the patient should be referred to a physician who is knowledgeable in the use of monoamine oxidase inhibitors (MAOI). One to two months may pass before neurovascular odontalgia responds to the MAOI.

## Eagle's Syndrome

The styloid process is considered elongated if it is longer than 30 mm, measured from the base of the temporal bone. In a study of 1771 panoramic radiographs, 319 styloid processes were elongated; only 8 patients in this study, however, had symptoms of Eagle's syndrome.[43] The symptoms are pain in the neck or throat that may radiate into the eye with turning the head when the external carotid is the affected artery. When the internal carotid is affected, the pain is located across the head from frontal to occipital regions.

This condition is rare but may be confused with temporomandibular joint dysfunction, migraine headache, glossopharyngeal neuralgia, cervical arthritis, and salivary gland disease. It can be diagnosed on the basis of radiographic evidence of an anterior-posteriorly broad, elongated styloid process and provocation of pain by palpation of a bony protuberance in the tonsillar fossa.

## Carotidynia

Patients experience episodic, throbbing, deep, dull neck pain that sometimes is associated with diffuse neck swelling over the carotid sinus regions. Dental trauma is a frequent precipitant of this syndrome. Palpation of the carotid sinus evokes excruciating pain, often referring to the face, jaw, and ear. This pressure test over the carotid artery is known as Fay's test.

Two types of carotidynia have been described: painful carotid associated with migrainous changes and painful carotid associated with arteritis.[44,45] The migrainous type was identified in a study of eight patients observed over 6 years.[46] These patients had episodic pulsatile neck pain with tender carotid arteries and soft tissue swelling over the carotid sinus. Sedimentation rates were normal and tests for antinuclear antibodies were negative in all eight patients. All the patients were women ranging in age from 37 to 77 years. In some patients, the pain radiated with sharp jabs into the eye and lower jaw. All patients responded to vasoactive drugs such as ergonovine, nortriptyline, methysergide, and propranolol.

The arteritis type of the disease resembles carotid system arteritis, with the most prominent symptoms noted in the neck and carotid artery. Nonsteroidal anti-inflammatory or steroid therapy is effective.[47]

## Examination of Head and Neck Arteries

To palpate the carotid arteries for tenderness, the index finger is positioned at the anterior margin of the sternocleidomastoid muscle just below the greater cornu of the hyoid bone. As soon as the pulsating artery is located, press inward and ask the patient to note the sensation elicited. The painless side is palpated first. The carotid on the painful side is then located and pressed inward. Again, ask the patient to compare the two sides. The artery typically is painful in patients with carotid system arteritis and carotidynia.

Next, with the index finger on the inferior border of the mandible at the anterior margin of the masseter muscle, pull back and forth, locating the facial artery as it flicks under the finger. The painless side is palpated first, then the other artery; and ask the patient to compare the two sides. The facial artery is painful in carotid system arteritis and also when the masseter muscle is painful to palpation, with trigger point pain.

Lastly, the pulse is located with the index finger over the posterior root of the zygomatic arch, just superior and posterior to the condyle lateral pole bilaterally. The pulse is often difficult to locate, because even light pressure results in collapse of the artery. The best technique is to press firmly, then to reduce the pressure until the occluded superficial temporal artery begins pulsating. The artery is painful, firm, and pulseless, like a matchstick, in patients with temporal arteritis. In association with carotid system arteritis, the artery is usually pulsating, but it is painful.

The results of this palpation, along with the history and findings from examination of the other head and neck tissues, help to determine whether other tests are needed to rule out vascular pain.

## References

1. Davis K.D. and Dostrovsky J.O.: Activation of trigeminal brain-stem nociceptive neurons by dural artery stimulation. Pain, 25:398, 1986
2. Itakura T., et al: Three-dimensional observation of the nerve fibers along the cerebral blood vessels. Histochemistry, 84:217, 1986
3. Edvinsson L., et al: Feline cerebral veins and arteries:

Comparison of autonomic innervation and vasomotor responses. J Physiol (Lond), 23:133, 1982

4. Wilkinson I.M.S. and Russell R.W.R.: Arteries of the head and neck in giant cell arteritis. Arch Neurol, 27:378, 1972

5. Meadows S.P.: Temporal or giant cell arteritis. Proc R Soc Med, 59:329, 1966

6. Mementhaler M.: Giant cell arteritis (cranial arteritis) polymyalgia rheumatica. J Neurol, 218:219, 1978

7. Whitfield R.A.: Temporal arteritis. Practitioner, 194:208, 1965

8. Sofferman R.A.: Lingual infarction in cranial arteritis. JAMA, 243:2422, 1980

9. Bowdler D.A. and Knight J.R.: Lingual claudication and necrosis as a complication of giant cell arteritis. J Laryngol Otol, 99:417, 1985

10. Henderson A.H.: Tongue pain with giant cell arteritis. Br Med J, 4:337, 1967

11. Das A.K. and Laskin D.M.: Temporal arteritis of the facial artery. J Oral Maxillofac Surg, 24:226, 1966

12. Pogrel M.A.: Necrosis of the upper lip from giant cell arteritis. J Oral Maxillofac Surg, 43:300, 1985

13. Ettlinger R.E., et al: Polymyalgia rheumatica and giant cell arteritis. Annu Rev Med, 29:15, 1978

14. Wilske K.R. and Healey L.A.: Polymyalgia rheumatica and giant cell arteritis: The dilemma of therapy. Postgrad Med, 77:243, 1985

15. Troiano M.F. and Gaston G.W.: Carotid system arteritis: An overlooked and misdiagnosed syndrome. J Am Dent Assoc, 91:599, 1975

16. Lance J.W. and Anthony M.: Some clinical aspects. A prospective survey of 500 patients. Arch Neurol, 15:356, 1966

17. Kallos P. and Kallos-Defner L.: Allergy and migraine. Int Arch Allergy Appl Immunol, 7:367, 1955

18. Bruyn G.W.: Complicated migraine. In Handbook of Clinical Neurology. Vol. 5. Edited by P.J. Vinken and G.W. Bruyn. New York, John Wiley and Sons, 1968

19. Epstein M.T., et al: Migraine and reproduction hormones throughout the menstrual cycle. Lancet, 1:543, 1875

20. Deubner D.C.: An epidemiologic study of migraine and headache in 10–20 year olds. Headache, 17:173, 1977

21. Carey H.M.: Principles of oral contraception. 2. Side effects of oral contraceptives. Med J Aust, 2:1242, 1971

22. Murphey F.: The scotomata of carotid artery disease as I remember them. J Neurosurg, 39:390, 1973

23. Bickerstaff E.R.: The basilar artery and the migraine-epilepsy syndrome. Proc R Soc Med, 55:167, 1962

24. Basser L.S.: The relation of migraine and epilepsy. Brain, 92:285, 1969

25. Raskin N.H. and Appenzeller O.: Headache, Vol. XIX, Major Problems in Internal Medicine. Philadelphia, W.B. Saunders, 1980

26. Ehyai A. and Fenichel G.M.: The natural history of acute confusional migraine. Arch Neurol, 35:368, 1978

27. Eggleston D.J.: Periodic migrainous neuralgia. Oral Surg Oral Med Oral Pathol, 29:524, 1970

28. Dexter J.D. and Weitzman E.D.: The relationship of nocturnal headaches to sleep stage patterns. Neurology, 20:513, 1970

29. Pearce J.M.S.: Chronic migrainous neuralgia, a variant of cluster headache. Brain, 103:149, 1980

30. Ekbom K.: A clinical comparison of cluster headache and migraine. Acta Neurol Scand (Suppl), 46:41, 1970

31. Kudrow L.: Lithium prophylaxis for chronic cluster headache. Headache, 17:15, 1977

32. Biber M.P. and Warfield C.A.: Headache: The spectrum. Hosp Prac (Off), 19:41, 1984

33. Leao A.A.P.: Spreading depression of activity in cerebral cortex. J Neurophysiol, 7:359, 1949

34. Olesen J., et al: Focal hyperemia followed by spreading oligemia and impaired activation of rCBF in classic migraine. Ann Neurol, 9:344, 1981

35. Lauritzen M. and Olesen J.: Regional cerebral blood flow during migraine attacks by xenon-133 inhalation and emission tomography. Brain, 107:447, 1984

36. Raskin N.J.: Migraine. In Disease of the Nervous System: Clinical Neurobiology. Edited by A.K. Astbury, G.M. McKhann, and W.I. McDonald. Philadelphia, W.B. Saunders, 1986

37. Martin E.A.: Headache during sexual intercourse. Irish J Med Sci, 143:342, 1974

38. Carson R.P., et al: Symptomatology, pathophysiology, and treatment of acute mountain sickness. Fed Proc, 28:1085, 1969

39. Raskin N.H. and Appenzeller O.: Headache, Vol. XIX, Major Problems in Internal Medicine. Philadelphia, W.B. Saunders, 1980

40. Rees R.T. and Harris M.: Atypical odontalgia. Br J Oral Maxillofac Surg, 16:212, 1979

41. Brooke R.J.: Atypical odontalgia, a report of twenty-two cases. Oral Surg Oral Med Oral Pathol, 49:196, 1980

42. Kreisberg M.K.: Atypical odontalgia: Differential diagnosis and treatment. J Am Dent Assoc, 104:852, 1982

43. Sivers J.E. and Johnson G.K.: Diagnosis of Eagle's syndrome. Oral Surg Oral Med Oral Pathol, 59:575, 1985

44. Murry T.J.: Carotidynia: A cause of neck and face pain. Can Med Assoc J, 120:441, 1979

45. Roseman D.M.: Carotidynia. A distinct syndrome. Arch Otolaryngol, 85:81, 1967

46. Raskin N.H. and Prusiner S.: Carotidynia. Neurology, 27:43, 1977

47. Orfei R. and Meienberg O.: Carotidynia: A report of eight cases and prospective evaluation of therapy. J Neurol, 230:65, 1983

Examination of the patient with craniofacial pain is based on thorough knowledge of the anatomy of the somatosensory nerves that innervate the head and neck.

## Innervation of the Head and Neck

Four cranial nerves, three spinal (cervical) nerves, and visceral afferents from the upper thoracic cord innervate the head and neck.

### Trigeminal Nerve

The trigeminal nerve, with its three divisions, innervates the anterior one half of the head (Fig. 14–1). The ophthalmic or first division innervates the forehead and scalp as far back as the vertex of the skull, the upper eyelids, and the bridge of the nose to its tip. The maxillary or second division innervates the anterior temple, lower eyelid, ala of the nose, upper lip, and cheek. The mandibular or third division innervates the posterior temple, lower cheek, lower lip, and chin. The trigeminal nerve does not innervate the angle of the mandible.

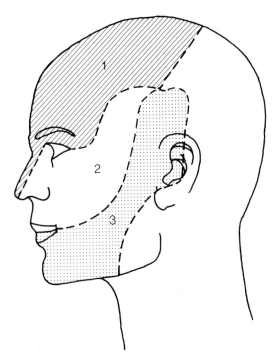

*Fig. 14–1.* Innervation of the face by the trigeminal nerve: 1. Ophthalmic division; 2. Maxillary division; 3. Mandibular division.

### Facial Nerve

The facial nerve sensory component, nerve intermedius, and the vagus nerve innervate the external auditory meatus, parts of the pinna of the ear, and a small zone of skin beneath and behind the lobe of the ear (Fig. 14–2). Geniculate or VII nerve neuralgia pain is localized in the external ear, external auditory meatus, and deep, lateral face. In a small percentage of Bell's palsy patients, pain is located just beneath the lobe of the ear. This pain persists for weeks and must be controlled with narcotic or synthetic narcotic medication until the neuropathy in nerve intermedius has resolved.

### Glossopharyngeal Nerve

The glossopharyngeal nerve provides sensory innervation to the posterior one third of the tongue, soft palate, the oral pharynx (Fig. 14–3), and the external auditory meatus. The glossopharyngeal neuralgia trigger area is located in the throat and base of the tongue. Localization of this trigger area by the patient and the clinician is difficult, and it is often erroneously localized in the floor of the mouth, which leads to a misdiagnosis of trigeminal neuralgia rather than glossopharyngeal neuralgia. Mechanical stimulation of the external auditory meatus often results in a cough reflex or "scratchy feeling" in the oral

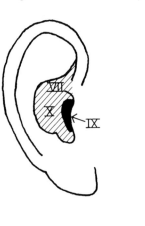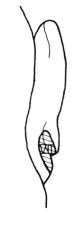

*Fig. 14–2.* Innervation of the ear by the facial (VII), glossopharyngeal (IX), and vagus (X) nerves. Innervation by the mandibular division of the trigeminal nerve is not represented here. Note the small zone below and behind the ear lobe where pain may occur in Bell's palsy.

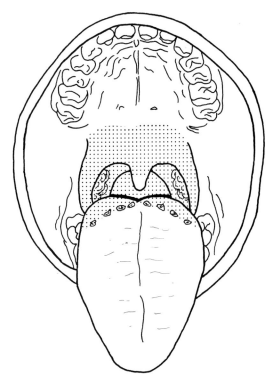

*Fig. 14–3.* Glossopharyngeal (IX) innervation of the dorsal third of the tongue, soft palate, palatine tonsil, and oral pharynx. Note that the lower half of the uvula has no small fiber innervation and is anaesthetic.

pharynx. Stimulation of the cough reflex is observed when one palpates the mandibular condyle by inserting the little finger into the patient's external auditory meatus.

## Vagus Nerve

A small branch from the vagus nerve provides sensory innervation to a small area in the deep pinna of the ear.

## Cervical Nerves

Sensory fibers of the first cervical nerve do not reach the skin, but rather innervate the deep upper, posterior neck tissues. The second cervical nerve innervates the occipital skull forward to the vertex, the pinna of the ear, the angle of the mandible, and the upper neck (Fig. 14–4). The third cervical nerve innervates the occipital skull, pinna of the ear, angle of the mandible, and the middle and lower neck (Fig. 14–5). The fourth cervical

nerve innervates the lower neck and upper shoulders (Fig. 14–4).

## Cervical Sympathetic Trunk

Visceral afferents may exist in the cervical sympathetic trunk and follow the external carotid artery branches to innervate the deep mandible, teeth, and ear regions of the head. If these afferents are not present, pain receptors in the regions of the head just mentioned must be responsive to activation by sympathetic nerves. Direct stimulation of the superior cervical ganglion produces strong pain in the lower teeth and behind the ear on the ipsilateral side.[1,2] Pinching the carotid sinus also produces these pains in teeth and the ear. Little is known about the relationship between sympathetic nerves and pain perception.

## Convergence of Sensory Nerves

Most of the large-diameter sensory fibers in the trigeminal nerve project to the main sen-

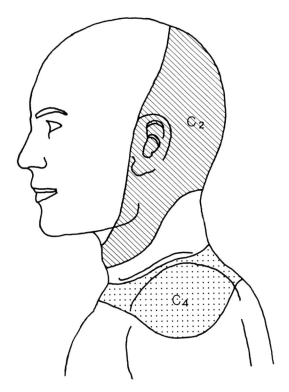

*Fig. 14–4.* Sensory innervation by the second and fourth cervical nerves. Note that C2 innervates the angle of the mandible.

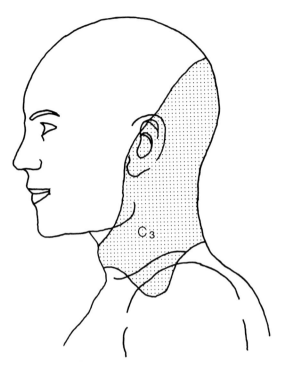

**Fig. 14–5.** Sensory innervation by the third cervical nerve. Note that C3 innervates the angle of the mandible.

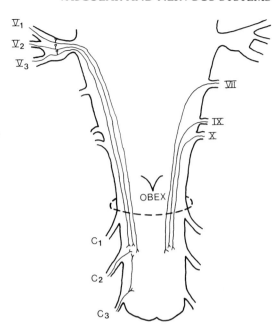

**Fig. 14–6.** Convergence of primary small fibers subserving pain at the level of C2 in the cervical spinal cord. Trigeminal, C2, and C3 fibers are shown on the left and facial (VII), glossopharyngeal (IX), and vagus (X) nerves are shown on the right.

sory nucleus, but about 50% of them send a collateral down the spinal trigeminal tract, descending as far caudally as the level of C2. Most of the small-diameter fibers subserving pain project down in the descending trigeminal tract to synapse in a pool of neurons at the level of C2 (Fig. 14–6). Complete facial analgesia sparing touch and proprioception is produced by sectioning the spinal trigeminal tract at the level of the obex. This procedure is known as the Sjöquist tractotomy.

Somatosensory fibers of the facial, glossopharyngeal, and vagus nerves follow the spinal trigeminal tract and project into the trigeminal spinal nucleus at the level of C2. Small fibers in C2, C3, and C4 ascend in Lissauer's tract into this same pool of secondary neurons. This extensive convergence of the nerves that innervate the head and neck provide the anatomic substrate for widely distributed referred pain patterns. The referred pain patterns described in this text are based on the convergence of nerve pathways.

## Nociceptors

The two major types of specialized nociceptive receptors are the high threshold mechanoreceptor and the polymodal nociceptor.[3] The high threshold mechanoreceptors with A delta axons respond only to strong pressure. They have large overlapping receptive fields. The polymodal nociceptors with unmyelinated C axons respond to pressure, heat, cold, and irritant chemicals. They have small or single-spot receptive fields. The polymodal nociceptor units are the most numerous single class of afferent units from skin. Other types of cutaneous nociceptors include a heat nociceptor and a receptor with A delta axons that respond to heat, pressure, and irritant chemicals.

These nociceptive receptors are stimulated by strong pressure or release of chemical substances into the extracellular fluid as a result of tissue damage. These substances can be an excess of hydrogen ions, histamine, bradykinin, serotonin, acetylcholine, or substance P (an undecapeptide that is also released by primary afferent pain fibers at their first central synapse in the spinal cord and brain stem). The release of potassium ion and prostaglandins in the tissues greatly increases the intensity of the pain.

The brain and pituitary gland contain at least nine different peptides that reduce pain with opiate-like properties.[4] These peptides are two enkephalins, three endorphins (alpha, beta, and gamma), dynorphin, anodynin, and two pituitary peptides of unknown structure. These peptides are quickly hydrolyzed by two aminopeptidases in the body fluids, so they produce analgesia only briefly when injected into animals experimentally. Enkephalins have epileptogenic effects and intracerebral injection of beta-endorphins into brain cortex leads to catatonic posturing.

Endorphin-containing neurons are located in parts of the brain stem that make up a pain control system. These neurons reduce the level of excitation of the pain sensory relay neurons when they are activated by painful stimuli, opiate drugs, electrical stimulation, and the placebo effect. Substance P is the neurotransmitter that excites the relay neurons that subserve pain. The release of substance P by these fibers is reduced by enkephalin.

## Pain Theory

For many years, clinical experience has shown that large fiber input inhibits pain perception in the head and neck. If the clinician, for example, squeezes the upper lip just before inserting a needle into the upper vestibule mucosa for a middle superior alveolar infiltration of anesthetic, the pain of the injection is obtunded. In 1965, the gate control theory of pain perception was proposed.[5] This theory stated that large fiber input (that accompanies a noxious stimulus) activates substantia gelatinosa cells to shut off the small fiber input via presynaptic inhibition of the transmission cells (Fig. 14–7). This theory was heuristic and the research it stimulated has modified the theory significantly. It is true, however, that if one can stimulate large fibers in excess of small fibers, pain is suppressed. On the other hand, if the ratio of large fiber to small fiber input is reduced by the loss of large axon receptors from a noxiously stimulated area, the pain is amplified.

With this brief review of the innervation of the head and neck and of some basic concepts of the pathophysiology of pain, the subsequent sections focus on neuropathy in the head and neck.

## Trigeminal Neuralgia

An estimated 15,000 patients in the United States develop trigeminal neuralgia every year.[6] It usually affects patients 40 years of age or older, and women more than men (2:1). The pain is an excruciating, electric-like sensation that is usually located in the middle face, shooting up into the cheek or eye. The pain is triggered by a light touch or puff of cold air on the nose and mouth region. The explosions of pain are brief or instantaneous in the beginning and may go into complete remission after a few days. The first remission may last for months or 1 year. The second exacerbation is more intolerable than the first,

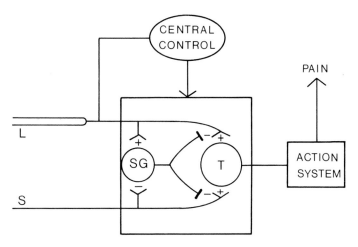

*Fig. 14–7.* The Gate control theory showing: SG–substantia gelatinosa cell, T–transmission cell, L–large fiber axon from the periphery, S–small fiber axon from the periphery, + –excitatory post-synaptic potential at the synapse, – at the SG cell indicates inhibitory postsynaptic potential and – at the primary nerve terminals indicates presynaptic inhibition.

because the pain explosions are not instantaneous but have a brief duration. The patient will usually identify a definite trigger location. The pain may last for months and then go into remission again. As time passes, the periods of remission get shorter and the pain increases in intensity and duration. Patients have committed suicide when they did not believe the pain could be controlled or eliminated. The authors have seen many trigeminal neuralgia patients with all maxillary and mandibular posterior teeth removed in a vain hope to eliminate the excruciating pain; usually, the removal has been from only one side. These patients had coerced dentists to extract tooth after tooth, thinking that the pain was a toothache. Investigators have shown that trigeminal neuralgia patients have demyelinated microneuromas in the rootlets of their trigeminal nerves on the affected side.[7] Figure 14–8 is a cross-section of a normal myelinated nerve. Figure 14–9 illustrates a plexiform microneuroma in the trigeminal rootlets of a patient with trigeminal neuralgia. Demyelinated microneuromas are common in the trigeminal rootlets as an incidental finding in all adults after exfoliation of the primary dentition. It is believed that the patient with trigeminal neuralgia has more extensive neuropathy than the patient without pain.

In many patients, the superior cerebellar artery, an aberrant vein, or a strand of connective tissue presses into the rootlets of the trigeminal nerve at the entrance zone into the pons. When the superior cerebellar artery compresses the rootlets, it loops downward from its origin at the basilar artery and curves back up to pass over the rootlets. Decompression of the rootlets by moving the loop of artery lateral to the rootlets and placing an alloplastic pad or muscle tissue between the rootlets and artery usually stops the pain.[8] The decompression procedure, percutaneous radiofrequency lesions of the affected nerves, rhizotomy of the mandibular division rootlets, and other neurosurgical procedures are used to treat this neuralgia when it does not respond to phenytoin (Dilantin), carbamazepine (Tegretol), baclofen (Lioresal), and/or other medications.

In the early stages of trigeminal neuralgia,

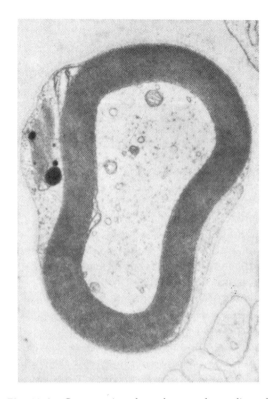

*Fig. 14–8.* Cross section through normal, myelinated nerve fiber. The myelin sheath's parallel dense lines surround the lightly speckled axon. To the upper left and lower right are seen portions of the Schwann's cell cytoplasm applied to the outer layer of myelin. (From H. deF. Webster, Progress in Brain Research, Elsevier Publishing Co., Amsterdam 1964. Courtesy of author and the publisher.)

local anesthetization of the branches of the trigeminal nerve involved often puts the disease into remission for months or years. In some elderly patients, local anesthetization of the involved nerve every 8 to 12 months controls the pain well enough to avoid surgical intervention. When the trigger is in the mandibular division, a maneuver of opening the mouth maximally and deflecting the mandible laterally toward the painful side often controls the attacks of pain.[9] The mandible is held laterally to stretch the neurovascular bundle from foramen ovale to the mandibular foramen maximally for 1 minute, three or four times per day. The authors have seen the pain

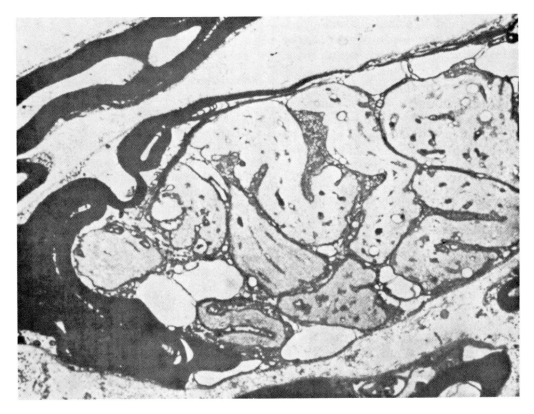

*Fig. 14–9.* Tortuous hypertrophic axis cylinder giving the appearance of a plexiform microneuroma. Degenerating Schwann cell cytoplasm seen between folds of axis cylinder. Note extreme thinness of myelin sheath on lower aspect of neuroma and absence of myelin above. ×9000. (From D.L. Beaver, J Neurosurg, 1967. Courtesy of the editor.)

controlled for 2½ years with use of this maneuver.

If the patient is wearing an ill-fitting denture with collapsed occlusal vertical dimension, opening the occlusal vertical dimension with a new denture often puts the neuralgia into remission for months or years.[10] When these dental procedures and then medication with phenytoin (up to 100 mg three times daily) do not control the attacks of pain, carbamazepine is usually prescribed by a physician who treats trigeminal neuralgia. If these medications are not effective, neurosurgical measures are indicated. A neuralgia-like condition has been related to bone cavities in the mandible and maxilla. This condition and its treatment are discussed in Chapter 18.

Intracranial tumors may be related to the onset of trigeminal neuralgia.[11] In one 10-year study, 16 of 2000 patients with facial pain had symptoms of trigeminal neuralgia or atypical facial pain associated with an intracranial tumor. Peripheral tumors were associated with atypical facial pain and sensory loss, middle fossa tumors were associated with atypical facial pain or trigeminal neuralgia, and posterior fossa tumors were associated with trigeminal neuralgia and subtle neurologic deficits. Initial relief of pain with carbamazepine does not rule out the diagnosis of tumor.

## Multiple Sclerosis Trigeminal Neuralgia

When a young patient 20 to 40 years of age demonstrates the symptoms of trigeminal neuralgia as just described, a diagnosis of multiple sclerosis (MS) warrants consideration.[12] When the demyelinating effects of this disease involve the trigeminal rootlets, they develop sclerotic plaques that are similar to the demyelinated microneurons seen in the 60-year-old patient with trigeminal neuralgia. Most cases of MS remit and relapse; only 20% of cases are progressive from onset. The history includes weakness of the limbs and other signs and symptoms of MS, and the pain is bilateral more often than occurs in patients with idiopathic trigeminal neuralgia. The T2 weighted (second echo) magnetic resonance image across the cortex of the brain has a cotton patch blotchiness that is now considered pathognomonic of demyelinating disease. The authors have examined a 63-year-old woman who had just developed MS trigeminal neuralgia, but her disease had been diagnosed at age 28 years. Her motor nerves were so affected she had to use a walker.

## Glossopharyngeal Neuralgia

The patient with glossopharyngeal neuralgia experiences an electric-like pain in the ear or throat region. The trigger is usually located in the throat and the pain is typically triggered by eating or drinking cold beverages. These patients often do not eat in public, because they throw the head to the side opposite the trigger when they swallow to try to avoid setting off the pain. They often jam their finger into the auditory meatus or against the tragus of the ear when the pain occurs. This procedure activates touch and pressure (large fiber) nerves and tends to reduce pain. The patient usually points to the lesser cornu of the hyoid bone and reports that the pain starts at this point and shoots up into the throat or ear, or the patient may say the pain starts in the ear and shoots down into the throat. The anterior, inferior cerebellar artery compresses the rootlets of the ninth and tenth cranial nerves in these patients. The neurosurgeon often ligates this artery and removes the section compressing the rootlets. The authors have also seen carcinoma of the larynx associated with glossopharyngeal neuralgia. The condition was also reported in a patient with muco-epidermoid carcinoma of the lateral tongue at the junction of the middle and posterior thirds.[13] A 1.5-cm mass was removed and the pain disappeared.

Some patients experience trigeminal and glossopharyngeal neuralgia simultaneously. One cannot expect to find only one type of pain in a patient at one time. Several diseases or conditions can cause pain in the head and neck simultaneously.

## Trigeminal Herpes Zoster

When the herpes zoster virus affects the trigeminal nerve, it affects the first division (ophthalmic) 95% of the time. The viral infection is usually self-limiting, but a small percentage of patients develop postherpetic neuralgia. It usually is unilateral and follows the distribution of the trigeminal division involved. The history of the vesicles on the forehead with initial pain and the persisting raised, reddened ulcers that develop an excruciating burning pain provide a diagnosis (see Fig. 14–10). The surface of the cornea may be involved, placing the patient's sight in jeopardy. When the cornea is involved, the patient should be referred promptly to an ophthalmologist.

Elderly patients are more prone to develop postherpetic neuralgia, and it may last as long as 1 year or more. Fifty percent of patients 50 years of age and older with acute herpes zoster develop postherpetic pain.[14] In cases of repetitive herpes zoster infections, biopsy reveals that with each infection, the axons in the nerve affected by the virus become smaller in diameter. Either the herpes zoster virus destroys large-diameter neurons more than small axons or the large neurons regenerate at a smaller diameter. The initial viral lesion not only involves the trigeminal ganglion, but also can extend to the thalamus.

When the virus affects the maxillary or mandibular divisions of the trigeminal nerve,

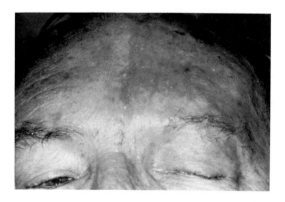

*Fig. 14–10.* Postherpetic neuralgia of the left ophthalmic division of the trigeminal nerve of 6 months duration. Note the erythematous and ulcerated skin from the midline of the forehead across the left forehead and including the upper left eyelid. (Courtesy of Dr. Marco Rand, Jacksonville VA Dental Clinic.)

it may be associated with odontalgia.[15] Some authors postulate that because the dental pulp contains terminal sensory nerves and herpes zoster may produce extensive fibrosis and scarring at nerve terminals, the teeth may be affected by the infection.[16] Cases of unilateral, internal resorption of teeth after herpes zoster infection of the nerve that innervates them have been described. Calcified pulp chambers and abnormal, shortened roots in lower posterior teeth were noted in a 15-year-old girl who contracted herpes zoster of the mandibular nerve at age 7 years.[17] She also had scarring of the chin and lip on the affected side.

Postherpetic neuralgia may respond to application of capsaicin, 0.025% topical cream (Zostrix) to the skin or oral mucosa.[18] Capsaicin depletes the small fibers of substance P, an endogenous neurotransmitter and important mediator of nociception in the peripheral nervous system. Pretreatment of the affected skin or mucosa with a topical anesthetic may help to prevent the pain that usually occurs with early applications of capsaicin. After repeated applications, the pain usually subsides. The application of aspirin dissolved in ether to affected skin may also reduce postherpetic neuralgia of the forehead.[19] This condition usually diminishes, even though it may take 1 year or more.

## Trotter's Syndrome

An extracranial tumor that develops in the infratemporal fossa, lateral to the palatine tonsil, produces a symptom complex called Trotter's syndrome.[20] This tumor is typically a carcinoma, and it grows into the lateral pterygoid muscle, anterior fibrous wall of the eustachian tube, and against the palatine tonsil. The syndrome includes numbness and pain in the distribution of the trigeminal mandibular division, excruciating headache, loss of hearing on the affected side, stuffiness in the ear, edema of the soft palate, bulging of the palatine tonsil, and deflection of the soft palate to the opposite side. The prognosis is poor, because the tumor is inoperable and is typically treated with antimetabolite and radiation therapy. The authors examined a patient who sought help because an unsightly round mound developed above and lateral to the left orbit. The mound was soft like a lipoma, and was actually a herniation of the buccal fat pad at the anterior margin of the temporalis muscle. Pressure from the growing tumor had forced the fat out into the subcutaneous tissue. The patient had difficulty occluding the left posterior teeth, and biting down became painful soon after the initial examination.

## Eosinophilic Granuloma of the Sphenoid Bone

Patients with eosinophilic granuloma of the greater wing of the sphenoid develop pain and paresthesia in the mandible and cheek on the affected side. One in 30,000 dental patients has eosinophilic granuloma affecting facial bones. A submentovertex radiograph often shows an irregular, eroded foramen ovale on the affected side. Biopsy of the lesion establishes the diagnosis. The condition responds to local surgical curettage and irradiation. In a 15-year-old girl, the symptoms of eosinophilic granuloma were obscured by and treatment was delayed because of an abscessed lower second molar.

## Metastatic Carcinoma

In a study of 2000 patients with cancer, including 300 with breast cancer, 15 individuals developed numbness of the chin.[21] Of these 15 patients, 13 had breast cancer and the other two had lymphoma. All but one had metastatic disease at the time the numbness developed. Pain associated with the numbness was minimal, and it was located in the skin adjacent to the tip of the jaw. Necropsy findings revealed dural involvement of the trigeminal nerve at the base of the brain in some of the patients. Survival of the patients ranged from 2 weeks to more than 4 years. The reason for the peculiar predilection of breast cancer for the mandibular branch of the trigeminal nerve is not known.

## Cerebellopontine Angle Tumor

Acoustic neuromas and gliomas growing in the cerebellopontine angle can exert pressure on the mandibular division of the trigeminal nerve as it passes into foramen ovale. These patients develop numbness, tingling, paresthesia, and pain in the distribution of the mandibular nerve. If the tumor is growing rapidly, they report excruciating headache. When local factors that cause such pain and paresthesia are not found, the patient should be referred for imaging of the cranial cavities without delay. These tumors are often benign and are operable, if they are not too large.

## Ramsay Hunt Syndrome

Ramsay Hunt syndrome is a herpes zoster infection of the sensory and motor branches of the facial nerve (cranial nerve VII) and sometimes the vestibular branches of the auditory nerve (cranial nerve VIII). It results in deafness, vertigo, and severe facial paralysis, with herpetic lesions in the external auditory meatus, external ear, mastoid area, anterior tongue, soft palate, and the fauces. Loss of the stapedial reflex also results. Treatment of the acute infection of herpes zoster is limited to the use of analgesics for pain. Supportive nutritional programs are useful.

## Raeder's Syndrome

Raeder's syndrome is a severe unilateral frontal headache followed by ipsilateral Horner's syndrome (ptosis and miosis) that usually affects men in the fifth decade. It is transitory and is caused by a disorder of the pericarotid sympathetic plexus in the cavernous sinus.

## Acute Angle Closure Glaucoma

Patients with acute glaucoma often have pain in the eye so severe that they vomit as though they have intestinal obstruction or cholecystitis. They have a red eye with a fixed, semidilated, vertically oval pupil, as well as corneal edema, manifested by an irregular reflection of light on a cloudy cornea. The authors have found that pain emanating from the temporomandibular joint is often referred to the eye. This pain may be sharp, like an "icepick," but the eye shows no changes such as are noted in association with acute glaucoma. Patients with chronic glaucoma usually experience little or no pain. Their first sign of disease may be loss of vision from degeneration of the retina.

## Tolosa-Hunt Syndrome

This chronic inflammatory process usually involves the cavernous sinus, carotid artery, and the orbit, and it produces a painful paralysis of the ocular muscles (ophthalmoplegia). Its etiology is unknown, but it responds to steroid therapy. The erythrocyte sedimentation rate (ESR) is elevated and Horner's syndrome may be present. Computed tomographic scanning of the orbit is helpful in diagnosing this condition.

## Bell's Palsy

The incidence of Bell's palsy in the general population is approximately 21 adults and 2 children per 100,000 persons per year (Fig. 14–11).[22,23] In children, 90% of patients spontaneously regain normal function, whereas only 71% of the population at large spontaneously normalize.[24]

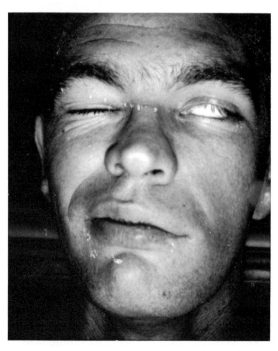

*Fig. 14–11.* Patient with Bell's palsy affecting the left facial nerve. Note the sagging appearance of the left corner of the mouth and inability to close the left eyelid.

Three simple tests are helpful in diagnosing Bell's palsy. First, the patient tightens the lips and blows against the cheeks. When the patient attempts this maneuver, air leaks out of the corner of the mouth on the affected side. Next, the clinician places the index and third finger on the patient's cheeks in the infraorbital regions, pushing gently downward on the skin. The patient is then instructed to close the eyes forcefully. The eye on the affected side remains open and the opposite side closes completely. Lastly, the clinician asks the patient to "look upward in wonder and amazement, raising the eyebrows." The forehead stays smooth on the affected side and wrinkles on the healthy side.

With decompression of the facial nerve in the internal auditory canal, veins and venules are dilated and engorged, the facial nerve is swollen, and, sometimes, hemorrhage is noted in the internal auditory canal, extending distally to the geniculate ganglion.[25] The narrowest point in the facial canal is at the meatal foramen; the diameter averages only 0.68 mm. With dilation and engorgement of tissues, the most likely site of compression is at this point in the canal. Compression dams up the axonal flow in the motor neurons, resulting in paresis of the muscles of facial expression. Histopathologic findings from biopsies of the greater superficial petrosal nerve in Bell's palsy patients reveal degeneration and demyelination of the large fibers and lymphocytic cellular infiltration in the nerve. This wallerian degeneration is indicative of a compressional injury at a site proximal to the geniculate ganglion, i.e., the meatal foramen.

Granulation tissue around the geniculate ganglion could indicate viral geniculate ganglionitis as the etiology of Bell's palsy. Decreased tearing and/or salivary flow within 3 days of onset of complete paralysis predicts incomplete recovery of the palsy if the nerve is not decompressed. One third of a group of patients with a compression block proximal to the geniculate ganglion had normal tear flow, indicated by using Schirmer's test. This finding can be explained in that the preganglionic parasympathetic, unmyelinated fibers are affected by compression and ischemia in the canal to a lesser extent than the large motor nerves to facial muscles. If paralysis is complete, some clinicians elect to decompress the facial nerve as soon as possible. If the degeneration exceeds 90% (measured by electroneurography) and the difference on minimal nerve excitability testing is 3.5 mA, decompression is indicated.

Bell's palsy patients often have numbness on the paretic side of the face, which makes one suspect that the trigeminal nerve is affected. The idea that Bell's palsy is a mononeuropathy affecting only the facial nerve has been questioned.[26,27] In a study of 30 patients with acute facial palsy, in which investigators used a trigeminous-evoked potential test, blink reflex test, and auditory brain stem response, 18 of the patients (60%) suffered polyneuropathy.[28] As many as 18 patients (60%) had evidence of pathologic involvement of the trigeminal nerve, and 8 (28%) had evidence of brain stem involvement.

## Painful Neuromas

The normal response to damage to a peripheral nerve is the formation of a neuroma. In some patients, these neuromas become painful. Sprouts that grow from the distal end of the nerve may course back along the nerve for long distances and become the site of spontaneous discharges.[29] "Cross-talk" between demyelinated or abnormally myelinated nerves may be the seat of spontaneous ectopic discharges. Fiber sprouts in neuromas are usually highly sensitive to circulating noradrenaline.[30] These findings demonstrate that even minor damage to peripheral nerves produces profound peripheral and central effects.

The neuroma impulse generators have unusual properties in that they become silent after high frequency activity. Transcutaneous electrical nerve stimulation (TENS) has proven effective in the routine management of most painful neuromas. When TENS provides significant relief, a stimulator can be provided for home use by the patient. A high rate of stimulation (range of 60 to 1000 Hz) is usually most effective.[31] The mechanism by which TENS alters pain perception is not understood, so under the guidance of the therapist, the patient adjusts the frequency, amplitude, and duration of the TENS waveform to achieve the maximum effect.

In a series of 60 patients, 78 painful neuromas were excised and the proximal end of the nerve was implanted in the deep side of a large muscle, leaving a loose loop of nerve to prevent any tension on the nerve.[32] The results were good to excellent in 82% of the treated neuromas. In animal studies, with use of a similar procedure, findings showed no invasion of the muscle by the small neuroma that developed at the distal end of the transected nerve, and a random pattern of small nerve fascicles embedded in dense scar tissue usually seen in the painful neuroma did not develop.

Ultrasound applied to neuromas relieves the pain in less than one half of these patients, but local injection of steroids has no effect on the spontaneous pain. Alcohol blocks do not relieve the pain and may reduce the effectiveness of local anesthesia because of fibrosis.[33]

Painful neuromas in the oral cavity typically arise after a surgical procedure, usually a dental extraction, and produce atypical facial pain or paresthesia, with a stinging or burning sensation. They are usually palpable and measure as much as 8 mm in diameter. Palpation provokes pain, which may be relieved by local anesthesia. In one report of six cases, excisional biopsy revealed traumatic neuroma. All six patients showed immediate clinical improvement.[34] One to three years later, four of the six patients remained essentially painfree. If ultrasound is not effective, excision of oral neuromas is indicated, both to provide possible pain relief and to identify the tumor histopathologically.

## Auriculotemporal Syndrome

Preauricular surgical incisions often section branches of the auriculotemporal nerve that enter the parotid gland and provide parasympathetic, secretomotor innervation to the gland. Sympathetic neurons following branches of the superficial temporal artery that supply sweat glands in the temple area are also sectioned. A unique feature of the sympathetic nervous system is that the postganglionic endings on the sweat glands are cholinergic rather than adrenergic. Therefore, when the sectioned auriculotemporal nerves sprout after being sectioned and cross over into the tract of wallerian degeneration in the sympathetic nerves, they innervate the sweat glands, release acetylcholine, and stimulate sweat secretion rather than saliva secretion. This crossover is one of the explanations for gustatory sweating, Frey's syndrome, or auriculotemporal syndrome.

The patients sweat in the temple or preauricular area of the face when they eat. It is usually more profuse when they eat spicy foods and it varies from a minor annoyance to an embarrassing flow that requires constant mopping with a towel as the meal progresses. Gustatory sweating may be noted after temporomandibular joint surgery or injection, condylar neck fractures, auriculotemporal nerve blocks, and parotid gland surgery.[35] The authors observed gustatory sweating in a 56-year-old man who had cystic adenocarcinoma of the parotid gland that destroyed the temporomandibular joint and extended into the middle ear. This patient had no history of preauricular surgical intervention or trauma. The growth of this tumor produced enough neuropathy to effect a crossover or "cross talk" between the secretomotor fibers in the preauricular region.

Most cases of gustatory sweating are not serious enough to require treatment. When required, topical application of 3% scopolamine in aqueous cream is an effective form of treatment. Sectioning of the auriculotemporal nerve is also effective, when the condition is serious and is not responsive to local measures.[36]

## Referred Pain

Convergence of peripheral neurons is used to explain the referral of pain from a site of noxious stimulation to some distant site. Pain is often referred from a visceral or deep structure to a more superficial structure, such as an area of skin (Fig. 14–12). Extensive convergence of nerves that innervate the head make the referral of pain in this region complex and difficult to diagnose.

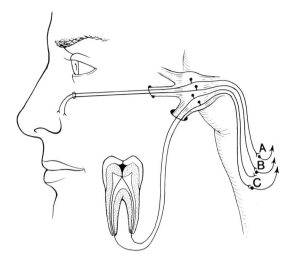

**Fig. 14–12.** The convergence theory of referred pain. Two cutaneous nerves from the skin of the ala of the nose project onto secondary neurons in the cervical cord A and B. Two nerves from a lower molar pulp project onto secondary neurons B and C. The cutaneous nerves have been active throughout life. The pulpal nerves have been inactive until the dental decay produces a microabscess in the coronal pulp. Since one of these nerves projects onto neuron B and, in the past, neuron B was activated by the cutaneous nerve from the ala of the nose, the pain is referred to the nose.

## Clinical Examples

The pain associated with otitis media in a pediatric patient is often referred to a mandibular molar. In one report, 8 children with otitis media had referred pain to lower primary or permanent molars.[37] The children usually had a history of recurrent upper respiratory infection. No dental cause of pain was found, the tympanic membranes were inflamed and/or bulging on the painful side, and patients had elevated temperatures. No complaint of pain in the ear was noted, except during examination with an otoscope. Otitis media was confirmed in every case and the "toothaches" were relieved within 24 to 36 hours with antibiotic and decongestant therapy.

In the older patient, the clinician must consider pain referred to the face from cardiac anoxia. These pains are sometimes difficult to diagnose, but they are typically clearly associated with physical exertion, exercise in cold weather, and the immediate postprandial state. Sometimes physical effort after food ingestion is required to initiate the pain. Many patients with cardiovascular disease carry nitroglycerine tablets or some other coronary vasodilator, but they do not like to take it because of the brief headache it causes. If the coronary vasodilator, placed under the tongue, immediately relieves the facial pain, it is probably referred from the heart, and appropriate measures should be initiated.

The authors examined a 63-year-old man who had loud crepitus and reciprocal clicking in both temporomandibular joints as well as generalized degenerative arthritis. His chief complaint was pain that began in the chin point and moved down the neck and into the chest. Jaw function produced loud crepitus and cracking sounds but no pain whatsoever. The history revealed the pain was initiated by walking in cold weather and was relieved by sitting down on a park bench. This patient did not suffer from arthralgia but had aberrant angina. His pain was controlled by wearing nitroglycerine patches and other medication for cardiovascular disease.

A recent report cited three well-documented cases of orofacial pain as the initial and major symptom of coronary insufficiency.[38] The patients were a 56-year-old woman, a 79-year-old man, and a 67-year-old man. The authors noted that facial pain of cardiac origin, although infrequent, does occur in young patients,[39] and should not be ruled out on the basis of age.

The pain was localized in the anterior maxillary and infraorbital area and radiated into the neck and shoulder regions in the female patient. Interestingly, her pain was not associated with exertion or food ingestion, but she had significant dyspnea while her history was obtained. In the third minute of a stress test, the facial pain developed, along with a 2-mm S-T segment depression in the electrocardiogram. Coronary angiography indicated an old inferior-wall myocardial infarction, complete obstruction of the circumflex artery and proximal one third of the right coronary artery, and partial obstruction of the left anterior descending artery. After a bypass operation, the patient became free of facial pain.

The 79-year-old man suffered pain in the jaws and short episodes of chest pain. He responded immediately to the sublingual administration of isosorbide dinitrate, but the

# Part VI

# Oral and Nasal Cavities and Salivary Glands

# *Odontalgia*

The teeth may be regarded as finely tuned sensory end organs ladened with position and pain receptors. Although the exact mechanisms are still not defined, we have a reasonable understanding of the clinical features of odontalgia.[1] Noxious stimuli to the dentin, cementum, pulp, or supporting structures may result in odontalgia, the noxious stimulus produced by primary diseases, abnormal metabolic states, and structural defects of either the enamel, dentin, cementum, pulp, periodontal ligament, or contiguous structures. Besides pain, teeth supported in their periodontal ligaments can signal such minute changes between occluding surfaces that even a baby's hair, too fine to feel between the fingers, can be detected by placing it between occluding teeth.

In terms of the quality of pain perceived, the odontogenic apparatus manifests a range, from annoying to mild to excruciating, crushing pain. Although the perception of pain depends on central nervous system functions, with modifications according to the personality and experiences of the patient, odontogenic pain usually cuts through the neural and psychologic processes and gives accurate sensory discriminative localization. Exceptions to such accurate clinical localization are noted in the following situations: when the somatosensory cortex begins to generate central pain;[2] when otherwise healthy teeth are afflicted with a metabolic alteration, as in the case of neurovascular odontalgia; when pain radiates from an affected tooth and the pain is sensed in adjacent teeth, which are diseased; and when pain is referred.

## Dentinal Pain

Pain may originate in dentin as a function of dentinal tubular fluid changes, which produce an osmotic shifting of fluid and stimulation of the nerve endings in the pulpal tissues.[3] When cementum is exposed in the cervical areas of teeth, it may be removed by toothbrush abrasion, and exposed open dentinal tubules respond to oral fluid osmotic pressures and chemicals, such as sugar and bacterial acids. Pains originating from dentin usually have evoking stimuli, such as thermal changes, chemical changes, pressure changes

when a loose restoration compresses the supporting dentin, and osmotic changes in the presence of sweets. A practical rule is that if sugar in the mouth produces a toothache, dentin is exposed. Dentinal pain is usually of short duration, associated with the noxious stimulus.

Thermal changes produce dentinal pain, manifested in teeth supporting metallic restorations, in dentin that has a loss of the coronal protection because of cracks or fractures in the enamel, in defects in margins of restorations, in dental caries, and in cervical areas exposed by periodontal disease. When testing for cold and hot thermal effects, a pellet of ice or a cone of solid nitrous oxide and a heated stick of impression compound, respectively, may be used.

## Pulpal Pain

Pulpitis is usually a secondary involvement of the pulp as a progression of the factors that produced the pain-evoking stimuli in the dentin. Pulpal pain is characteristically of long duration and excruciating intensity. Because of radiating pain and the intensity, localizing the pain to a given tooth may be difficult for the patient. The use of electrovitalometers, thermal tests, and periodontal ligament diagnostic anesthetic infiltrations may supplement the clinical and radiologic examinations.

Pulpal pain related to denticles is rare. In one case (Fig. 15–1), the patient had intermittent and recurring bouts of mild and severe pain in the side of the face. Previous treatment included removal of the third molars, injection of steroids in the temporomandibular joints and occlusal therapy, without success. In the letter of referral, the clinician wrote, " . . . a week ago, she developed a terrific pain on the lower right of the mandible." The musculoskeletal system of the head and neck was within reasonable ranges of normal, as were the regional respiratory, neurologic, and vascular systems. Diagnostic inferior alveolar nerve blocks relieved the pain. When sensation returned after the nerve blocks, periodontal ligament injections of the first and second molars gave prompt relief; these injections were repeated on two additional occasions, 10 days apart, with ces-

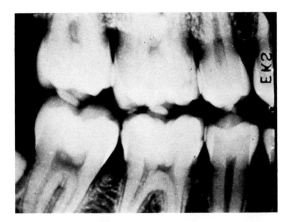

**Fig. 15–1.** Denticles in the pulp chambers of the mandibular first and second molars. These teeth had manifestations of pain varying from mild to severe on an irregular basis, with no apparent consistent exciting cause. The teeth received root canal therapy, and the pain was eradicated.

sation of symptoms for the duration of the local anesthesia. Endodontic treatment of these teeth demonstrated the pulpal horns were necrotic and the pulp chambers were essentially obliterated by the denticles. After endodontic treatment involving the first and second molars, the patient was free of pain. Fourteen years later, the patient remained painfree.

Maxillary sinal inflammatory processes may affect and cause pain in the maxillary dentition. We have seen incidences of "occlusal adjustments," and even removal of teeth, that were merely secondarily involved by an inflammatory process of the maxillary sinus (Fig. 15–2). Inflammation in the maxillary sinus may be asymptomatic in terms of the sinus per se. Diagnosis may not be possible until the study of radiographs or computed tomographic scans of the midface is completed. Barometric pressure changes within the sinuses, such as experienced by aviators, may directly affect the maxillary dentition, producing a sharp and overwhelming pain, particularly if defective restorations are present (Fig. 15–3). Likewise, barometric changes within the sinuses, in the event they are not patent to the nasal passages, may manifest as incapacitating pain elsewhere in the trigeminal nerve distribution because of the referral of pain.

Donlon presented a report of a patient with a presumptive diagnosis of trigeminal neuralgia. The patient had undergone extensive consultations and nonsurgical treatments, and the symptoms terminated after treatment of an irreversible pulpitis.[4]

## Nonodontogenic Odontalgia

Chronic or acute odontalgia may occur in otherwise normal teeth in response to regional and systemic maladies. Examples are noted in neurovascular odontalgia, herpes zoster affecting the trigeminal nerve, and mucormycosis of the upper respiratory tree.

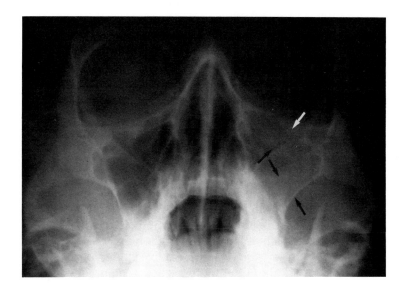

**Fig. 15–2.** Unilateral inflammatory process of the maxillary sinus that produced pain in the contiguous maxillary teeth. The inflamed and thickened sinal membrane is indicated by arrows. (Courtesy of Dr. Edwyn L. Boyd.)

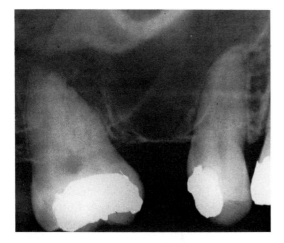

*Fig. 15–3.* Maxillary dentition with the apices in close proximity to the maxillary antrum. The patient, a passenger in a nonpressurized aircraft, reported excruciating dental and cranial pain, to the point that " . . . even the roots of the hair on my head hurt . . . " when the airplane rapidly lost altitude in a controlled spiral descent.

## Neurovascular Odontalgia (Atypical Odontalgia)

Severe pulpal pain that is continuous and is often of several months to years duration may arise from what we postulate is neurovascular instability of otherwise healthy dental pulps (Fig. 15–4). The patient describes exploding feelings, crawling sensations, a sense of pressure, or similar unusual interpretations of sensations in or around the tooth or teeth. In long-term cases, the history usually includes a spreading of the sensations from the initiating tooth or area to more and more teeth.

These symptoms are associated with a condition termed atypical odontalgia. The usual patient is a woman with a history of migraine headaches, one of the migrainous maladies, muscle contraction headaches, depression, and/or anxieties, and with manifestations of a pain-prone personality.

We have examined many patients with several years of extensive involvement of the dentition to the point that every tooth in both arches was painful. Previous forms of treatment included multiple restorations, endodontic procedures, otolaryngologic operations, coronoidectomies, removal of teeth, open and arthroscopic surgical intervention in the temporomandibular joint, and avulsion

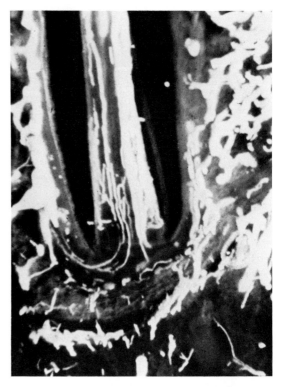

*Fig. 15–4.* Microcirculation study demonstrating the vascularity of the dental pulp and contiguous medullary spaces.

of peripheral nerves. Their history usually included multiple referrals to practitioners as well as the use of narcotic analgesics, antibiotics, and carbamazepine.

In 1974, Harris described the condition as an idiopathic periodontalgia, and suggested that its association with migraine indicated that vascular instability was a factor.[5] In 1979, Rees and Harris renamed the condition atypical odontalgia, because of an apparent relation to facial neuralgia.[6] Manifestations of depression were noted in 75% of the 44 patients in the Rees and Harris study (36 female and 8 male patients). In agreement with Rees and Harris, Brooke wrote, " . . . this condition is a form of atypical facial neuralgia and should be treated as such. It cannot be stressed too strongly that much mental anguish and unnecessary treatment can be prevented by recognition of this condition and the avoidance of dental treatment based on no findings other than the presence of pain."[7]

## Treatment

In our experience, the most reliable treatment of neurovascular painful disorders of the dental pulps is psychologic support and the prescription of tricyclic antidepressant medications (i.e., 10 mg amitriptyline bid, morning and bedtime, and gradually increasing every 2 weeks to qid, before meals and bedtime). The dosage of tricyclic antidepressant medications must be tailored to the individual patient; the effective dosage of amitriptyline, for example, may range from 10 mg bid to 20 mg qid.

Kreisberg summarized the literature on the actions of the tricyclic antidepressants: ". . . to account for the analgesic effects of the tricyclic antidepressants . . . it appears that pain relief is obtained . . . independent of antidepressant effects and is related to central enhancement of the biogenic amine serotonin."[8]

Chlorpromazine and the mood-elevating monamine oxidase inhibitors are effective when the pain does not respond to the antidepressants. The use of migraine-specific medications has been intermittently successful.

Antidepressant medication may be supplemented with minimal, but regular, doses of either ibuprofen (i.e., 200 mg qid) or indomethacin (25 to 50 mg per day) for 2 weeks. After 2 or 3 weeks, the ibuprofen or indomethacin course may be repeated.

The chemistry of diverse psychologic pathologies is altered with antidepressant medications. An effective antidepressant medication is fluoxetine. We have found effective responses with doses beginning with a 20 mg capsule in the morning and increasing, as necessary, to 20 mg morning and evening. Control of symptoms may require 2 to 3 weeks.

## Case Report

One of the most bizarre cases of neurovascular odontalgia in our experience involved an aviatrix, a crop-duster pilot, who had been subjected, on several different occasions over 5 years, to the removal of every tooth from both the maxillary and mandibular arches on the right side in a vain attempt to control pain. The pain was treated successfully with psy-chologic counseling supplemented, during the early phases of therapy, with prescriptions of tricyclic antidepressants.

## Herpes Zoster

Herpes zoster affecting the trigeminal nerve may result in severe, incapacitating odontalgia. Symptomatic relief of otherwise healthy dental pulps may be necessary with either endodontic or exodontic procedures, and, of course, in most situations, endodontic treatment is preferred. Good and Jacobsen have summarized the pathogenesis of herpes zoster as it may pertain to odontalgia.[9]

## Mucormycosis

Mucormycosis is a rapidly progressing fungal disease. Webb and associates described a patient who was not under control for her insulin-dependent diabetes on presenting with pain localized to a maxillary molar. Exodontic treatment, with accompanying antibiotics and analgesic, was performed. The mucormycosis was identified in a matter of hours, and orbital exenteration and maxillectomy were necessary.[10] We know of a similar case in which a central incisor was removed from a diabetic patient with ketoacidosis; several weeks later, there was a destructive rhinocerebral infection by mucormycosis. The plaintiff's lawyer won a pretrial settlement in a subsequent planned court contest in spite of the lack of medical relationship between the exodontic procedure and the mucormycosis.

## Periapical Inflammation

Periapical inflammation secondary to the dying and the death of dental pulp produces the classic signs of acute dental inflammation, including slight extrusion of the tooth from the alveolus owing to the periapical collection of products of inflammation. The usual periapical inflammation is regarded as an extension of the factors that lead to the pulpal death. Localization of the affected tooth is usually not a problem for the patient or the dentist, because light percussion elicits both extreme pain from the affected tooth as well as a dull sound. After the products of acute inflammation have invaded surrounding tissues, regional lymphadenopathy and systemic manifestations may occur (Fig. 15–5).

## Periodontal Inflammation

Periodontal inflammation secondary to periodontal disease is usually not characterized by the overwhelming type of pain that accompanies pulp and periapical acute inflammations. The mobility of the teeth usually permits the draining of acute inflammatory exudates and gives relief from the pain associated with the inflamed periodontal areas (Fig. 15–6). Nevertheless, dangerous dissecting extensions of periodontal inflammation may involve the adjacent facial spaces, demonstrating that pain is only one indicator, and not necessarily the most important, of the seriousness of infection.

## Fractured Teeth

The pulpal response to fracturing is similar to that described for pulp-originating pain; however, the tooth structure may open and close around the pulp, causing intermittent painful sensations with complete freedom from pain between episodes. The patient may become a unilateral masticator to avoid pain of biting on the fractured tooth. The pulpal response may be regional rather than specific to the tooth, and referral of pain may further obfuscate the area of noxious stimulus, the fractured tooth. The tooth may respond normally, on an intermittent basis, to pulp testing with thermal and electronic devices.

The fracture may be demonstrated in one or a combination of methods. Radiologic surveys with two or three different directions of the central ray may demonstrate a fracture line. Light beams directed at various angles detect reflective rays from fracture lines in the translucent enamel. Exploration of grooves, pits, fissures, and restoration margins with a dental explorer instrument also may demonstrate a fracture line. Percussion of the cusps of a fractured tooth may produce a dull sound rather than the crisp, resonant sound. If the clinician suspects a tooth has a fracture but it was not demonstrable by inspection,

radiography, or percussion, one may place a drop or two of a dye, e.g., methylene blue, on the occlusal or incisal surface of the suspected tooth and have the patient bite with the suspected tooth alternately easily and firmly on an elastic object. Pumping of the dye into the fracture often results, thus demonstrating the defect (Fig. 15–7). A necessary step may involve removing a restoration and placing the dye on the floor of the cavity preparation to identify an occult fracture.

Diagnostic blocks, especially periodontal ligament infiltrations, identify a fractured tooth by the relief of pain. If the pain of a fractured tooth is referred, the distant site is freed of pain.

## Impacted Teeth

Definitive oral and maxillofacial care of impacted teeth includes either the removal, long-term observation, or the management of useless teeth that may produce periodontal defects, cysts, tumors, structural weaknesses of the surrounding bone, obstruction of adjacent teeth, destruction of adjacent teeth, unhygienic areas, and inflammatory processes of contiguous tissues. Pain from any of these factors varies from the type that is characteristic of a pulpal etiology to that associated with acute inflammation of periapical abscesses. Any tooth may be embedded; however, the teeth most likely to be involved are the third molars and the canines. Treatment may include removal, moving the impacted tooth to the proper location in the dentoalveolar processes by orthodontic or surgical methods, removal of adjacent tissues for hygienic purposes, and autogenous transplantation of a tooth to a location at which it may be useful (Fig. 15–8).

In rare instances, long-term observation of an impacted tooth may be indicated. For instances in which no clinical pathologic process is present or pending, no discernible follicular space is observed by radiographic examination, and the tooth has been quiescent for many years, observation during the coming years, both clinically and radiologically, is a reasonable plan. We emphasize, however, that the eruption potential of embedded teeth may persist throughout life. A

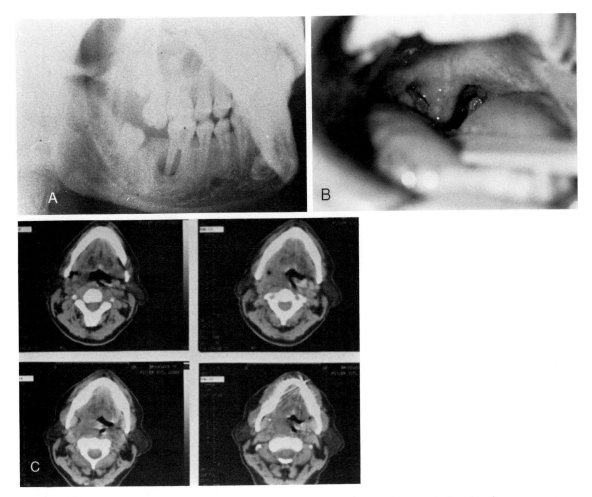

***Fig. 15–5.*** Periapical abscesses. A. Radiolucent lesion in the mandibular molar periapical region due to an acute inflammatory process originating from a carious lesion that invaded the pulpal tissues; B. The periapical inflammation dissected medially into the submandibular space and, by direct extension, into the lateral pharyngeal space; C. The airway and the patient's life were preserved by endotracheal intubation.

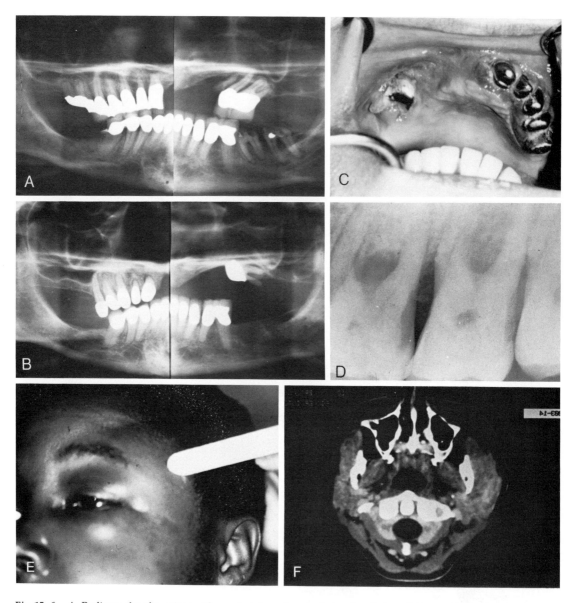

*Fig. 15–6.* A. Radiographs of a patient with an admixture of periapical and periodontal chronic inflammatory processes that were producing low grade, constant pain. She had received an overlay denture without appropriate therapy for the supporting dentition and was experiencing constant annoying pain. She refused recommendations for removal of the mobile teeth that were not reasonable candidates for root canal therapy; B. One year later, although some teeth had been removed when periapical abscesses became active, she continued to refuse definitive care of the remaining teeth that produced either no pain or were annoyingly painful, including the right maxillary molar. C. Attempts to institute proper oral hygiene were not successful. The overriding consideration in the retention of her bizarre oral condition was based on the amount of money she paid for the prosthesis, and, " . . . therefore, it must be all right!" D, E, and F. Periodontal abscesses, especially in the maxilla, usually drain and produce minimal pain and, rarely, extensions to contiguous tissues. In this patient, however, the extension of the microorganisms invaded the masticator space and manifested, quite painlessly but dangerously, in the temporal fossa.

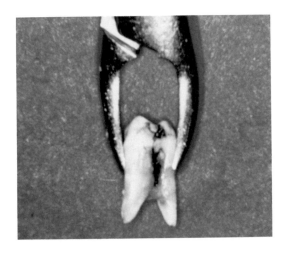

*Fig. 15–7.* A cracked tooth reassembled after removal. A bifurcation acute abscess was not visible on the preoperative radiographs. Identification of the tooth as the source of occasionally severe pains included the application to the occlusal surface of a dye that seeped into the fracture line on biting on a dental restoration rubber-polishing disk.

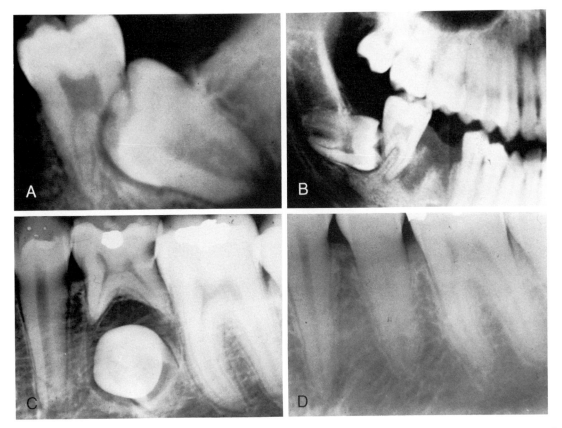

*Fig. 15–8.* A and B. Two cases of second molars becoming acutely painful because of erosion by the crown and follicle of the third molars; C and D. Preoperative and 5-year postoperative radiographic views of the transplantation of an impacted mandibular premolar after removal and enlargement of the alveolus of the retained deciduous molar. (Courtesy of Dr. Merle Hale, Indianapolis, Indiana.)

92-year-old patient in our practice demonstrated eruption potential; the left mandibular third molar, mesioangularly impacted against the second molar, attempted to erupt. Soft tissue changes associated with eruption of a tooth were noted in the retromolar trigone and acute pericoronitis developed. The treatment included removal of the third molar, and healing was normal.

## References

1. Krell K.V. and Walton R.E.: Odontalgia: Diagnosing pulpal, periapical, and periodontal pain. *In* Hardin J.F. (Ed.): Clark's Clinical Dentistry, Revised Edition. Philadelphia, J.B. Lippincott Co, 1989
2. Biedenbach M.A., Van Hassel H.J., and Brown A.C.: Tooth pulp-driven neurons in somatosensory cortex of primates: Role of pain mechanisms including a review of the literature. Pain, 7:369, 1979
3. Brannstrom M.: The hydrodynamic theory of dentinal pain: Sensations in preparations, caries, and the dentinal crack syndrome. J Endodont, 12:453, 1986
4. Donlon W.C.: Odontalgia mimicking trigeminal neuralgia. Anes Prog, 36:98, 1989
5. Harris M.: Psychogenic aspects of facial pain. Br Dent J, 136:199, 1974
6. Rees R.T. and Harris M.: Atypical odontalgia. Br J Oral Maxillofac Surg, 16:212, 1979
7. Brooke R.I.: Atypical odontalgia, a report of twenty-two cases. Oral Surg Oral Med Oral Pathol, 49:196, 1980
8. Kreisberg M.K.: Tricyclic antidepressants: Analgesic effect and indications in orofacial pain. J Craniomandib Dis Facial Oral Pain, 2:171, 1988
9. Good W.W.Y. and Jacobsen P.L.: Prodromal odontalgia and multiple devialized teeth caused by herpes zoster infection of the trigeminal nerve: Report of a case. J Am Dent Assoc, 116:500, 1988
10. Webb D.J.: Acute, life-threatening disease first appearing as odontogenic pain. J Am Dent Assoc, 109:936, 1984

# 16

# *Nasal Cavity and Paranasal Sinuses*

The nasal cavity and maxillary sinuses, because of their close proximity to the oral cavity, are frequently the origin of facial pain that mimics dental or oral pain. Pathologic processes in the other sinuses, the frontal, ethmoid, and sphenoid sinuses, may refer pain to other areas in the maxillofacial tissues. Comprehensive care of patients with facial pain requires a practical understanding and knowledge of the anatomy and function of the nasal cavity and paranasal sinuses.

## Anatomy of the Nasal Cavity

The nasal cavity extends from the anterior nasal aperture in the nose to the choana (posterior communication with the nasal pharynx) and from the base of the cranium superiorly to the roof of the mouth inferiorly. Its medial wall is the nasal septum, which consists of two bones, the vomer and perpendicular plate of the ethmoid bone, and three cartilages, the septal cartilage and the two medial crura of the alar cartilages (Fig. 16–1). The complex lateral wall consists of eight bones and the maxillary hiatus, which is a connective tissue membrane (Fig. 16–2). The major part of the lateral nasal cavity wall is the medial wall of the maxilla. The medial maxilla, however, has a large opening across which stretches a connective tissue membrane, the maxillary hiatus.[1] The hiatus is partially covered by four bones: anteriorly by the lacrimal bone, inferiorly by the base of the inferior turbinate, posteriorly by the perpendicular plate of the palatine bone, and superiorly by several processes of the ethmoid bone.

### Turbinates

Three scroll-shaped bony processes called turbinates or conchae project into the nasal cavity from the lateral wall. The inferior turbinate is a separate bone, whereas the middle and superior turbinates are processes of the ethmoid bone. The turbinates are covered with erectile tissue, the function of which is discussed in a subsequent section. The space below each turbinate is a meatus.

### Meati

The inferior meatus lies below the inferior turbinate and has one opening, the ostium of the nasolacrimal duct. This ostium is covered by a flap valve, the valve of Heissner. When nasal cavity pressure increases, as in blowing the nose, the flap valve closes to prevent the patient from blowing bubbles out the medial canthus of the eye.

The middle meatus contains most of the ostia that open into the nasal cavity (Fig. 16–3). The most prominent landmark in the middle meatus is the blister-shaped ethmoid

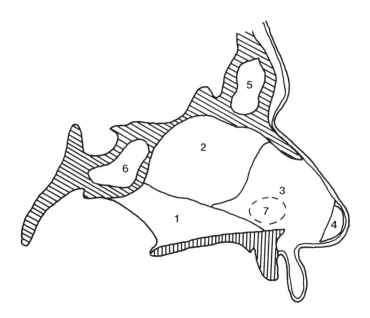

Fig. 16–1.  Medial wall of the nasal cavity showing: 1. Vomer; 2. Perpendicular plate of the ethmoid; 3. Septal cartilage; 4. Medial crura of the alar cartilage (only one shown); 5. Frontal sinus; 6. Sphenoidal sinus; and 7. Kiesselbach's area where 90% of nose bleeds occur.

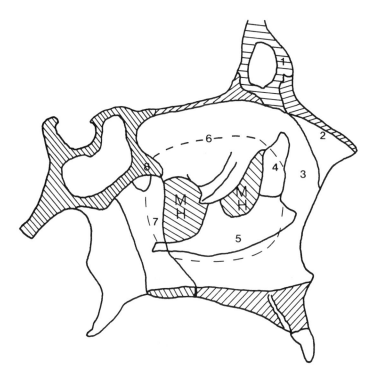

*Fig. 16–2.* Lateral wall of nasal cavity showing: 1. Frontal bone; 2. Nasal bone; 3. Maxilla; 4. Lacrimal bone; 5. Inferior turbinate (concha); 6. Ethmoid bone; 7. Palatine bone; and 8. Sphenoid bone, MH–maxillary hiatus. Note that four bones—palatine, ethmoid, inferior turbinate and lacrimal—partially cover the maxillary hiatus, whose outline is dashed across the four bones.

bulla. The anatomy of the middle meatus varies considerably, but one can be oriented by identifying the prominent bulla. The groove below the bulla is the hiatus semilunaris, into which opens the ostia of the frontal sinus, anterior ethmoidal air cells, and maxillary sinus. The anterior end of the hiatus semilunaris opens like a funnel, the infundibulum, beneath the base of the middle turbinate, into which the frontal sinus drains. The ostium of

the maxillary sinus, in its location in the middle meatus, is not positioned near the floor of the sinus. Because of its location high in the medial wall of the sinus, a patient must bend over and turn the head laterally to facilitate drainage of the maxillary sinus. Just below the hiatus semilunaris is the hook-shaped uncinate process of the ethmoid bone, and below this process, from anterior to posterior, is the lacrimal bone, the maxillary hi-

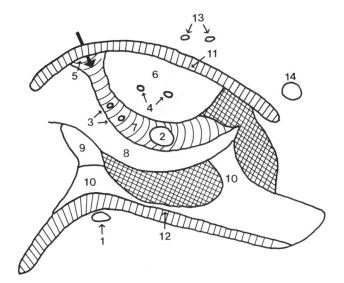

*Fig. 16–3.* Anatomy of the lateral nasal wall showing: 1. Ostium of nasolacrimal duct (in inferior meatus); 2. Ostium of the maxillary sinus; 3. Ostia of the anterior ethmoidal air cells (sinus); 4. Ostia of the middle ethmoidal air cells; 5. Infundibulum (arrow shows ostium of the frontal sinus); 6. Bulla of the ethmoid; 7. Hiatus semilunaris (a groove in the lacrimal bone); 8. Uncinate process of the ethmoid; 9. Lacrimal bone; 10. Base of inferior turbinate; 11. Cut surface of the middle turbinate; 12. Cut surface of inferior turbinate; 13. Ostia of posterior ethmoidal air cells in superior meatus; and 14. Sphenopalatine foramen.

atus, and the base of the inferior turbinate. The posterior ethmoidal air cells open into the superior meatus, and the sphenopalatine foramen is located just above and posterior to the base of the middle turbinate.

## Arteries

Branches of five arteries supply the nasal cavity. The anterior-superior lateral wall receives its supply by the anterior ethmoidal artery, the posterior-superior section by the posterior ethmoidal artery, the turbinates and meati by posterior lateral nasal branches of the sphenopalatine artery, and a small area of the posterior inferior meatus by a branch from the greater palatine artery (Fig. 16–4). The sphenopalatine artery passes medially across the sphenoid body just beneath the ostium of the sphenoidal sinus. Mechanical trauma to this artery during irrigation of the sphenoidal sinus may cause a serious nose bleed.

Five arteries supply blood to the nasal septum (Fig. 16–5). The anterior-superior part receives blood from the anterior ethmoidal artery, the posterior-superior part from the pos-

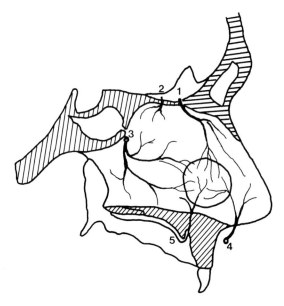

**Fig. 16–5.** Blood supply to nasal septum showing: Circle–Kiesselbach's area; 1. Anterior ethmoidal artery; 2. Posterior ethmoidal artery; 3. Sphenopalatine artery; 4. Septal branch of the superior labial artery; and 5. Incisal branch of greater palatine artery.

terior ethmoidal artery, the posterior-inferior area from the septal branch of the sphenopalatine artery, the middle-inferior area from the incisal branch of the greater palatine, and the anterior-inferior area from the septal branch of the superior labial artery. All of these arteries, with the exception of the posterior ethmoidal, supply Kiesselbach's area. This area is the site of 90% of nose bleeds. Note that minor nose bleeds sometimes stop after placing a finger against the upper lip to occlude the superior labial artery.

## Innervation

The olfactory nerve and the first and second divisions of the trigeminal nerve provide sensory innervation of the nasal cavity. The olfactory nerve supplies the most superior recess of the nasal cavity to provide the sense of smell. Somatosensory innervation to the anterior nasal cavity derives from the first division of the trigeminal nerve via the anterior ethmoidal nerve. The posterior-superior aspect of the lateral nasal wall is innervated by the lateral posterior-superior nasal nerves from the second division of the trigeminal

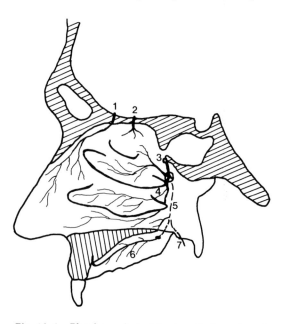

**Fig. 16–4.** Blood supply to lateral wall of nasal cavity showing: 1. Anterior ethmoidal artery; 2. Posterior ethmoidal artery; 3. Sphenopalatine artery; 4. Posterior lateral nasal artery; 5. Descending palatine artery; 6. Greater palatine artery; and 7. Lesser palatine artery.

nerve. The posterior aspect of the inferior meatus is innervated by branches from the greater palatine nerve. The posterior nasal septum is innervated by the nasopalatine nerve, which follows the septal branch of the sphenopalatine artery. The nasopalatine nerve continues through the incisal canal to supply the gingivae palatal to the upper incisors; in some individuals, the nasopalatine nerve brings sensory innervation to the maxillary incisor teeth.

The facial nerve via the greater superficial petrosal and vidian nerves provides parasympathetic innervation. The parasympathetic nerves activate secretions from the nasal glandular cells and the lacrimal glands. Sympathetic innervation derives from the cervical sympathetic trunk via the deep petrosal and vidian nerve. The sympathetic nerves activate constriction of vessels in the mucosa and erectile tissue in the nasal cavity.

## Anatomy of the Maxillary Sinus

The bilateral maxillary sinuses in adults are lateral to the nasal cavity, above the maxillary dentition, and below the eyes, and range in size from a capacity of 10 to 30 ml. Each sinus extends from the maxillary third molar region on the posterior to the premolar area at the anterior; the sinus rarely extends anteriorly to the normally positioned maxillary canine tooth.

The apices of the posterior teeth may project into the maxillary sinus, covered by a thin cortical bone and the mucous membrane of the sinus. An unerupted or impacted maxillary third molar may be separated from the posterior wall of the maxillary sinus by only a thin cortex of bone.

A few fibers of the inferior head of the lateral pterygoid muscle may originate from the maxillary tuberosity overlying the maxillary sinus adjacent to the lateral pterygoid plate. These fibers may be in the vicinity of an unerupted or impacted third molar tooth. Eruptive activity of this tooth may produce muscular spasms in the lateral pterygoid muscle, which may either cause temporary dysfunction of the temporomandibular joint or pain in the infratemporal fossa or retro-ocular region (Fig. 16–6).

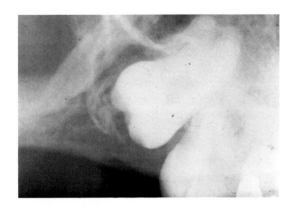

**Fig. 16–6.** Maxillary third molar erupting into the fibers of the pterygoid muscles. A 35-year-old female with complaints and findings commensurate with unilateral myofascial pain of the pterygoid muscles and an associated, recent in onset, monarticular clicking disk subluxation of the TM joint. An impacted maxillary third molar was present on the same side. A posterior superior alveolar local anesthetic injection relieved her chief complaint of pain, and 3 weeks after removal of the impacted third molar, the signs of TM joint disk subluxation subsided.

## Upper Airway Mucosa

### Nasal and Sinal Mucosa

The nasal cavity and paranasal sinuses are lined with pseudostratified, ciliated columnar epithelium with goblet cells. The goblet cells produce a mucous blanket that is moved in a specific pattern by beating of cilia beneath in a ratchet fashion. This blanket may move at a maximum rate of 16 mm per minute as the cilia beat 160 to 1500 times per minute. Cilia in the trachea and bronchioles beat up toward the larynx. Those of the nasal cavity beat back toward the oral pharynx, and those of the sinuses beat toward the ostium into the nasal cavity. These ostia must remain patent to avoid pain and congestion of the lining tissue. When an ostium is swollen shut or obstructed by a tumor, the gases in the sinus are absorbed into the capillary blood according to their solubilities in serum. This absorption reduces the pressure in the enclosed space and the pressure gradient is reflected across the vascular system. The capillary beds in the lining membrane then engorge with blood and the lining thickens with stasis, pain, and susceptibility to infection.

## Mucous Blanket of the Upper Airway

The mucous blanket of the nose and pharynx attaches to inhaled particles that are larger than 40 μm. Smaller diameter particles in inhaled air may pass into the bronchial tree. Aerosols as small as 1 μm can pass all the way into the alveola of the lungs. Air turbine handpieces produce infective aerosols in the dental operatory to as small a diameter as 1 μm. Their inhalation can be prevented only by wearing a mask.

The ideal relative humidity for functioning of the mucous blanket ranges from 35 to 50%. When the relative humidity drops significantly below 35%, the mucus becomes viscous because of water loss, and stasis may occur, with failure of its filtering function. This situation occurs in the winter in heated buildings when upper respiratory infection and sinusitis are most prevalent.

## Physiology of Nasal Vasculature

The turbinates or conchae in each nasal cavity are covered by erectile tissue similar to that found in the genitalia. The function of this tissue is to warm and humidify the inhaled air so the lining of the lung alveola remains moist and can absorb oxygen and expel carbon dioxide and other waste gases. When the erectile tissue is engorged with blood, it may occlude the nasal cavity. In cold weather, nasal cavity occlusion cycles at periods of approximately 30 minutes. When one cavity is chilled by breathing of dry, cold air, its erectile tissue engorges with warm blood and closes the cavity. The opposite cavity opens and transmits air while the mucous blanket in the obstructed side is warmed and rehydrated by the blood in the erectile tissue. This cycling back and forth helps to avoid nasal, sinus, and lung infection in frigid, cold weather.

Some teenage girls have nose bleeds at menarche and with menstruation. Another physiologic parallel in erectile tissue function is demonstrated by nasal obstruction with dyspnea that often occurs during sexual intercourse.

## Nasal and Sinal Disease

### Nasal Mucosa Contact Headache

Pathologic conditions involving the middle meatus may refer pain to the orbital and supraorbital areas;[2] such conditions include polyps, pneumatization of the middle turbinate, deviation of the uncinate process of the ethmoid bone, deviated septum, and enlarged ethmoidal bulla. These structural abnormalities cause contact of opposing mucosal surfaces. They are typically found in patients with long histories of rhinitis and maxillary sinusitis. The contacting mucosal surfaces cause stasis of the mucous blanket and may lead to polyp formation.

This condition is difficult to diagnose in that the identification of the causative pathologic process necessitates nasal endoscopy and coronal computed tomographic or magnetic resonance imaging through the middle meatus (Fig. 16–7).

Information regarding nasal mucosal contact referred pain is important in the differential diagnosis of ocular and supraorbital pain. For example, pathologic changes in the temporomandibular joint may refer pain to the orbit that the patient typically describes as piercing or lancinating. The differential diagnosis also includes cluster headache, which is usually described as a diffuse and often throbbing pain in and above the orbit. The pain referred from mucosal contact pathologic processes is typically a constant, diffuse, aching pain in the orbital and supraorbital areas.

### Sinusitis

Chronic sinusitis is usually not painful, but many patients complain of a noxious fullness or pressure sensation. Individuals with maxillary sinusitis may experience a vague ache in the upper posterior teeth that feels better when biting down with force. This sensation probably occurs when the superior alveolar nerves in the sinus wall become inflamed. Sinusitis can be serious, leading to cavernous sinus thrombosis or brain abscess. Maxillary sinusitis refers pain to the cheek and upper posterior teeth. Ethmoid sinusitis is usually referred to the orbits. Sphenoidal sinusitis refers pain most often to the vertex of the skull

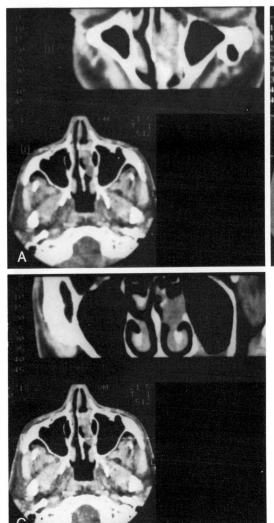

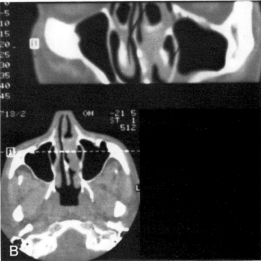

*Fig. 16–7.* Coronal CT views from anterior to posterior of a male patient with middle meatus mucosal contact headache referred to the forehead. A. View across anterior of the middle meatus. B. View across middle of the meatus. C. View across posterior of sinus.

or occiput. Frontal sinus pain is rare (Fig. 16–8).

## Maxillary Sinusitis

Sinus pain or a pressure sensation tends to increase with jarring, as occurs when walking downstairs, stooping, and coughing. Panoramic and Waters view radiographs and other images may reveal maxillary sinus wall thickening, fluid, or cysts. Many cysts are found on routine radiographic examination and are asymptomatic.

Examination by transillumination in a completely darkened room reveals an opaque frontal or maxillary sinus. The frontal sinus is transilluminated by holding the light against the sinus floor while covering the back glare with a finger. Transillumination of the maxillary sinus is accomplished by applying the light along the infraorbital rim while viewing the palate through the open mouth. The frontal sinus can be palpated through the skin and the maxillary sinus can be palpated along the upper buccal vestibule.

## Sphenoid and Ethmoid Sinusitis

Infections of the sphenoid sinus can cause intense deep facial pain and are potentially dangerous. The first six cranial nerves all contact the sphenoid body, as does the pituitary

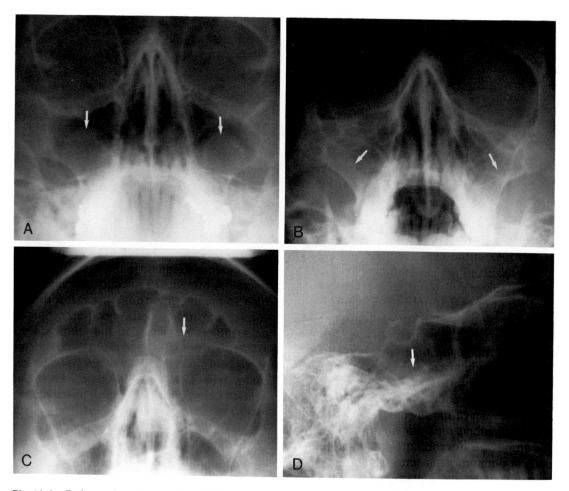

*Fig. 16–8.* Radiographic evidence of sinal inflammatory and related processes. A. Bilateral maxillary sinal polyps; B. Thickened maxillary sinus membranes; C. Unilateral frontal sinusitis as demonstrated by the fluid level; D. Sphenoid sinusitis as demonstrated by the fluid level. (Courtesy of Edwyn L. Boyd, M.D., Otorhinolaryngologist, Birmingham, Alabama.)

gland and the cavernous sinus. All of these structures can be injured by sphenoid sinusitis. Ethmoid and sphenoid sinus disease should be evaluated with laminagraphy, magnetic resonance imaging, or computed tomography.

### Neoplasms

When carcinoma of the maxillary sinus erodes bone, it usually destroys the lateral or posterior wall of the sinus or the palatine process of the maxilla. A screening panoramic film frequently shows the absence of a radiodense line extending superiorly from the maxillary tuberosity on the affected side when the posterior wall is eroded. When the lateral wall is affected, loose maxillary teeth or a malignant growth in the vestibule are signs of a maxillary sinus neoplasm. If the presentation of the malignancy is through the palatine process of the maxilla, a nonfluctuant, soft tissue in the oral palatine vault or loosening of a denture may be the clinical signs.

Unilateral nasal and sinal polyps in an adult with no history of rhinitis or sinusitis may be indicative of an intranasal melanoma, maxilloethmoidal carcinoma, or an intrasinal malignant growth. Polyps should always be considered for continued observation or biopsy.

Neoplasms in the ethmoidal air cells often obstruct the nasolacrimal duct and cause tears to flow across the patient's face. Nasopharyngeal carcinoma often causes a sixth nerve palsy with diplopia during lateral gaze, because the lateral rectus muscle does not function to make the eyeball track laterally. The most common tumor to metastasize to the sinuses is renal cell carcinoma, followed by breast and lung neoplasia.

## Case Histories

### Odontogenic Pain from Maxillary Sinusitis

A 22-year-old dental assistant, employed by a recently graduated dentist, had intermittent, acute pain in her right midfacial region localized in the right maxillary second molar. The pain began during the midwinter season. All of the posterior teeth had been restored with crowns. The second molar tooth was sensitive to percussion. A root canal procedure was performed, to no avail. As the symptoms increased, the tooth was removed. The patient then sensed pain in the first molar, and, subsequently, the same treatment, including extraction, was performed on the first molar and, later, on the second premolar. Erythromycin (low dose) was administered throughout the 4-month history of care as described. At this juncture, the patient was referred to our office for evaluation. Our diagnosis was chronic sinusitis on the basis of a history of stuffiness and of pain in the midface when jarring the head during athletic events, and by palpation over the maxillary sinal anterior wall. These clinical findings were confirmed by a paranasal sinal radiograph that demonstrated a fluid level in the sinus. The patient responded promptly to effective antibiotic therapy, and a Caldwell-Luc procedure, which produced copious amounts of purulent exudate, providing complete relief of pain (Fig. 16–9).

### Pain from Alveolar Extension of Maxillary Sinus

A 56-year-old woman had, for 2 years, experienced intermittent, vague, annoying pain in the right side of the face. Because of a language barrier, taking a history was difficult,

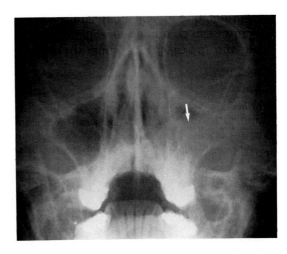

*Fig. 16–9.* Waters paranasal sinus x-ray view of purulent fluid level in the right maxillary antrum. This 22-year-old female patient had several months of dental care culminating in the removal of 3 posterior teeth before odontalgia caused by maxillary sinusitis was diagnosed.

but a relationship could not be established between activities, weather, or habits. She had normal range of motion of the mandible, loss of posterior teeth had been managed by a partial denture, and no signs or symptoms of sinusitis were apparent. An alveolar extension of the maxillary antrum was noted in the posterior edentulous area, and palpation with a finger in this location was distinctly uncomfortable for the patient. Local anesthetic diagnostic blocking of the area provided relief. A decision was made to insulate the maxillary sinus from the oral cavity by placing an autogenous cancellous bone graft in the concavity created by the alveolar extension of the sinus (Fig. 16–10). The procedure utilized bone from the iliac crest. Within weeks postoperatively, the pain ceased, and the 2-year postoperative findings included radiographic evidence of a successful bone graft that was maintaining an osseous barrier between the sinal and oral cavities.

### Sinal Carcinomas Invading the Oral Cavity

Close questioning of patients with oral manifestations of sinal malignant neoplasms usually does not elicit mention of acute pain, and the discomfort is often tolerated by the patient. We believe these patients sense that

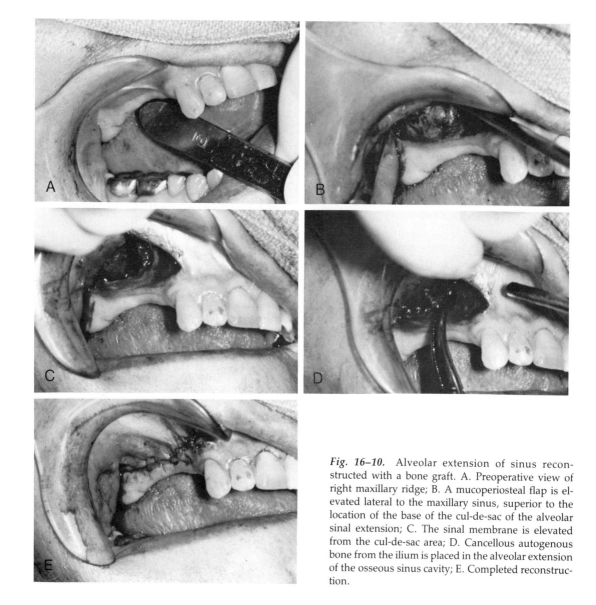

*Fig. 16–10.* Alveolar extension of sinus reconstructed with a bone graft. A. Preoperative view of right maxillary ridge; B. A mucoperiosteal flap is elevated lateral to the maxillary sinus, superior to the location of the base of the cul-de-sac of the alveolar sinal extension; C. The sinal membrane is elevated from the cul-de-sac area; D. Cancellous autogenous bone from the ilium is placed in the alveolar extension of the osseous sinus cavity; E. Completed reconstruction.

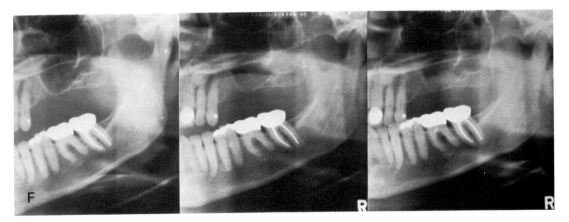

*Fig. 16–10 Continued.* F. Left, preoperative radiograph; Middle, 1 week postoperative; Right, 10-year follow-up radiograph. The patient's original complaints of diffuse facial pain have not returned.

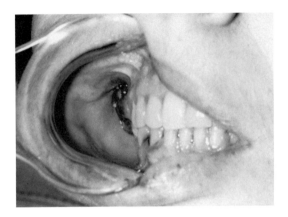

*Fig. 16–11.* Sinal carcinoma invading the posterior maxillary oral vestibule.

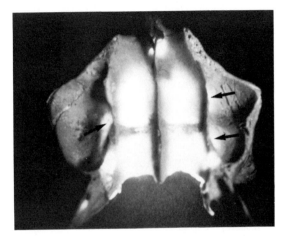

*Fig. 16–13.* Transluminated specimen of the maxilla as viewed from above demonstrating the thin bone between the maxillary sinus and the palatal vault of the oral cavity (arrows).

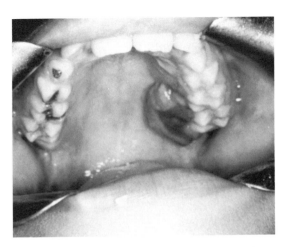

*Fig. 16–12.* Malignant lymphoma invading the oral cavity palatal to the upper left molars.

they are afflicted by a serious problem and a subconscious, protective denial of its existence is the basis for the lack of complaints and acknowledgment of pain for which they ultimately seek relief.

The asymptomatic growth of lesions out of the sinus and into surrounding areas was observed in a 45-year-old man referred with a presumptive diagnosis of "pyorrhea." Biopsy of an asymptomatic, exophytic mass in the posterior maxillary buccal vestibule yielded results indicative of a squamous cell carcinoma (Fig. 16–11).

The invasion of the oral cavity by sinal lesions was observed in a 13-year-old girl palatal to the upper left molars. Biopsy of the lesion disclosed a malignant lymphoma. The patient was referred to the oncology team (Fig. 16–12).

The thinness of the bone between the maxillary sinus and the hard palate provides an avenue for invasion of the oral cavity by neoplasms from the maxillary sinus (Fig. 16–13).

## References

1. Paff G.H.: Anatomy of the Head and Neck. Philadelphia, W.B. Saunders, 1973.
2. Stammberger H. and Wolf G.: Headache and sinus disease: The endoscopic approach. Ann Otol Rhinol Laryngol (Suppl), 97:134, 1988.

# 17

## Salivary Glands

The oral cavity receives its necessary and distinctive moist characteristics from six major and hundreds of minor salivary glands. If the oral cavity has, quantitatively, too little or too much moisture, or qualitatively, an improper ratio of mucous and serous fluids, a series of unpleasant complaints may arise, the mastication of food may be impossible, the oral climate may permit rapid and destructive caries, and an osteomyletic infection of the associated skeleton may follow. Devastating osteoradionecrosis, with the loss of sections of the mandible, may occur in patients who receive cancericidal radiation with subsequent loss of function of salivary glands and the associated qualitative and quantitative change in the saliva.

Pain originating in the glands may accompany inflammatory infectious afflictions and blockades of the ductal structures. Blockage is associated with sialolithiasis, mucous plugs, tumors, trauma that sections major ducts or produces scar contracture closure of ducts, and infection.

## Clinical Evaluation

The evaluation of the salivary glands begins with the clinical inspection and evaluation of the function of the minor salivary glands. The evaluation proceeds to the paired sublingual, submandibular, and parotid glands (Fig. 17–1).

### Minor Salivary Glands

The oral cavity mucosa contains minor salivary glands extending from the tip of the uvula anteriorly to the line of demarcation between the oral mucous membrane and the normally dry vermilion of the lips. The minor salivary glands are designated by anatomic location: labial (a combination of mucous and serous glands with a predominance of mucous glands); buccal (a continuation of the labial glands and, in the vicinity of the parotid orifice, may be designated molar glands); palatine (about 250 pure mucous glands in the hard palatal mucosa, 100 in the soft palate, and 12 in the uvula); lingual (glands on the dorsum of the tongue near the vallate papillae area, the von Ebner glands, are of the serous type); anterior (the gland of Blandin or the gland of Nuhn is on the ventral surface of the tongue and excretes principally mucous saliva through three to five ducts near the lingual frenum); incisive (in the anterior floor of the mouth behind the mandibular incisor teeth); and glossopalatine (pure mucous glands in the mucosa of the glossopalatine fold, the anterior faucial pillar with possible blending with the palatine glands, and on the medial aspect of the mandibular retromolar area).

The usual maladies of minor salivary glands involve loss of function owing to age, irradiation, medications, and psychologic factors. The glands frequently are involved in traumatic closure of the orifices or ductal portions, producing mucoceles.

The minor salivary glands are evaluated in the usual clinical outpatient clinic by inspection and palpation and, when indicated, by biopsy. The inferior and superior lips and the buccal tissues are retracted gently and rolled over the finger. The mucosal surface is wiped and then inspected for the normally prompted reappearance of beads of saliva arising from the individual glands; secretion can be stimulated by having the patient rinse with an astringent mouthwash; the clinician then blots the area with gauze, and, with adequate lighting, observes while waiting for the shiny beads of saliva to form. Palpation of the buccal or labial tissues gives the sense of a slippery smooth membrane when lubricated by normally functioning glands. Biopsy to obtain a histologic observation and estimate of functioning glands may be indicated when examining for Sjögren's disease.

### Sublingual Glands

The bilateral sublingual glands are predominantly mucous glands, with a few serous glands. The glands are located below (ventral) to the oral mucosa and superior (dorsal) to the mylohyoid muscle. The mylohyoid muscle is the muscular floor of the mouth, thus, these glands are often considered part of the environment of the oral cavity. The ductal system of the sublingual glands may take one of several, or a combination, of routes. The glands may excrete, bilaterally, into the floor of the mouth through two to seven ducts of

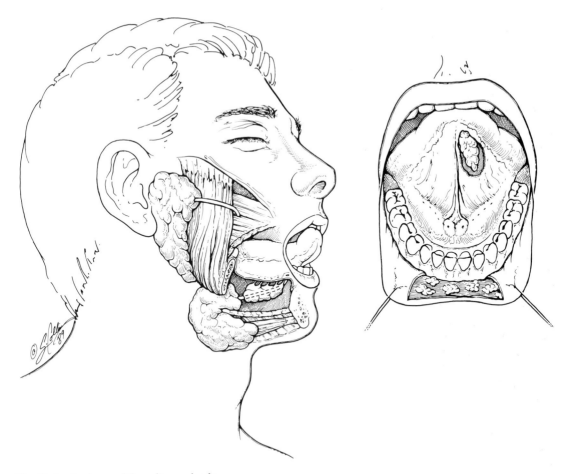

*Fig. 17–1.* Anatomy of the salivary glands.

Rivinus exiting in the ridge-like plica sublingualis in the anterior floor of the mouth; through a single duct parallel to the submandibular duct (Bartholin's duct); or into the submandibular duct (Wharton's duct).

Clinical inspection of the sublingual gland begins by having the patient open the mouth and raise the tip of the tongue. The mucosa of the anterior floor of the mouth "bulges" below and posterior to the plica sublingualis. The plica is dried with a 10 × 10 cm gauze pad and the floor of the mouth is caressed with a palpating finger, passing from posterior to anterior. Careful use of light pressure avoids inclusion of the submandibular gland in the sweeping palpating strokes. A normal sublingual gland produces droplets or a stream of saliva in the plica area. Saliva appears from the ducts of Rivinus along the crest of the plica, from the submandibular duct orifice, from the orifice of a submandibular duct, or from a combination of orifices.

Anterior pressure by a sublingual gland from unknown causes may produce an osseous defect in the cuspid or incisor area, or the medial aspect of the mandible. This asymptomatic lesion is an incidental radiographic finding presenting, in variations, as a sharply circumscribed radiolucency to a diffuse area, depending on the degree of penetration of the lobule of the gland.

### Submandibular Glands

The submandibular glands consist predominantly of serous glands; about 20% are mucous glands. The glands are located, bilaterally, in the submandibular space, below (ventral) to the mylohyoid muscle. The submandibular space communicates posteriorly with the lateral pharyngeal space, an area of potential morbid consequence if invaded by an acute inflammatory process. The excretions of the gland pass through the submandibular duct (Wharton's duct), which curves posterior to the mylohyoid muscle, and then passes anteriorly, superior to the mylohyoid muscle, to terminate at its orifice in the anterior aspect of the plica sublingualis, lateral to the frenum of the tongue.

The bilateral submandibular glands are palpable in healthy subjects and are best appreciated through bidigital palpation. The patient is asked to swallow, open the mouth, and relax; during the moment of relaxation, the index or middle finger "slides" down the alveolar ridge to rest in the lateral posterior floor of the mouth. With the palpating fingers of the other hand, the submandibular gland is examined. In healthy individuals, the gland is firm, about the consistency of a wet sponge, and free of pain, masses, and nodules. To evaluate the salivary flow, the external fingers squeeze the gland posteriorly and then stabilize the gland while the intraoral finger milks the saliva in the duct from posterior to anterior. The normal response is the flow of a mucoserous, clear fluid, sometimes as a stream or spray from a small fountain.

A sialogram may be performed by instilling 1.0 to 2.0 ml of contrast medium (Fig. 17–2). Sialography requires cannulating the duct with either a polyethylene tube or the introduction of a rounded, smooth 18-gauge needle that is attached to a syringe or to a plastic tubule leading to a syringe. The contrast solution is instilled until the patient feels "fullness," and then an additional 0.25 ml is instilled. If a plastic or polyethylene cannula is used, it may be clamped; a metallic needle is

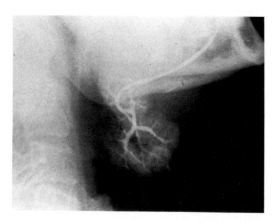

*Fig. 17–2.* Normal sialogram of the submandibular gland.

withdrawn. Radiography, or another form of imaging is immediately performed before the solution is either absorbed or excreted. Overfilling may result in rupture of the tubules, causing the dye to extravasate. The dye usually is absorbed, although oil-based dyes may persist, without apparent problems, for a matter of years in the extraglandular tissues.

Lateral pressure by a submandibular gland, from unknown causes, may produce an osseous defect in the posterior body of the mandibular area. This asymptomatic lesion is an incidental radiographic finding presenting, in variations, as a sharply circumscribed radiolucency to a diffuse area depending on the degree of penetration of the lobule of the gland.

## Parotid Glands

The parotid glands, composed of pure serous glands, are located in a vertical position, much like a bunch of grapes (hence the label racemose [grape-like] glands), bilaterally below the ears. Each gland is cone shaped, with a curvilinear superior margin anterior to the ear and the rounded apex extending from anterior to the mandibular gonial angle posteriorly around the masseter muscle and the mandibular ramus to the sternocleidomastoid muscle region. The excretions of the gland pass through the parotid duct (Stensen's duct) that courses lateral to the masseter muscle, parallel and about 15 mm below the zygomatic arch. The duct terminates medially anterior to the masseter muscle and has an orifice in the buccal tissues, lateral to the maxillary second molar tooth. Accessory glands may extend from the parotid duct.

The delicate structure of the parotid glands is not distinctly palpable in healthy subjects; however, the serous secretions may be readily observed flowing from the parotid orifice. The mouth is opened 15 or 20 mm, and the buccal tissues anterior to the parotid orifice are retracted. While inspecting the orifice, a sweeping motion of the palpating fingers is performed, beginning over the upper one fourth of the sternocleidomastoid muscle. The movement of the fingers passes into the valley behind the mandible and below the external ear and then superiorly and anteriorly toward the middle of the zygomatic arch. In healthy individuals, the saliva appears at the parotid orifice as a clear, serous solution.

A sialogram may be performed by instilling 1.0 to 2.0 ml of contrast medium (Fig. 17–3). Sialography requires cannulating the duct with either a polyethylene tube or the introduction of a rounded, smooth 18-gauge needle that is attached to a syringe or a plastic cannula connected to a syringe. The direction of the cannula or needle at the orifice of the parotid duct is slightly lateral so as to pass anterior to the masseter muscle. In some patients, the needle then passes horizontally and posteriorly lateral to the muscle, sometimes up to the hub of the needle. Likewise, in many patients, a polyethylene cannula passes around the masseter muscle to the area of the gland anterior to the ear. Cannulas may be sutured into position. The contrast medium is instilled until the patient reports the sensation of fullness below the ear, and an additional 0.25 ml is instilled. If a metallic needle is used, it is withdrawn. Radiography and/or other imaging methods are immediately performed before the solution is either absorbed or excreted. The consequences of overfilling were detailed in the section concerning the submandibular glands.

### Differential Diagnostic Signs

Certain clinical signs may assist in the clinical differential diagnosis of afflictions of the parotid gland, the submandibular gland, the masticator space, and the lateral pharyngeal space. A diagnostic sign of involvement of the parotid gland is the lifting of the ear lobe when the parotid gland is affected by an inflammatory or obstructive process (Fig. 17–4). A diagnostic sign that differentiates between inflammatory processes of the submandibular gland and the masticator space is that, though near normal mandibular movements, although painful, are possible when the submandibular space is affected; afflictions of the masticator space, which includes all four of the major muscles of mastication, produce a trismus that limits mandibular movements. When the salivary glands are involved in an inflammatory process, either the stimulus of ingestion of citrus fruits or the mere suggestion of their ingestion produces pain in the afflicted gland; such pain does not occur if the inflammatory process involves the masticator space or the lateral pharyngeal space. The potential for spread of infection from the submandibular space posteriorly to the lateral pharyngeal space is ever present. In addition to possible systemic findings, involvement of the lateral pharyngeal space may be noted by bulging of the pharyngeal wall, and the patient may have difficulty speaking louder than with a raspy whisper.

## Infectious, Obstructive, and Inflammatory Disorders

With the exception of mucoceles of the minor salivary glands, a common clinical de-

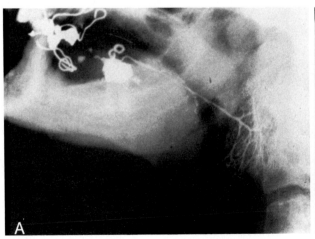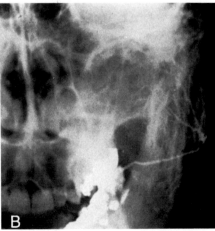

*Fig. 17–3.* Parotid gland sialograms. A. Lateral view; B. Anterior view.

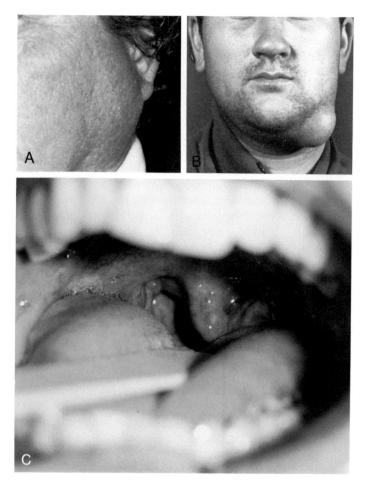

*Fig. 17–4.* Inflammatory processes. A. Parotid gland inflammation; B. Submandibular space; C. Lateral pharyngeal space involved by extension from the submandibular space.

nominator for inflammatory and obstructive disorders of the salivary glands is pain. Interruption of glandular flow may occur from viral infections, bacterial infections, sialolithiases, neoplasms, and trauma.

Bacterial infections of the salivary glands occur frequently in patients who are debilitated. The patient reports a bitter taste. A purulent exudate or cloudy saliva is expressed from the duct orifices, and lymphadenopathy and lymphadenitis are apparent. If scant to no saliva is expressed from the orifices, an obstruction has occurred. If the condition becomes chronic, a sialogram may reveal the extent of sialodochitis by showing enlarged pools of contrast medium in areas of degenerated ducts.

Bimanual palpation of the submandibular and sublingual glands, with the fingers inside the oral cavity and over the submandibular and submental areas, is necessary to differentiate between lymphadenopathy, lym-

phadenitis, and salivary gland enlargement. In lymphadenopathy, as noted with metastatic disease, palpation reveals discrete, firm, usually asymptomatic nodules. In lymphadenitis, such as occurs in response to an inflammatory process, the mass is softer and is tender to palpation. Salivary gland enlargement owing to an obstruction is a more diffuse involvement, and excretion of salivary fluids may be abnormal or absent. Similar findings are noted in the parotid gland areas, but the intraoral aspect of the palpation is not possible. We recommend simultaneous palpation of both parotid glands to provide a comparison in the physical findings.

### Viral Infections

#### Mumps (Epidemic Parotitis)

The most common cause of salivary gland diseases is viral infection, and the parotid gland is typically affected by the mumps virus more often than the other glands. Disease onset is most common in the winter and spring, and children constitute 85% of the patient population. The infection is transmitted by aerosol droplets and produces a painful swelling, usually bilateral, of the parotid glands, accompanied by malaise, pharyngitis, chills, and fever. The secretions of the glands remain clear. The incubation period is 2 to 3 weeks, with the maximum signs and symptoms occurring 36 to 48 hours after the onset and persisting for 7 to 10 days. The contagious period lasts from 2 or 3 days before development of the acute signs and symptoms until the swelling subsides.

The diagnosis is usually based on history and clinical findings, but medical laboratory tests are confirmatory. Treatment is symptomatic. Complications may include residual sialectasis, sensorineural hearing loss, orchitis or oophoritis, and meningoencephalitis.

*Other Viral Diseases*

Cytomegalic viral diseases may include clinical manifestations of the salivary glands along with signs and symptoms of hepatosplenomegaly, thrombocytopenic purpura, and jaundice. Other viral diseases affecting the salivary glands include para-influenza virus, choriomeningitis, coxsackie A, and ECHO virus.[1] These disorders are usually treated on a symptomatic basis, with an objective of preventing stasis, obstruction, and secondary infections of the salivary glands.

*Bacterial Infections*

*Acute and Chronic Suppurative Sialoadenitis*

Stasis or decreased salivary flow may predispose to an invasion of microorganisms through the excretory tubules to lodge and flourish in the salivary glands. The most common bacterial infections are caused by *Staphylococcus aureus*, *Staphylococcus pyogenes*, *Streptococcus viridans*, and *Streptococcus pneumoniae* (Fig. 17–5). Conditions that may predispose to a bacterial invasion include medications that produce xerostomia, trauma to the glands, trauma to the ductal orifice, dehydra-

tion, and sialolithiasis. The parotid gland is affected more than the sublingual or submandibular glands because it is less active during resting phases; also, the submandibular and sublingual glands have a high mucus content in the excreted saliva that tends to protect the glands because of the consistency of the saliva and of a bacteriostatic effect within the mucus.

Treatment includes general systemic metabolic supports of hydration and nutrition, penicillinase-resistant antistaphylococcal antibiotic (until culture and sensitive findings are available), sialogues, dilatation of the excretory duct, and incision and drainage.

The presence of an acute infection alters the architecture of the gland and predisposes it to subsequent acute suppurative infections. If the process progresses to abscess formation in the glands, incision and drainage is performed, with appropriate antibiotic therapy. The inflammatory process may spread from the submandibular gland to the lateral pharyngeal space or the fascial spaces of the anterior cervical regions. An inflammatory process in the parotid gland may spread into the external auditory canal or the parapharyngeal spaces before any clinical evidence of an abscess formation is apparent.

Definitive treatment may include excision of the gland if the condition becomes chronic, is intermittent and recurring, or threatens contiguous areas.

*Necrotizing Sialometaplasia*

This condition manifests as an ulcer, usually in the minor salivary glands. It is rapid in onset and growth, with an ulcerated center and well-demarcated margins (Fig. 17–6). The ulcer may be mistaken for a carcinoma. Treatment is surgical excision and long-term observation.

*Sialolithiasis*

The most common obstruction of salivary glands is by sialolithiasis, with the submandibular gland most commonly affected (Fig. 17–7). Kralls reported that 92% of the stones occur in the submandibular gland, 6% in the parotid, and 2% in the sublingual and minor

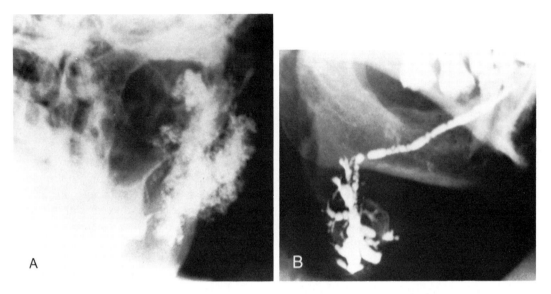

*Fig. 17–5.* Sialograms of sialoadenitis. A. Chronic sialoadenitis of the parotid gland demonstrating destruction of the architecture of the gland; B. Chronic sialoadenitis and sialodochitis of the submandibular gland.

salivary glands; 20% of patients have multiple calculi.[2] At a National Dental Institute of Research conference, Blitzer reported that approximately 80% of stones occur in the submandibular gland, 19% in the parotid, and 1% in the sublingual gland. He observed that two thirds of patients with chronic sialodenitis produce stones, which consist of hydroxyapatite with traces of magnesium carbonate and ammonia with an organic matrix of amino acids and carbohydrate. The stones usually appear in areas of ductal directional changes, as in the submandibular duct, where it curves around the posterior aspect of the mylohyoid

muscle, and in areas of previous infection or trauma.

If the stone has not crystallized, and the blockage of the saliva is secondary to a mucous soft tissue plug, the patient may have complaints commensurate with blockage by a crystallized stone but without the radiographic finding of a radiopaque mass. A mucous plug may occur in association with dehydration, and treatment would include massaging the gland and restoration of fluid and electrolyte balances.

Bahn and Tabachnick found in a literature search and in their patients that the distri-

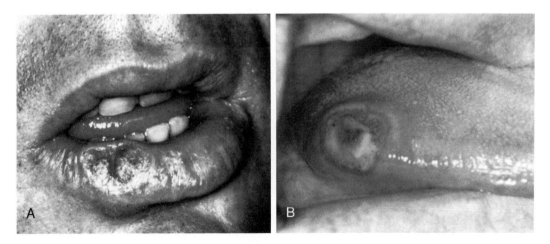

*Fig. 17–6.* Necrotizing sialometaplasia. A. Lip lesion; B. Tongue lesion.

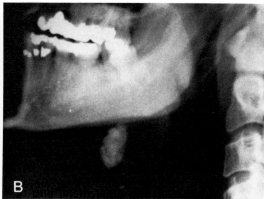

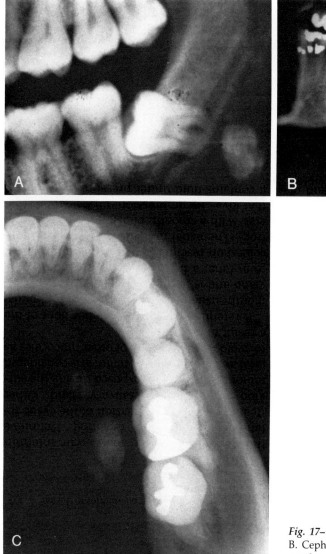

*Fig. 17–7.* Sialoliths. A. Panoramic radiographic view; B. Cephalometric radiographic view; C. Occlusal radiographic view.

bution of sialoliths centered in the buccal mucosa near the commissure; they also noted a probable association with calcifications elsewhere in the body.[3] Kralls observed that the most common site for minor salivary gland calculi is the superior lip, and sialolithiasis may occur in any of the minor salivary glands. Treatment of minor salivary gland sialolithiasis is excision under local anesthesia.

Submandibular salivary gland sialolithiasis is diagnosed, primarily, by history, inspection, and palpation, with confirmation by diagnostic imaging techniques. The history includes pain when anticipating foods or during eating. The pain is usually accompanied by a submandibular swelling related to the retention and back-up of saliva that cannot pass the stone. Radiography, usually an occlusal, lateral mandible, and/or a panoramic view, reveals one or more stones as spherical, linear, or lobulated radiopacities.

Sialolithiasis of the sublingual gland is extremely rare. When a stone is identified, it may be excreted spontaneously or it may be removed during an intraoral procedure under regional anesthesia.

Sialolithiasis of the parotid gland poses surgical and anatomic problems. The route of the duct, from the collecting ducts within the parotid gland to the major duct that passes parallel and below the zygomatic arch over and around the masseter muscle, is such that only a short segment is available for a transoral approach. Hence, if a stone or a collection of stones is causing blockage of salivary secretions in the proximal parts of the ductal system, an extraoral approach is necessary for surgical removal. The deeper and the more posterior the stones are located within the gland, the more likely the operation will involve branches of the seventh cranial nerve, the facial nerve. Two or more exposure localization sialograms or three-dimensional computed tomographic sialograms are helpful in identifying the precise location of the calculi.

### Neoplasms

The salivary glands may be the site of benign and malignant neoplasms. Often the benign neoplasms, growing slowly, are accommodated by the glands and, thus, do not disturb the functions of the gland or, in the case of the parotid gland, of the motor activity of the facial nerve (Fig. 17–8). Often the earliest point at which a benign tumor is suspected is after the lesion had attained considerable size. Malignant neoplasms may invade or destroy the ductal apparatus and, in the case of the parotid gland, the facial nerve. A benign tumor, on the other hand, rarely causes a facial palsy. The patient's chief complaints may relate to an obstructive phenomenon of the gland, sensory nerve pain, and facial paralysis. The parotid gland is the site of most neoplasms of the salivary glands.

### Benign Neoplasms

The most common benign tumor is the pleomorphic adenoma, a benign mixed salivary gland tumor. The pleomorphic adenoma is usually a firm, discrete, 1 cm in diameter nodule in the lower pole of the parotid gland; a medial lobule may extend into the pharyngeal area. If the tumor is in the parotid gland, the facial nerve is usually pushed aside by the slow growth of the tumor and the motor activities to the muscles of facial expression are not compromised. If the tumor originates in the minor salivary glands, the clinical presentation, by inspection, may resemble a

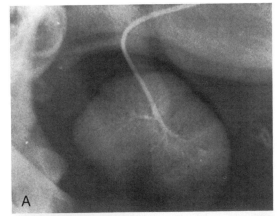
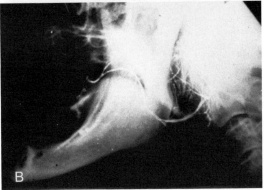

*Fig. 17–8.* Sialograms demonstrating displacement of normal tissues by benign tumors. A. Submandibular gland sialogram; B. Parotid gland sialogram.

chronic dentoalveolar abscess or a palatal torus (Fig. 17–9). Treatment involves surgical resection with wide margins. Malignant transformation may occur in a small percentage of cases.

Papillary cystadenoma lymphomatosum, Warthin's tumor, is the second most common benign neoplasm of the parotid gland. Warthin's tumor may be bilateral, grows slowly, and may become painful when inflamed. These tumors are treated by surgical excision.

### Malignant Neoplasms

Malignant neoplasms of the salivary glands range from those that carry a reasonable prognosis after excision to those that have a poor prognosis, even after surgical excision, neck gland dissections, and radiation. Facial paralysis and painful sensory nerve dysfunction may be indicative of a malignant lesion as opposed to a benign neoplasm. Neoplasms arising in the submandibular, sublingual, and

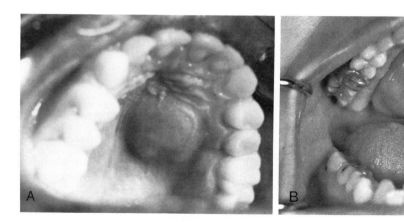

*Fig. 17–9.* Mixed salivary gland tumors of the minor salivary glands. A. Lesion in the lateral anterior vault of the palate; B. Lesion in the central portion of the maxilla.

minor salivary glands are more likely malignant than neoplasms arising in the parotid gland.

Mucoepidermoid carcinomas account for approximately 40% of malignant tumors arising in children.[4] These carcinomas, in all age groups, may range from a low order of malignancy to high-grade malignant neoplasms. Examples of a low-grade malignant neoplasm include acinic cell carcinoma and malignant oncocytoma; these low-grade malignant neoplasms may not be noted by the patient in the earliest stages if no obstruction of the glands or interference with nerve function results. The acinic cell adenocarcinoma occurs most frequently in the parotid gland and rarely in the other major salivary glands and the minor salivary glands. The clinician's index of suspicion, however, must ever be high for the unusual. Acinic cell adenocarcinoma has been reported in minor salivary glands of the superior labial vestibule and the buccal tissues.[5,6]

An adenoid cystic carcinoma may produce paralysis and pain owing to early nerve involvement. The primary treatment is surgical excision, with long-term follow-up evaluations to observe for possible recurrences. Poorly differentiated neoplasms and adenocarcinomas destroy the ductal architecture and nerves. The prognosis is guarded, even with surgical removal of the affected gland, contiguous tissue, and cervical lymph nodes, and radiation therapy.

## Metastatic Neoplasms

Metastatic tumors may lodge in the salivary glands. The clinical presentation depends on the gland afflicted and the degree of malignancy. For example, a high-grade malignant metastatic tumor may cause obstruction of the salivary secretions by damaging the ductal system.

## Other Tumorous Lesions in the Salivary Glands

Children may have hemangiomas and lymphangiomas in the salivary glands, typically in the parotid. The area usually occupied by the affected gland may enlarge as much as fivefold. Hemangiomas usually replace the normal glandular tissues, and lymphangiomas displace and partially surround normal glandular tissues. Hemangiomas may spontaneously regress, but lymphangiomas usually do not. Thus, certain indications, depending on many other physical and metabolic factors, favor nonsurgical management of hemangiomas and surgical excision of lymphangiomas. These benign lesions frequently appear in children, and often surgical excision is delayed until the adolescent years. If, however, the lesion arises in the minor salivary glands or the sublingual or submandibular gland, it may threaten the airway, and removal is mandatory, regardless of the age of the patient.

A high index of suspicion and the recall of general knowledge of physiology and anatomy permits the clinician to note unusual findings that may be indicative of a tumorous process. For example, Buckspan and Rees described a situation in which an aneurysm presented as a parotid mass. Conversely, as mentioned elsewhere in the text, an inflammation of the parotid gland may be misdiagnosed as an acute arthritis of the temporomandibular joint.

## Cysts

### Congenital Cysts

Dermoid cysts, branchial cleft cysts and deformities, and retention cysts may arise in or near the parotid gland. These lesions may manifest during infancy or, in some cases, are identified in the adolescent or, even, adult years.

Dermoid cysts may appear in the parotid gland and, as with dermoid cysts elsewhere in the body, have an inclusion of one or more of the skin structures: hair follicles, sweat glands, and sebaceous glands. These cysts are managed by surgical excision.

Branchial cleft abnormalities may be as minor as a small cyst or pit anterior to the tragus of the ear (Fig. 17–10). The abnormality may be more extensive, involving structures extending from the cutaneous areas to the external and middle ear, the parotid gland and facial nerve, and into the pharyngeal area. Inflammatory responses related to infection may occur; treatment is by surgical excision.

### Serous Retention Cysts

Infants with retention cysts of the parotid demonstrate asymptomatic enlargement of the gland. The lesions are confirmed by computed tomographic imaging and/or sialography, and often regress without surgical or nonsurgical intervention.

### Mucous Retention Cysts

Mucous retention cysts, mucoceles, of the minor salivary glands occur most often on the inferior lip (Fig. 17–11). The etiology is probably a traumatic or other type of closure of the ductal orifice. Saliva may accumulate within the ductal tissues, in the main part of the small duct, or in the most distal end of

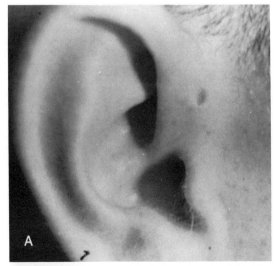

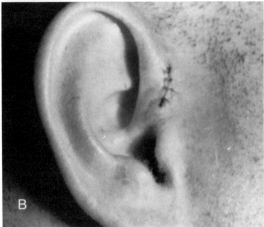

*Fig. 17–10.* Branchial cleft pit anterior to the ear. A. Preoperative; B. After excision.

the duct. A mucocele may occur intermittently, rupturing and repairing. Definitive treatment is surgical excision of the cystic region and the minor salivary gland. Other minor glands may be exposed during the surgical excision, and their removal is considered to avoid the production of other mucoceles as a result of the operation.

A retention cyst in the anterior floor of the mouth usually arises from the sublingual gland and is termed a ranula (a term derived from rana, a frog, because the contours and coloration resembled the ventral surface of a frog). The usual ranula is 2 to 3 cm in diameter, with a smooth, bluish mucosal covering that gives the impression, on palpation, that it contains fluid under pressure (Fig. 17–12).

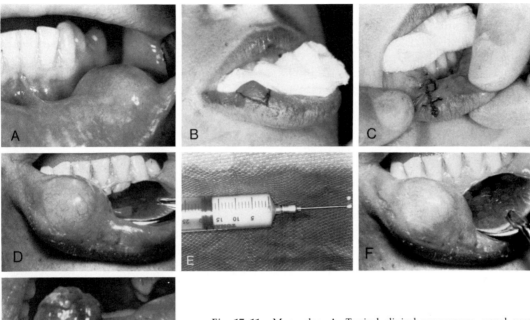

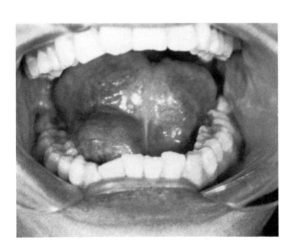

*Fig. 17–11.* Mucoceles. A. Typical clinical appearance, usual surgical management; B. The incisional line is outlined; C. The specimen is controlled with a suture, and the affected gland is excised. Other accessory glands exposed by the surgery are removed. The area is closed. A variation in surgical management: D. Preoperative view; E. The cyst is aspirated of its contents and then filled with alginate. F and G. After the alginate has set, the cyst is excised. The alginate prevents rupture and disorientation of the cyst.

The usual treatment is marsupialization with biopsy of the overlying tissue; the biopsy findings usually display the cuboidal epithelium of an excretory duct. Some ranulas may dissect deeply into the cervical area with multiple compartments. Treatment consists of combinations of marsupializations and surgical excisions.

## Trauma

After trauma to the submandibular gland, the patient may have the signs and symptoms of blockage of the excretion of saliva resulting from damage to the excretory ductal structures. The trauma may be local, such as from the flange of a denture, and correction of the underlying problem should permit the duct to function. If the major duct was damaged by a laceration or intraoperatively, in some cases it may be repaired by using microsurgical and macrosurgical techniques. If the damage involves the collecting ductal structures, however, excision of the gland may be

*Fig. 17–12.* Usual appearance of ranula.

necessary to either prevent or correct infections in the accumulations of saliva. Trauma to the parotid gland may interrupt, distort, or block the excretory ducts, producing salivary retention in the gland. If the trauma resulted from an intraoral occurrence, e.g., by biting or from a dental prosthesis or orthodontic appliance directly to the parotid papilla, the problem is usually readily corrected by controlling the trauma. If the trauma is laceration of the major duct, the immediate surgical repair is directed at restoration of the duct, often by placing a polyethylene tube and repairing the lacerated duct (Fig. 17–13). If the injury involves the major portion of the parotid gland, the major concern is directed toward identifying and repairing the major branches of the facial nerve. If a sialocele forms within

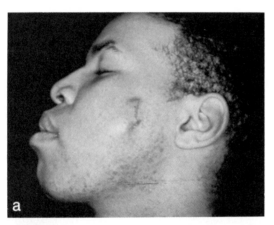
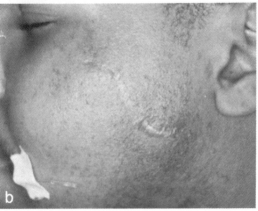

*Fig. 17–13.* Management of a laceration of the parotid duct. A. Serous parotid fluid collected in the buccal tissues 4 weeks following a laceration; B. The area was opened, the duct was reconstituted around a polyethylene tube (which can be seen exiting from the mouth with salivary fluid in it), and the laceration was revised.

the parotid gland, it often resolves spontaneously, aided by aspiration, pressure dressings, and the prescription of an antisialagogue; this treatment is usually effective, even if a fistula has formed. In patients that do not respond to these nonsurgical approaches, removal of the parotid gland may be necessary.

## Xerostomia

The lack of or a decrease in salivary gland function produces xerostomia. Xerostomia may result from emotional stress, medications, irradiation, various metabolic and disease processes including Sjögren's syndrome, and loss of major salivary glands by surgical excision.

In patients with xerostomia, the mucous membranes appear dry and either pale or red, in response to inflammation. The dorsal surface of the tongue may have a decreased number of papillae. Encrustations of dried mucus are evident in the oral cavity, and the breath is fetid. In time, multiple carious lesions of the teeth form, including surfaces that are usually self-cleansing.

Local therapy is directed toward prescription of salivary substitutes, salivary stimulants, and the application of fluoride gels.

Katz and colleagues investigated the bacterial colonization of and the flow rate from the parotid ducts in 10 control subjects and in 17 patients who were to undergo sialography. None of the control subjects had bacterial colonies. Nine of the 17 patients, those with the lower flow rates, had bacterial colonization of the parotid duct with staphylococci and other gram negative anaerobes.[8] We recommend oral prophylactic measures and systemic antibacterial agents be prescribed for xerostomic patients who are to undergo sialography of any of the salivary glands.

### Xerostomia-Producing Medications

Sreebny wrote, "The intake of xerogenic drugs is the most likely cause of xerostomia."[9] The hyposalivation associated with the ingestion of xerogenic drugs does not result from damage or destruction of the salivary glands. Although the xerostomic effect usually is reversible with the cessation of intake of a xerogenic drug, a dry mouth induced by a pharmaceutical product is usually a side action. Therefore, modifying the dosage of a xerogenic agent depends on the primary need for the drug. Table 17–1 is a list of the xerogenic classes of drugs.

Xerostomia is a major problem in the elderly. These individuals consume more drugs than younger individuals, and they are less able to withstand the effects of normal physiologic demands as well as the effects of medicines. In addition, as noted by Handleman and associates, institutionalized elderly patients may receive more than one xerogenic agent.[10]

## Metabolic Disorders

Xerostomia may be a diagnostic sign in certain disease processes or it may be a symptom reported by patients with other conditions. The most common clinical disorder associated with a dry mouth is primary or secondary Sjögren's syndrome.

### Sjögren's Syndrome

As summarized by Screebny, Sjögren's syndrome is a triad of exocrine gland dysfunction, serologic gland dysfunction, and organ system abnormalities. The principal histopathologic finding in the salivary glands is a lymphoepithelial lesion. Because the minor salivary glands are affected in the same histologic manner as the major glands, biopsy of the labial salivary glands may be diagnostic. In the early stages, general hyperplasia is accompanied by a proliferation of lymphoreticular cells and metaplasia of the ducts. In the later stages, atrophic changes are prominent, including acinar degeneration and obliteration of the ducts. In the generalized exocrinopathy, similar changes produce xerophthalmia and dryness of the vagina and the upper airway.

One third of patients with Sjögren's syndrome have the primary or sicca form, of which xerostomia and xerophthalmia are prominent signs and symptoms. It affects women more commonly than men (9:1). The symptoms are usually more severe with the primary than with the secondary forms of the syndrome.

A study by Çelenligil and colleagues investigated the peripheral blood immunoregulatory lymphocytes in the peripheral blood and in affected salivary glands in 14 patients with primary Sjögren's syndrome. They identified differences in affected salivary glands and the peripheral blood in the number of T cells, antigen positive cells, and B cells. They discussed further studies to identify the pathogenesis of primary Sjögren's syndrome.[11]

The other two thirds of patients experiencing Sjögren's syndrome have the secondary form, in which the xerostomia and xerophthalmia are part of the sign and symptom complex of a connective tissue or collagen disease. The most common condition producing a secondary xerostomia and xerophthalmia is rheumatoid arthritis, with about one half of the patients manifesting evidence of Sjögren's syndrome. Other conditions that are associated with a secondary Sjögren's syndrome are systemic lupus erythematosus, scleroderma, Raynaud's phenomenon, biliary cirrhosis, atrophic gastritis, pancreatic insufficiency, and type V hyperlipoproteinemia.[9]

## Surgical Removal of Salivary Glands

The loss of one or two major salivary glands by surgical removal or trauma alters the quantity of saliva available to provide a normal oral environment. The other major glands and the minor glands, however, usually are sufficient to forestall the morbid effects of xerostomia (Fig. 17–14).

## Irradiation of Salivary Glands

The loss of function of the salivary glands by irradiation, as a part of the definitive treat-

**TABLE 17–1.** *Selected Classes of Drugs That Induce Xerostomia*[8]

Anorectics
Anticholinergics
Antispasmodics
Antidepressants
Antihistamines
Antihypertensives
Antiparkinsonian agents
Antipsychotics
Diuretics
Sedatives
Hypnotics

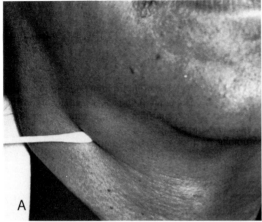

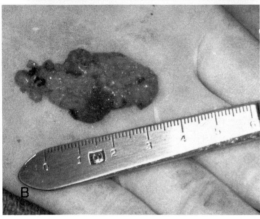

*Fig. 17–14.* Submandibular gland with chronic sialoadenitis. A. The patient was experiencing recurring bouts of acute inflammation; B. Atrophied gland after surgical excision.

ment of a malignant neoplasm, may produce early neurovascular physiologic changes in gland function and irreversible destruction of the parenchyma of the glands. The parotid gland is the most susceptible to irradiation changes, followed by the submandibular and the sublingual glands.

The changes often begin with rampant dental caries, so-called irradiation caries, that may produce periapical and periodontal abscesses. The acute inflammatory attack by the abscesses may be devastating to the surrounding soft and osseous tissues, which have been deprived of their defensive mechanisms by the irradiation treatment. The result may be osteoradionecrosis, an osteomyelitis that is difficult to control. Osteoradionecrosis afflicts the mandible almost ex-

clusively, as compared to the maxilla (Fig. 17–15).

*A Management Protocol*

A protocol for a patient who has reasonable healthy oral cavity and is to undergo cancericidal radiation to the oral cavity area is as follows.

1. *In-depth consultation with the patient and the patient's family.*

The patient and the patient's family receive instruction regarding the changes expected in the oral cavity that result from decreased salivary gland function.

The patient may experience soreness and dryness 10 to 20 days after the initiation of therapy by x-irradiation and chemotherapy.

If x-irradiation was used, the dryness may be permanent.

Teeth tend to degenerate in a dry environment, leading to such extensive losses of tooth structure that restoration is not possible. Abscessing may follow, which in turn may cause a rampant infection of the surrounding bones that have been exposed to radiation.

A point of emphasis is that the personal care is not complicated; the usual home care of plaque control is supplemented by the use of topical fluorides.

2. *Special professional and self care is necessary for the remainder of the patient's life.*

On awakening, before retiring at night, and after eating, brush all surfaces of teeth, gingiva, and dorsum of the tongue with either (as prescribed by the dentist) soft brush or disposable foam stick.

Rinse the mouth with normal saline or prescribed mouthwash after brushing.

If prescribed by the dentist, daily application of a gel of topical fluoride with a toothbrush or other applicator helps in caries control.

Do not use dental floss, unless prescribed and demonstrated by the dentist.

Avoid abrasive, fried, spicy, or acidic foods and foods served in high or low extremes of temperature.

Add sauces to foods.

Drink extra water with and between meals, if fluid intake is not restricted. Artificial bal-

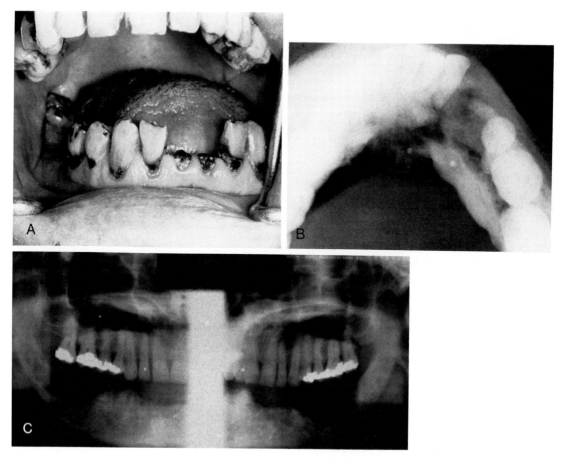

*Fig. 17–15.* Effects of cancericidal irradiation. A. Rampant caries and loss of dental structures; B. Osteoradionecrosis secondary to a dentoalveolar abscess. The patient incurred a pathologic fracture. Concurrent with hyperbaric oxygen and other supportive therapy, the teeth were removed. A pedical bone graft from the clavicle to restore the mandible and support the tongue was successful after two major surgical attempts and multiple hospitalizations and great morbidity; C. Osteoradionecrosis secondary to bone exposures after the removal of teeth and conservative contouring of the alveolar ridges. The osteoradionecrosis began in bilateral areas of exposed alveolar interdental bone and resulted in great morbidity, but without progressing to pathologic fractures.

anced saliva, as a spray or as a liquid, may be prescribed by the dentist.

Sugar-free chewing gum and sugar-free lemon candies may give comfort.

Use lanolin-based moisturizing creams on the lips, prescribed by the dentist, as necessary. Avoid dehydrating the lips by moistening with the tongue and by using agents that feel cool.

In the event of an inflammation of the soft tissues of the mouth, fracturing of a tooth, or any questions, contact the dentist at once.

*Keep all appointments with the dentist for monitoring the oral cavity.* Visits may be weekly during the early phases of treatment and,

then, every 3 or 4 months for an extended, indefinite period.

3. *Typical professional care.*

Initiate preventive dental disease program of plaque control and fluoride therapy.

Perform restorative dentistry procedures.

Any surgical procedures must be completed in time for early repair to occur before the initiation of cancericidal radiation to the area, because repair practically ceases when the radiation therapy begins.

Intraoral anesthetic injections and surgical procedures follow proper preparation of the oral cavity by drying and application of an antiseptic solution.

Remove retained root segments and teeth that have either nonrestorable conditions, extensive periodontal bone loss, or periapical pathologic involvement not amenable to endodontic therapy.

Initiate periodontal therapy, as indicated, to include scaling, curettage, and planing.

Initiate endodontic therapy, as indicated, for teeth essential for abutments, mastication, and esthetics.

## Prevention of Osteoradionecrosis

Prevention of osteoradionecrosis may include a protocol for the removal of teeth. If preirradiation exodontia is planned, the focus of the procedure should be the removal of the superior one half of the residual alveolar processes, a surgical procedure that may go against the grain of a doctor trained to perform alveoloplasties to prepare the oral cavity for conventional dentures. In this case, the objective is to remove possible oral communications with the body of the mandible and produce a mucoperiosteal repair in the shortest possible time. We observed a patient who underwent radiation for management of a malignancy of the posterior floor of the mouth in which her dentition was ravaged by several decades of minimal care. Preirradiation removal of the mandibular teeth was recommended. Unfortunately, the mandibular arch was prepared with a conservative alveoloplasty, commensurate with preparation for artificial dentures. A subsequent osteoradionecrosis began in an interdental crest of bone that was exposed to the oral cavity, and the process progressed to the point a mandibular fracture occurred. Of interest, this particular patient received an iliac bone graft to the mandible, accompanied by hyperbaric oxygen and, eventually, artificial dentures.

## Replacement and Stimulants for Deficient Saliva

For palliative therapy of xerostomia, the patient is advised to sip water during waking hours, to hold crushed ice in the mouth, and to hold sugarless citric fruit candies in the mouth. Salivary substitutes can be provided by a pharmacy as prepared liquid or sprayed

substances or on prescription for a generic agent as follows.

Rx: Sodium carboxymethyl cellulose, 0.5% aqueous solution

Dtd: 250 ml

Sig: Oral retention prn

A time-honored stimulant for salivary flow, providing the salivary glands have some function and use in certain patients is not contraindicated, is pilocarpine, as follows.

Rx: Pilocarpine HCl solution, 1 mg/ml

Dtd: 500 ml

Sig: 1 teaspoonful (5 ml) qid

## Nutritional Factors

Benign enlargement of the parotid glands may occur in patients with diabetes, a history of heavy alcohol consumption, anorexia nervosa, malnutrition secondary to unusual eating habits of bulimia and vomiting, nutritional deficiencies, and the use of certain medicines. Individuals, usually young women, who practice bulimia may have significant parotid enlargement, often accompanied by pain. Parotid hypertrophy associated with heavy alcohol consumption is painless.

## Bulimia

Bulimia is a behavioral eating disorder. The condition is characterized by episodes of excessive eating followed by self-induced vomiting and/or the abusive use of laxatives. The patients characteristically exhibit a generalized pattern of enamel erosion, except for the lingual surfaces of the mandibular anterior teeth, which are preserved because the tongue is braced forward against these teeth as the acidified stomach contents are expelled across the oral cavity. Restorations, as though they were growing out of the teeth, project above the dissolved teeth surfaces. Petechial hemorrhagic areas may be evident on the soft palate secondary to the vomiting phases of the disorder. Reportedly 5% of female high school and college students demonstrate bulimic behavior.[12]

Bulimic patients may suffer electrolyte imbalance with hypokalemia, alkalosis, hypochloremia, edema, renal dysfunction, and cardiac arrhythmias. The painful parotid enlargement may represent a malnutritional mumps or the enlargement of the parotid as seen in association with starvation states. Differential diagnoses are Sjögren's syndrome, sarcoidosis, hepatic disorders, parotid disease, and parotid-masseter hypertrophy-traumatic occlusion syndrome.

The patient may not volunteer or admit that he or she practices bulimia. Unfortunately, the resumption of a normal eating behavior may not reverse the parotid swelling. Because it is unsightly, the parotid swelling may further decrease the patient's level of self-esteem and lead to perpetuation of the practice.

Treatment of bulimia involves psychologic behavior modification and psychiatric counseling, including the use of appropriate psychotropic medications. Bilateral superficial parotidectomies may be performed to correct the parotid hypertrophy.[12,13] Restoration with full coverage of the partially destroyed teeth is usually indicated.

## Psychopathologic Factors

The environment and health of the oral cavity is directly affected by the quality and quantity of saliva. In a definitive literature review, Morse and associates noted the relationship of stress and saliva production,[14] and included an interesting account demonstrating the age-old recognition of the relationship between saliva and stress.

For centuries we have known that stress inhibits salivary flow, and this has been used to determine guilt and innocence in individuals. The ancient Bedouins gave an individual suspected of a crime a hot iron to lick; evidence of guilt was noted if the tongue was burnt from lack of protective saliva. Hundreds of years ago in Asia, rice powder would be given to a suspect, and guilt was assumed if the individual subsequently expectorated dry powder. Centuries ago in Europe, a suspect would be given bread and cheese to masticate, and an indication of guilt was noted if the salivary quantity was too low to permit swallowing.

Saliva produced during stress is not only less watery and copious, but also it contains more oral bacteria[15] and an increased number of glycoproteins,[16] conditions that could result in increased caries formation and, probably, fetid breath. In a patient experiencing long-term, unresolved facial pain, the complaints could include foul breath and a dry mouth. Furthermore, a patient with decreased salivary flow may have the setting for an opportunistic infection, most commonly, *Candida albicans*. Thus, a somatic explanation for the invasion of *Candida albicans* in patients under emotional stress would include xerostomia that permits overgrowth of the normal oral flora by the fungal infection.

A patient subjected to chronic stress of living factors may have a long-term decrease in the quantity and quality of salivary flow. This decrease could result in foul breath, increased formation of dental caries, and inflammatory processes, e.g., erythema multiforme, *Candida albicans* invasion, and acute necrotizing gingivitis.

## References

1. Blitzer A.: Inflammatory and obstructive disorders of salivary glands. J Dent Res, 66:657, 1987
2. Kralls S.O.: Sialolithiasis of the minor salivary glands. Ear Nose Throat J, 67:296, 1988
3. Bahn S.L. and Tabachnick T.T.: Sialolithiasis of minor salivary glands. Oral Surg Oral Med Oral Pathol, 32:371, 1971
4. Myer C. and Cotton R.T.: Salivary gland disease in children: A review. Clin Pediatr (Phila), 25:353, 1986
5. Miller R.I. and Houston G.D.: Acinic cell adenocarcinoma arising from minor salivary gland tissue. J Oral Maxillofac Surg, 45:543, 1987
6. Triantafillidou E., Karnezi E., and Tsamis I.: Acinic cell adenocarcinoma of minor salivary gland: Report of a case. J Oral Maxillofac Surg, 45:450, 1987
7. Buckspan R.J. and Rees R.S.: Aneurysm of the superficial temporal artery presenting as a parotid mass. Plast Reconstr Surg, 78:516, 1986
8. Katz J., et al: Bacterial colonization of the parotid duct in xerostomia. Int J Oral Maxillofac Surg, 19:7, 1990
9. Sreebny L.M.: Dry mouth in salivary gland hypofunction. Part I: Diagnosis; Part II: Etiology and patient evaluation; Part III: Treatment. Compendium, 9:569, 630, 716, 1988
10. Handleman S.L., et al: Prevalence of drugs causing hyposalivation in an institutionalized geriatric population. Oral Surg Oral Med Oral Pathol, 62:26, 1986
11. Çelenligil H., et al: Characterization of peripheral blood and salivary gland lymphocytes in Sjögren's

*We thank Dr. Iradj Sooudi, Brookwood Medical Center, Birmingham, Alabama, for information pertaining to management of oral cavities subjected to cancercidal radiation.

syndrome. Oral Surg Oral Med Oral Pathol, *69*:572, 1990

12. Burke R.C.: Bulimia and parotid enlargement—case report and treatment. J Otolaryngol, *15*:49, 1986

13. Berke G.S. and Calcaterra T.C.: Parotid hypertrophy with bulimia: A report of surgical management. Laryngoscope, *95*:597, 1985

14. Morse D.R., et al: Stress, relaxation and saliva: Re-lationship to dental caries and its prevention, with a literature review. Ann Dent, *42*:47, 1983

15. Morse D.R., et al: The effect of stress and meditation on salivary protein and bacteria: A review and a pilot study. J Human Stress, *8*:31, 1982

16. Morse D.R., et al: Examination-induced stress as measured by changes in total salivary protein and salivary glycoprotein. Stress, *3*:14, 1982

# Selected Painful Maladies

Certain soft tissue, osseous, and related nerve system lesions that may produce pain also may cause problems in arriving at a final diagnosis. This chapter includes a summary of selected soft tissue lesions and manifestations of biologic changes of special interest in differential diagnoses.

The most common local, painful osseous event after removal of teeth is the production of a dry socket. This postextraction neuralgia usually follows mandibular third molar extraction, but it may occur after the removal of any tooth. The pain results from the inflammation of the reparative process involving a localized osteomyelitis.

On rare occasions, dentoalveolar surgical intervention may be a factor in the etiology of a painful osseous inflammatory process characterized by either reactive bone hyperplasia, a monostotic fibro-osseous type lesion, or chronic osteomyelitis, or inflammation of the periosteal tissues.

Long-term dysfunction of nerves may manifest as neuritis or neuralgia after dentoalveolar procedures, surgical intervention involving the nerve, and regional anesthetic regimens.

## Lichen Planus

Lichen planus of the oral cavity may occur independent of or concomitantly with cutaneous and genital lesions. The etiology of this entity, which may be autoimmune, is unknown, but many authors cite a predilection for individuals subjected to unusual emotional stress and for aggressive individuals who usually conduct their lives at a high level of stress. The disease may have a predilection for patients with general catabolic conditions, infections, and sensitivity to medications. The disease occurs in adulthood with no pronounced predisposition for either gender.

Lichen planus of the oral mucosa features lesions usually on the buccal tissues, to a slightly lesser extent on the labial tissues, and occasionally on the tongue and palate. Lacy, white striations are distributed in a random manner (Fig. 18–1). On the cutaneous surface, these striations are termed the stria of Wickham. A raised nodule is often noted at the intersection of the striations, as though the striations were additive to one another where they crossed. Areas of normal-appearing mucosa between the striations are irregularly circular. The patient's chief complaints are related to burning sensations in the lesions, fears of malignancy, and concerns of spreading an infection.

Lichen planus is not considered a premalignant lesion. In rare cases, however, squamous cell carcinoma developed in or from oral lichen planus lesions, usually the erosive lichen planus.[1]

Variations of the disorder include atrophic, hypertrophic, bullous, and erosive lichen planus. Atrophic lichen planus, with faint, poorly developed stria, is asymptomatic. The hypertrophic variety is associated with dense, white, well-established plaques that seem to

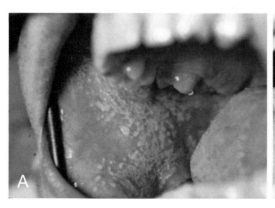
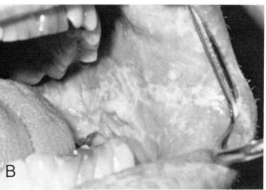

*Fig. 18–1.* Lichen planus. A. White, lacy striations on the buccal mucosa of a typical manifestation of lichen planus. In this patient, these lesions would recur following periods of remission with no apparent etiology; B. Confluence of dense, thick plaques of a hypertrophic lichen planus; in this patient, these lesions were asymptomatic and did not resolve during a 3-year period of observation.

be enlarged and pronounced striations; biopsy may be necessary to distinguish it from leukoplakia. The bullous variation manifests as vesicular lesions that rupture and leave painful ulcerated areas. The erosive form may be a progression from other forms or may begin directly in the erosive mode; it typically is painful.

Treatment of lichen planus is directed toward making a positive diagnosis by history and physical examination and, occasionally, by biopsy, if premalignant or malignant features are present. The usual treatment plan consists of establishing sound nutrition, application of steroids, and removal of stress from the patient's life by counseling and prescription of tricyclic antidepressant agents, not major tranquilizers. Removal of the usual lesions or the atrophic and hypertrophic variations by defocused laser beams may be considered.

Sample regimen of topical steroidal medication is as follows:

Rx: Dexamethasone elixir, 0.5 mg/5 ml

Dtd: 100 ml

Sig: Retain 5 ml (1 teaspoonful) over oral lesions for 2 to 3 minutes (by the clock), qid. Expectorate; do not swallow the solution.

A sample prescription of a tricyclic antidepressant medication is as follows:

Rx: Nortriptyline HCl, 25 mg

Dtd: 60 caps

Sig: 1 cap hs × 7 days; 1 cap bid × 7 days; 1 cap qid × 7 days

We recommend evaluating the patient weekly, and adjusting the dosage as indicated depending on response and tolerance. The example is of a minimal dose level; doubling the dose level may be indicated.

## Moniliasis

Moniliasis (candidiasis, thrush) is a superficial infection of the mucosa by a fungus with yeast characteristics that is a normal inhabitant of the oral cavity. The risk of producing monilial infection is increased in a variety of circumstances: in an individual with a debilitating disease and in patients with immune mechanism abnormalities, such as in Addison's disease; in a localized unhygienic area, as under a denture; and as a consequence of antibiotic therapy, which may reduce microorganisms that combat yeast in the oral cavity.[1]

Monilial infections may occur any place in the oral cavity. The whitish lesions resemble areas of thick cream splashed on the affected surface. The lesions usually are easily lifted, wiped, or stripped off of the mucosal surface, revealing macular, inflamed mucosa (Fig. 18–2).

The major concern of the patient, in addition to the itching, burning, and sometimes

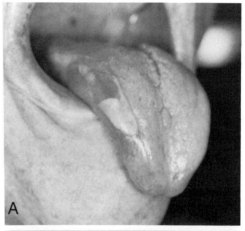

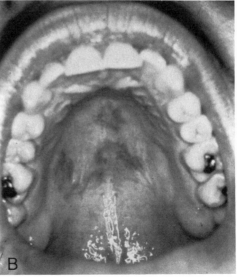

*Fig. 18–2.* Moniliasis. A. Moniliasis of the tongue. Note that the lesion has been partially wiped away revealing an inflamed area on the surface of the tongue. B. Moniliasis of the palatal mucosa.

throbbing pain, is the possibility that the lesions are indicative of a malignancy or other dreaded problem. The clinician must give priority to determining if the patient has a noxious habit, such as permitting a nonhygienic prosthodontic device to be in place; the pattern of usage of oral topical or systemic antibiotics; and the status of the patient's general health. In the oral cavity, proper hygiene, including, where applicable, correct dental restorations and properly maintained prostheses, is essential to decrease the areas that may harbor *Candida albicans* and permit the proliferation of these organisms.

The treatment plan encompasses the provision of suitable oral and systemic care, the initiating of indicated referrals, and planning for follow-up observation and care. Although usually confined to the oral cavity, the organisms could invade the respiratory tree or the gastrointestinal system and produce a life-threatening problem.

The organisms of moniliasis, *Candida albicans*, are resistant to antibiotics. In fact, the use of oral topical antibiotics may destabilize the balance of the oral flora, helping to produce an environment that is conducive to an overgrowth of the *Candida albicans*. Nystatin, a specific antifungal agent, is held in contact with the lesions and is indicated in controlling and, in most cases, eradicating the infection. The oral lesions usually resolve rapidly with topical applications of nystatin as either a suspension, a powder, an ointment, or a troche held in contact with the affected area. The oral suspension of nystatin is held in the mouth for several minutes several times each day. Nystatin as a powder or an ointment is placed on a denture and thus is held in contact with a lesion. The troches developed for vaginal use are convenient for oral use.

Chronic moniliasis involving the cutaneous and mucosal surfaces may be treated from a systemic approach with ketoconazole as follows:

Rx: Ketoconazole, 200-mg caps

Dtd: 15 caps

Sig: 1 cap po per day

Examples of nystatin prescriptions are as follows:

Rx: Nystatin, oral suspension, 100,000 units/ml

Dtd: 100 ml

Sig: 5 ml (1 teaspoonful) qid. Retain and rinse oral cavity for 3 minutes by the clock; then either expectorate or swallow.

Rx: Nystatin ointment

Dtd: 15-g tube

Sig: Apply to lesion and denture pc

Rx: Nystatin troches, 100,000 units

Dtd: 40 troches

Sig: Use as oral lozenge qid

## Erythema Multiforme

Erythema multiforme is primarily a cutaneous disease that usually occurs in young adults, but it may afflict patients of any age. The etiology is unknown, but as with other oral mucosal inflammatory processes, we believe a basis of antecedent personal stress may be a factor in producing the disease.

The disorder is characterized on the skin by painless macular, papular, and sometimes vesicular lesions. The lesions are principally on the limbs, head, and neck, and often appear as a series of concentric circles about 15 mm in diameter in varying shades of inflammation. The lesions are quite painful when on the oral mucosa and other mucous membranes of the body (Fig. 18–3).

The oral manifestations may be severe and prevent the patient from maintaining a normal diet. The lesions are characterized by erosive areas on the intraoral tissues and encrustations of the vermilion. Weeping hemorrhagic exudates, easily seen on the vermilion areas, are common.

The major variation of erythema multiforme is the Stevens-Johnson syndrome, which is characterized by widespread involvement of cutaneous areas and multiple mucous membranes, namely the oral cavity, genitalia, and conjunctiva.

Erythema multiforme is usually a self-limiting disease that tends to recur. The disease is managed by steroid therapy or a combination of steroid and azathioprine therapy. The azathioprine in the combination therapy,

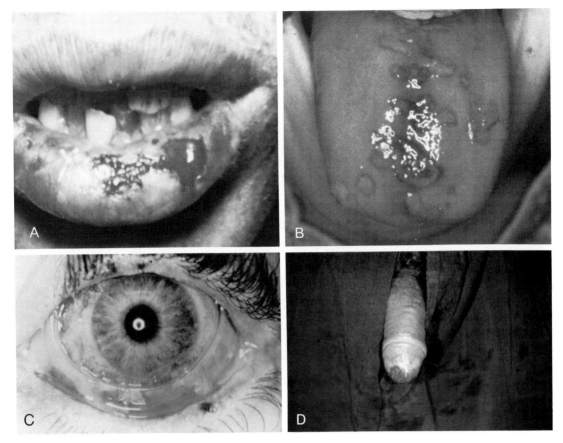

*Fig. 18–3.* Erythema multiforme. Hemorrhagic erosive lesions of a patient with erythema multiforme with manifestations A. on the vermilion of the inferior lip; B. on the tongue; C. as ocular lesions and D. as penile lesions.

as described by Lozada,[2] enhances the corticosteroid activity and permits lower doses of the steroid medication with a reduction of possible side effects. With all regimens, the use of topical prednisone suspension mouth retentions may be useful.

Examples of a prednisone prescription follow:

   Rx: Prednisone, 50-mg tabs

  Dtd: 10 tabs

   Sig: 1 per day

   Rx: Dexamethasone elixir, 0.5 mg/5 ml

  Dtd: 300 ml

   Sig: Rinse oral cavity with 5 ml (1 teaspoonful) for 2 minutes, by the clock, qid; expectorate.

An example of the combination regimen follows:

   Rx: Prednisone, 20-mg tabs

  Dtd: 20 tabs

   Sig: 1 tab per day

   Rx: Azathioprine, 50-mg tabs

  Dtd: 10 tabs

   Sig: 1 tab every other day

   Rx: Dexamethasone elixir, 0.5 mg/ml

  Dtd: 100 ml

   Sig: 5 ml (1 teaspoonful) and retain in oral cavity for 2 minutes, by the clock, qid; expectorate.

## Cheilitis Glandularis

A disease of unknown etiology, cheilitis glandularis manifestations may range from simple hyperactivity of the salivary glands, usually of the lower lip, in which the ductal orifices become enlarged and have a hyperemic halo, to suppurative stages that are destructive and extremely painful. In the advanced suppurative stages, hemorrhagic encrustations may be noted. Although the disease attacks the superior lip of adult male patients, both genders and both lips may be afflicted (Fig. 18–4).

The condition must be monitored by clinical and histopathologic examinations for malignant transformations. Surgical excision is definitive in terms of eradicating the pathology, although in patients with disease in the advanced suppurative stage, excision may be crippling to the function of the lips.

The patient should receive a thorough general physical examination, with special emphasis on evaluations for sarcoidosis. The use of antibiotic therapy when the condition is in an advanced stage, with a suppurative component, as well as systemic corticosteroid therapy may be indicated.

## Pemphigus

Although this dermatologic disease carries a grave prognosis, 25 to 50% of pemphigus patients have the earliest manifestation of several of the types of pemphigus in the oral cavity with cutaneous tissues that appear normal. These oral manifestations may precede the cutaneous lesions by 3 to 5 months. The etiology of the disease is unknown; in the vulgaris type, the most common, and in the vegetans type, 74% of patients were Jews as reported by Rosenburg and associates.[3] The eventual mortality rate associated with the disease is greater than 50%, with the vulgaris variety approaching 100%.

Pemphigus lesions of the oral cavity are especially painful when secondarily infected, and they may resemble erythema multiforme or types of lichen planus. The earliest appearance is multiple vesicular, blistering formations in sheets of inflamed area, with adjacent tissues that appear normal. Secondary local infections usually occur, and the lesions fill with purulent sanguineous exudates. When wiped away, the moist base appears as a macular, raw, eroded inflamed surface that is painful (Fig. 18–5).

The cutaneous lesions begin as vesicles

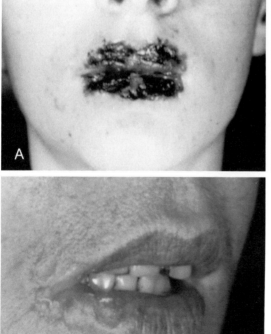

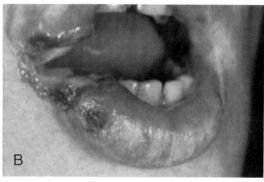

*Fig. 18–4.* Cheilitis glandularis. A. Painfully disabling, hemorrhagic encrusted cheilitis glandularis lesions of the inferior and superior lip. These were nonresponsive to management by pharmacotherapeutic agents, and excisional operations were performed. B. Painful lesions of the inferior lip and commissure that, C., responded to corticosteroid therapy without recurrence during 3 year postoperative observation.

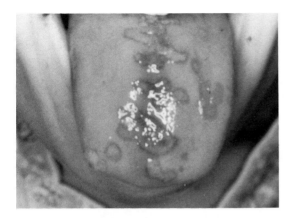

*Fig. 18–5.* Pemphigus. Oral manifestations of pemphigus demonstrating sheets of vesicular lesions on the tongue.

with a clear fluid that rapidly becomes purulent and sanguineous. In the surrounding, apparently normal tissues, a loss of junction may occur between the squamous epithelium and the subcutaneous tissues, a prevesicular stage. Wiping away this normal-appearing skin leaves a raw base, termed Nikolsky's sign.[1]

No specific treatment is available for this disease, aside from the administration of corticosteroids and protecting the patient from secondary infections with antibiotics, because regression occurs in some patients and remission in others. The treatment of oral lesions is similar to that described for erosive lichen planus.

## Leukoplakia

The word leukoplakia is used, variously, to designate the clinical appearance of lesions, a deleterious process, and a histologic diagnosis. Three percent of leukoplakic lesions in a series reported by Waldron and Shafer[4] were infiltrative squamous cell carcinomas, and Kramer and associates[5] reported a rate as high as 6%. The histologic characteristics of hyperkeratotic lesions with a premalignant or malignant potential are distinct from those of other hyperkeratoses. Hyperkeratotic lesions were described by Wood and Goaz according to their clinical appearances: homogeneous white plaques, white and red speckled patches, combination of white and red patches, and verrucous leukoplakias.[6] They

wrote that the lesion may be classified as reversible or irreversible, depending on the resolution of the lesion after removal of the noxious stimulus. In addition, they observed that, " . . . obviously reversible leukoplakias are not malignant, but a significant number of irreversible leukoplakias are premalignant or frankly malignant." The following clinical features often are indicative of a premalignant or malignant diagnosis: hyperemia, red speckles or patches, verrucous appearance, ulcers, and fissures.

The lesions are usually nonpainful, although patients may have great and understandable concern as to the implications of the diagnosis, the type of treatment that is planned, and the prognosis. The clinical keys to leukoplakia are knowing the kind of stimulus that excited the original hyperkeratotic response and understanding the natural history of the particular type of hyperkeratosis that ensued. The authors have observed leukoplakia that has become irreversible and, in some cases, undergone malignant transformation in all sectors of the oral cavity in both men and women of all ages, from the teens through the eighth decade of life.

Although not the only noxious stimulus that may lead to leukoplakia, tobacco, in all of its forms, is the most prevalent etiologic agent. The tobacco products include cigarettes, cigars, pipe tobacco, chewing tobacco, and dipping tobacco (snuff) (Fig. 18–6).

The treatment of leukoplakia must include removal of the noxious stimulus, and immediate biopsy if the lesion has red patches or speckles, a verrucous appearance, fissures, or ulcers. A biopsy of tissue from a homogeneous leukoplakia is performed 3 weeks after the noxious stimulus is removed, if the lesion does not reverse and begin to resolve. Definitive management must await the biopsy results, and then, it may consist of a range of therapies, from long-term observation to removal or destruction by surgical stripping, electrosurgery, defocused laser beams, and cryosurgery.

## Geographic Tongue

Geographic tongue (benign migratory glossitis), a benign, chronic condition of unknown

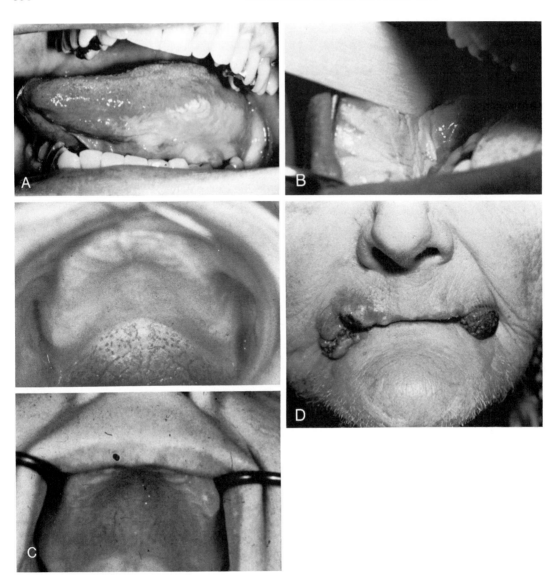

**Fig. 18–6.** Leukoplakia. A. A sheet of white hyperkeratosis on the ventral surface of the tongue of a female patient who had a several decade history of placing tobacco in the area; histopathologic findings were of a hyperkeratosis without dyskeratosis. She discontinued the use of tobacco in all forms. B. Hyperkeratosis of the buccal mucosa of a male patient with a 5-year history of placing tobacco in the area; histopathologic findings were of a hyperkeratosis with dyskeratosis. He discontinued the use of tobacco in all forms. C. Top shows hyperkeratosis of the soft palate with red punctate spots indicating the orifices of the minor salivary glands in an edentulous patient with a several decade history of cigarette smoking; the denture has protected the hard palate mucosa from the effects of the cigarettes. Below: An interesting contrast is seen in the manifestations of an inflammation of the mucosa of the hard palate, sometimes with a monilial infection, in an edentulous patient who practically never removed her denture even for daily hygiene. D. Leukoplakia overtaken with obvious squamous cell carcinoma in a female patient with a multiple decade history of placing tobacco in her mouth. After treatment by an oncology team, she continued to use tobacco and was lost to follow-up evaluations.

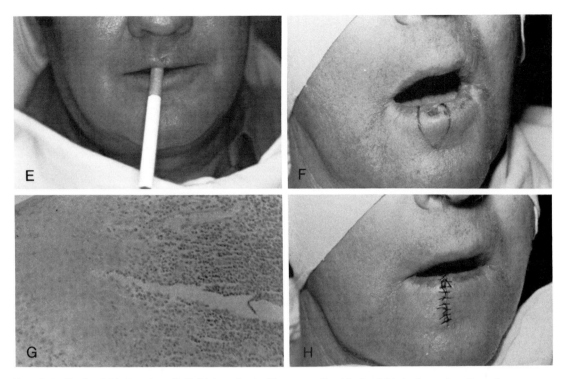

*Fig. 18–6.* Leukoplakia (continued). E. Male patient with a generalized leukoplakia in the oral cavity and a squamous cell carcinoma on the vermilion following several decades of smoking filter tip, low tar cigarettes. The patient habitually placed the cigarette on the area where the carcinoma occurred; F. excisional biopsy produced the, G., histopathologic findings of squamous cell carcinoma, and, H., following repair the patient abstained from tobacco in all forms and was free of recurrence at 15-year postoperative evaluation.

etiology, manifests as irregular reddish patches on the dorsum of the tongue. The red areas are regions of desquamation of the filiform papilla. The filiform papilla, which persist in the reddened areas as small papillations, reform from time to time and return to their normal size and appearance; in adjacent areas, the loss of height and characteristics of the filiform papillas occurs. The margins of the desquamated areas appear to have a pronounced border, which provides a definite outline, thus giving the tongue the appearance of being a map, hence, the name geographic tongue. The moving of the desquamated areas has prompted a more accurate designation as benign migratory glossitis (Fig. 18–7).

Patients complain of a burning sensation, a sensitivity to spicy food and those hot in temperature, and concern of a possible grim prognosis. The authors have seen extreme diagnostic measures instituted, including multiple biopsies over several years in one patient and subjecting another patient to a complete radiographic analysis of the gastrointestinal tract.

Treatment consists, primarily, of reassurance and advice for nutritional requirements for both the quality of the diet and avoidance of foods that are uncomfortable to the tongue.

## Recurrent Aphthae

Recurrent aphthae comprise two forms: major and minor aphthae. The clinical characteristics are similar to those of recurrent herpes simplex; however, particular clinical findings aid in differential diagnoses.

The positive, single etiologic factor for recurrent aphthae has not been established. The onset has been associated with ingestion of certain foods: nuts, chocolate, acidic vegetables; psychologic disturbances; trauma to the mucosa; an autoimmune response; and an endocrine disturbance.

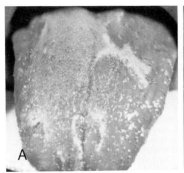
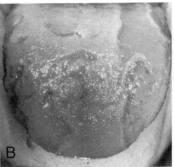
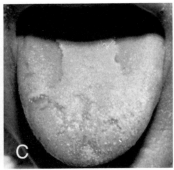

*Fig. 18–7.* Geographic tongue. A, B, and C, Three examples of geographic tongue.

## Minor Aphthae of the Oral Cavity (Canker Sores)

The lesions begin as single hyperemic macules that become papular in a matter of about 24 hours. Within another 24-hour period, the central part of the papule ulcerates, progressing to a shallow ulcer that is, typically, less than 1.0 cm in diameter. Some ulcers, however, are 2 cm or more in diameter. The usual manifestation is a single ulcer or a maximum of two or three ulcers in different locations on the freely movable, nonkeratinized mucosal surfaces of the oral cavity. The ulcerations, which may be painful, resolve in 7 to 10 days. Topical anesthetic agents, such as lidocaine, may be used as retentions, especially before meals.

## Major Aphthae of the Oral Cavity (Periadenitis Mucosa Necrotica Recurrens and Recurrent Scarring Aphthae)

The lesions of the major aphthae of the oral cavity are ulcerations 1 to 3 cm in diameter that may appear singly or, more likely, in large numbers on the freely movable, nonkeratinized mucosa of the oral cavity.

The ulcerations are extremely painful and persist for a matter of weeks to a few months; the history reveals that the patient is never free of having one or more ulcerations. The afflicted areas repair with scar tissue.

Brown and Bottomley summarized the etiologic classification of the major aphthae as autoimmune and originating " . . . from an antibody response to the tissue's mucopoly- saccharide encapsulation of the L form of alpha hemolytic *Streptococcus.*" They described a successful treatment using the purine analog, azathioprine, an investigational medicine for autoimmune diseases, and topical dexamethasone.[7] Multiple treatments have been advocated, including systemic and topical steroid agents, topical antibiotics, excision, and removal by cryosurgical techniques.

Examples of prescriptions follow:

Rx: Dexamethasone elixir, 0.5 mg/ml

Dtd: 200 ml

Sig: Rinse and retain in oral cavity for 2 minutes, by the clock, qid; expectorate

Rx: Prednisone, 5-mg tabs

Dtd: 105 tabs

Sig: 2 tabs qid × 5 days, then 2 tabs tid × 5 days, then 2 tabs bid × 5 days, then 1 tab bid × 5 days, then 1 tab per day × 5 days.

## Recurrent Herpes Simplex

Similar to recurrent aphthous ulcers, multiple etiologies for recurrent herpes simplex have been proposed, including responses to foods, psychologic upsets, trauma, and an oral manifestation of a systemic malady.

Recurrent herpes simplex is a result of activation of latent herpes viri producing clusters of vesicles without a hyperemic halo. The vesicles, which rupture in 4 or 5 hours, produce clusters of ulcers with individual diameters of less than 1.0 cm. The ulcerations may coalesce, with a variable hyperemic border. The ulcerations appear on the fixed, keratinized mucosa of the oral cavity (Fig. 18–8). The ulcers, which are painful, have a life cycle of 7 to 10 days.

The topical treatment may include 5-minute retention, five times per day, with a warmed supersaturate baking soda solution to relieve pain and, perhaps, shorten the course of the viral infection. Topical anesthetic agents and the systemic use of vitamin C compounds and antiviral chemotherapeutic medicines are suggested.

Examples of prescriptions follow:

Rx: Ascorbic acid, 400-mg tablets

Dtd: 20 tabs

Sig: 2 tabs stat, then 1 tab qid for 4 days

Rx: Acyclovir, 200-mg caps

Dtd: 50 caps

Sig: 1 cap 5 times/day

## Postextraction Neuralgia

The most common neuralgia secondary to tooth removal is a localized osteomyelitis or osteitis, referred to as a dry socket. This designation has been recognized as inadequate, and terms descriptive of aspects of the complex of symptoms, or noting various phases of the pathologic process, or an occasional reference to the overall process, have been used: dry socket, painful socket, alveolagia, necrotic alveolar socket, alveolar osteitis, so-called dry socket, degeneration of the blood clot, delayed repair of the extraction site, painful delay in repair, and postextraction osteomyelitic syndrome.

Usually, the clinical presentation is of a postextraction tooth socket that is nearly or completely devoid of an organized vital blood clot; a foul odor and taste emanate from the socket. Neuralgia is localized to the area of the involved bone, but it may radiate or refer to another area. The vital signs may indicate a systemic response arising from an associated bacteremia. Some patients manifest trismus and cellulitis.

Delay in the repair of an extraction site is usually related to one or more of three factors: local infection, loss of parent tissues to vitalize the coagulum, and systemic factors (Fig. 18–9). The presence of an acute or chronic oral and pharyngeal inflammatory process often assures the loss of coagulum by being overwhelmed by microorganisms.

Trauma to the surrounding alveolar bone is a predisposing factor in loss of the blood clot, because damage to the residual periodontal membrane limits its role as a source for fibroblasts and angioblasts to organize the coagulum during the initial reparative stages. The incidence of production of a localized postextraction osteomyelitic process may be higher in patients with mitigating systemic factors, such as advanced age; sockets that are in areas that have received irradiation therapy; poorly controlled diabetes; and long-term corticosteroid therapy; however, we have had many patients with these systemic factors, and in the vast majority, repair was normal after removal of teeth, including mandibular third molars.

The neuralgia accompanying a postextraction delay in repair may be intense, and it is usually promptly attenuated by local treatment. The local treatment consists of two distinct steps: gentle, thorough irrigation with copious amounts of warm normal saline and placement of an anodyne dressing. Several applications of the preparation may be necessary until granulation tissues form on the socket walls, usually about 7 days after the onset of symptoms. After cessation of the symptoms and reparative tissues are evident, the bony defect may be cleansed by the pa-

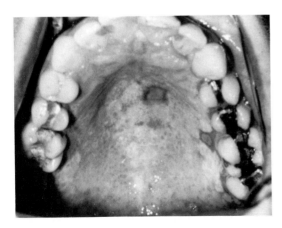

*Fig. 18–8.* Recurrent herpes simplex. The viral infections of recurrent herpes simplex occur on the keratinized, fixed mucosa of the oral cavity.

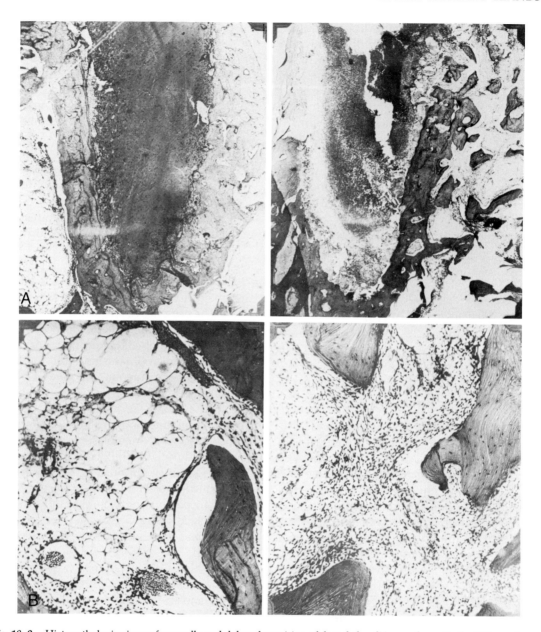

*Fig. 18–9.* Histopathologic views of normally and delayed repairing of dental alveoli in monkeys. Each of 25 monkeys in this series had one molar tooth removed from the left and the right mandibular arches. This study evaluated the repair of alveoli following the removal of teeth (as controls) without burnishing the remaining periodontal ligament compared with burnishing the alveoli (and, hence, the remaining periodontal ligament) on the affected sides. A. One week postoperative. Left: control side disclosed presence of a dense, organized coagulum and high power magnifications revealed the periodontal ligament to be orderly in appearance, and the cells in the coagulum had arrangements consistent with early fibroplasia. Right: affected side disclosed minimal periodontal ligament and the friable coagulum is only partially retained. High power magnifications revealed the periodontal ligament to appear disrupted with multiple cystic spaces. B. One week postoperative. Left: on the control side, the adjacent marrow spaces are normal with only a few scattered inflammatory cells. Right: on the affected side, the adjacent marrow spaces had the characteristics of an osteomyelitis with the marrow heavily infiltrated with inflammatory cells.

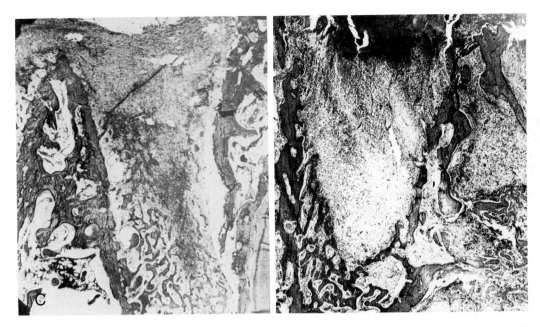

*Fig. 18–9.* (Continued). C. Two weeks postoperative. Left: on the control side, new bone formation is evident from the apical area to nearly top of the alveolus. No evidence of osteomyelitis in the surrounding marrow spaces. Right: on the affected side, regeneration bone is minimal, the coagulum is friable and supports a mass of cell debris and colonies of microorganism. The surrounding marrow spaces are filled with inflammatory cells of osteomyelitis.

tient after meals by using a plastic syringe; the area is inspected periodically by the dentist until it becomes self cleansing.

In some cases, repairing mucosa covers the socket, but the alveolus does not have a vital blood clot. In these instances, opening the alveolus with a cotton pliers permits the escape of purulent exudate, and the alveolus is then dressed with a sedative dressing.

## Reactive Bone Hyperplasia

A group of osseous lesions with painful manifestations that usually include in the history of the present illness the extraction of a tooth or other routine intraoral surgical procedure has been labeled reactive bone hyperplasia. Similar lesions have been termed fibro-osseous lesions of the mandible mimicking chronic osteomyelitis.[8,9] Maladies with similar clinical and histologic findings, including an unknown or an innocuous onset, are focal or diffuse sclerosing osteomyelitis, bone enostoses, sclerosing cementomas, gigantiform cementomas, and sclerotic cemental masses.

The mandible is the usual site of reactive hyperplasia of bone. An unpublished review of 300 cases disclosed a high incidence in women in the fifth, sixth, and seventh decades of life; the larger, and the most painful, lesions were observed in young women between 15 and 30 years of age.[10]

The process is characterized by the proliferative stage of inflammation, with a result initially of an increase of fibrous connective tissue in the medullary bone and, later, by an increase in size of the cancellous architecture by osseous deposition. The clinical impression is of sclerotic bone, and the histopathologic findings resemble those of other types of fibro-osseous diseases. Intermittent and recurring severe pain and occasional inflammation of the overlying cutaneous tissues may occur. No microorganisms or exudate are noted, and periosteal osseous production is not prominent (Fig. 18–10).

Treatment often is frustrating to both the patient and the clinician. Use of narcotic analgesics is not indicated, because of the chronicity of the disease, and pain control centers on the intermittent use of nonsteroidal anti-inflammatory agents and simple analgesics. Relief of pain, on selected occasions during painful exacerbations, is sometimes achieved

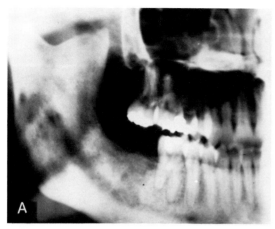
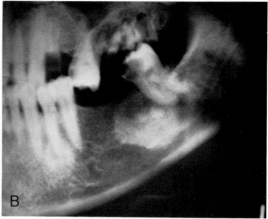

**Fig. 18–10.** Reactive bone hyperplasia. A. Reactive bone hyperplasia affecting the ramus and posterior body of the mandible. This painful process followed the removal of a mandibular third molar and a typical "dry socket." During the 10 years the patient was followed, the process was nonresponsive to pharmacotherapeutic measures and to surgical decortication of the lateral cortex of the mandible. B. Reactive bone hyperplasia of the mandible limited to an area of a chronic inflammatory process anterior to the mandibular molar. Roots were retained in the area of bony sclerosis and the remaining molar was nonvital because of nonrestorable caries.

by the systemic administration of corticosteroids, with due regard for the effects of the long-term use of these potent agents. In some cases, antibiotics are helpful in reducing painful exacerbations. Surgical excision, neurectomies, and decortication procedures have been unreliable in providing either consistent pain relief or alteration of the course of the disease. The process may run its course for as much as a decade.

## Postoperative Trigeminal Neuralgia

Neuralgia in the distribution of the trigeminal nerve may follow, on rare occasions, routine use of local anesthetics, dentoalveolar surgery, transoral surgery, and restorative dentistry. Multiple specific etiologies are possible, but a common denominator involves chemical, biologic, or mechanical challenges to the peripheral nerves.

### Traumatic Neuralgias

Gregg reported investigations in which he identified 3 sites of pathosis for posttraumatic maxillofacial pain and 4 symptom complexes of traumatic neuralgias.[11,12] He proposed that the predominant loci for the pathophysiology of traumatic neuralgias in the maxillofacial region were traumatic neuromas, cutaneous

and autonomic collateralization, and central nervous system deafferentation loci. The symptom complexes were anesthesia dolorosa, sympathetic mediated pain, hyperalgesia, and hyperpathia.

Gregg described traumatic peripheral neuromas as amputation neuromas associated with severed nerves, lateral neuromas that were adherent to periosteum, exophytic neuromas lateral to the nerve trunk, and either hypertrophic or compressed neuromas in continuity with the nerve. He observed that collateral nerves from the injured nerve, from other sensory branches, and from autonomic nervous system nerves were seen in zones of previous trigeminal nerve injury. The re-innervation may be successful in returning normal sensation, or abnormal pain reflexes may ensue. Central nervous system trigeminal deafferentation is influenced by both peripheral injuries and input from the higher centers. Profound pathologic symptoms of lowered pain tolerance and behavioral changes may result.[11,12]

*Anesthesia dolorosa,* often associated with phantom sensations or spontaneous paresthesias, is a painful or annoying sensation in an area of subjective numbness and objective anesthesia or hypesthesia. It is related to pathology of the central nervous system and to amputation neuromas. *Sympathetic mediated pain,* similar to causalgia, is a nerve injury pain aggravated by increased sympathetic tone, cold, and emotional stimuli, and reduced by sympathetic nerve anesthetic blockage. It is attributed to autonomic C-fibers in areas of injury. *Hyperalgesia,* similar to hyperesthesia or allodynia, is a rapid painful reaction to a normally nonpainful stimulus. It is related to mechanosensitive A-fibers in the nerves that are linked to related irritable central nervous system neurons. *Hyperpathia* is characterized by an increased threshold and delayed response to mechanical pressure, and involves ephaptic transmissions between adjacent nerve tissues.

Among surgeons, ongoing discussions center on the timing of the microsurgical repair for injured trigeminal nerves; these discussions are assisted by an understanding of the pathophysiology of the trauma. As Gregg points out, diagnostic trigeminal anesthetic blocks are sound predictors for the pain relief that may be expected from microsurgical repairs. In a study of 84 patients with traumatic neuralgias, he observed microsurgical repairs benefited 60.5% of the patients with hyperalgesia, 56.3% of the patients with hyperpathia, 20.7% of the patients with sympathetic mediated pain, and 14.6% of the patients with anesthesia dolorosa.[11,12]

Campbell and colleagues summarized persistent phantom pain after surgery associated with endodontic periapical curettage, apicoectomy, root resection, retrofilling, hemisection, and root amputation. The following mechanisms were identified to account for the phantom pain phenomenon: deafferentation hypersensitive, in which areas in the gingiva or bone act as spontaneous impulse generators because the normal balance of sensory input is gone; a central nervous system deficit is present, and minor noxious stimuli in the oral cavity become the focus of constant pain; post-traumatic dysesthesia associated with either traumatic microneuromata or ephaptic union of the ingrowth of sympathetic and other nerves into the severed sensory nerves.[13]

In general, as soon as a nerve injury has been diagnosed, the treatment plan evolves in 3 phases: immediate, 6 to 18 months, and long term. The immediate phase should include a continuum of observation, elimination of infection, prescribing sound nutrition, and medicines with peripheral vasoactivity and central catecholamine mechanisms, specifically, antidepressant and monamine-oxidase inhibitors. In a matter of months, if it is determined that progress toward recovery by an injured nerve has ceased, and if a physical interruption of the nerve occurred, consider the options of surgical exploration, decompression, and repair of the nerve. To approach the inferior alveolar nerve, we prefer, when indicated, an osseous sagittal splitting at the intersection of the ramus and body of the mandible which will provide access for microsurgical techniques as well as macrosurgical decompression. A decision for surgery should be tempered by the many clinical reports that indicate recovery of reasonable nerve function is the rule, not the exception, in the maxillofacial region.[14-16] Long-term treatment options include psychologic supports to aid in patient understanding and acceptance; the use of topical analgesic agents, for example, 0.025% capsaicin cream; prescription and monitoring of antidepressant agents or monamine oxidase inhibitors and intermittent prescriptions of nonaddicting analgesia medicines; and, rarely, either differential coagulation, avulsion, sectioning, or other destructive procedure to a peripheral nerve.

## Bone Cavitations

An etiology for trigeminal neuralgia as well as atypical neuralgias was described by Ratner and colleagues.[17] They reported infected localized, devitalized bone cavitations that persisted after dentoalveolar surgery and were instrumental in producing an ascending neuropathy of the peripheral nerves with accompanying transganglionic degeneration and deafferentation. This concept, although not widely accepted, was confirmed by Roberts and colleagues.[18] Treatment included identifying and debriding the bone cavities within the maxilla and mandible.

## References

1. Shafer W.G., Hine M.K., and Levy B.M.: A Textbook of Oral Pathology. 3rd Ed. Philadelphia, W.B. Saunders, 1974

2. Lozada F.: Prednisone and azathioprine in the treatment of patients with vesiculoerosive oral disease. Oral Surg Oral Med Oral Pathol, 52:257, 1981

3. Rosenberg F.R., Sanders S., and Nelson C.T.: Pemphigus: A 20-year review of 107 patients treated with corticosteroids. Arch Dermatol, 112:962, 1976

4. Waldron C.A. and Shafer W.G.: Leukoplakia revisited. Cancer, 36:1386, 1975

5. Kramer I.R.H., El-Labbon N., and Lee K.W.: The clinical features and risk of malignant transformation in sublingual keratosis. Br Dent J, 144:171, 1978

6. Wood N.K. and Goaz P.W.: Differential diagnosis of oral lesions. St. Louis, C.V. Mosby, 1985

7. Brown R.S. and Bottomley W.K.: Combination immunosuppressant and topical steroid therapy for treatment of recurrent major aphthae: A case report. Oral Surg Oral Med Oral Pathol, 69:42, 1990

8. Jacobsson S., et al: Fibro-osseous lesion of the mandible mimicking chronic osteomyelitis. Oral Surg Oral Med Oral Pathol, 40:433, 1975

9. Alling C.C. and Martinez M.G.: Comment on reactive hyperplasia of bone. Oral Surg Oral Med Oral Pathol, 40:445, 1975

10. Martinez M.G.: Personal communication, 1988

11. Gregg J.M.: Studies of traumatic neuralgia in the maxillofacial region: Symptom complexes and response to microsurgery. J Oral Maxillofac Surg, 48:135, 1990

12. Gregg J.M.: Studies of traumatic neuralgia in the maxillofacial region: Surgical pathology and neural mechanisms. J Oral Maxillofac Surg, 48:228, 1990

13. Campbell R.L., et al: Chronic facial pain associated with endodontic therapy. Oral Surg Oral Med Oral Pathol, 69:287, 1990

14. Girard K.: Considerations in management of damage to the mandibular nerve. J Am Dent Assoc, 89:65, 1979

15. Alling C.C.: Nerve dysfunction after third molar surgery. J Oral Maxillofac Surg, 44:454, 1986

16. Hayward J.R.: The triumphant trigeminal nerve. J Oral Maxillofac Surg, 44:2, 1986

17. Ratner E.J., et al: Jawbone cavities and trigeminal and atypical facial neuralgias. Oral Surg Oral Med Oral Pathol, 48:3, 1979

18. Roberts A.M., et al: Further observations on dental parameters of trigeminal and atypical facial neuralgias. Oral Surg Oral Med Oral Pathol, 58:121, 1984

# Index

Page numbers in *italics* indicate illustrations; numbers followed by "t" indicate tables; numbers followed by "n" indicate notes.

## DATE DUE

| | | | |
|---|---|---|---|
| | | | |
| | | | |
| | | | |
| | | | |
| | | | |
| | | | |
| | | | |
| | | | |
| | | | |
| | | | |
| | | | |
| | | | |
| | | | |
| | | | |
| | | | |
| | | | |
| | | | |
| | | | |
| | | | |